ALLERGIC DISEASES

CURRENT ◊ CLINICAL ◊ PRACTICE

ALLERGIC DISEASES

DIAGNOSIS AND TREATMENT

2ND EDITION

Edited by

PHIL LIEBERMAN, MD

Allergy Associates, Cordova, TN

and

JOHN A. ANDERSON, MD

VIVRA Asthma and Allergy, Tucson, AZ

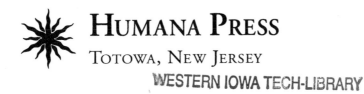

HUMANA PRESS
TOTOWA, NEW JERSEY

© 2000 Humana Press Inc.
999 Riverview Drive, Suite 208
Totowa, New Jersey 07512

For additional copies, pricing for bulk purchases, and/or information about other Humana titles, contact Humana at the above address or at any of the following numbers:
Tel: 973-256-1699; Fax: 973-256-8341; E-mail: humana@humanapr.com or visit our website at http://humanapress.com

Due diligence has been taken by the publishers, editors, and authors of this book to assure the accuracy of the information published and to describe generally accepted practices. The contributors herein have carefully checked to ensure that the drug selections and dosages set forth in this text are accurate and in accord with the standards accepted at the time of publication. Notwithstanding, as new research, changes in government regulations, and knowledge from clinical experience relating to drug therapy and drug reactions constantly occurs, the reader is advised to check the product information provided by the manufacturer of each drug for any change in dosages or for additional warnings and contraindications. This is of utmost importance when the recommended drug herein is a new or infrequently used drug. It is the responsibility of the treating physician to determine dosages and treatment strategies for individual patients. Further it is the responsibility of the health care provider to ascertain the Food and Drug Administration status of each drug or device used in their clinical practice. The publisher, editors, and authors are not responsible for errors or omissions or for any consequences from the application of the information presented in this book and make no warranty, express or implied, with respect to the contents in this publication.

All articles, comments, opinions, conclusions, or recommendations are those of the author(s), and do not necessarily reflect the views of the publisher.

Cover design by Patricia F. Cleary.

This publication is printed on acid-free paper. ∞
ANSI Z39.48-1984 (American National Standards Institute)
Permanence of Paper for Printed Library Materials.

Photocopy Authorization Policy:
Authorization to photocopy items for internal or personal use, or the internal or personal use of specific clients, is granted by Humana Press Inc., provided that the base fee of US $10.00 per copy, plus US $00.25 per page, is paid directly to the Copyright Clearance Center at 222 Rosewood Drive, Danvers, MA 01923. For those organizations that have been granted a photocopy license from the CCC, a separate system of payment has been arranged and is acceptable to Humana Press Inc. The fee code for users of the Transactional Reporting Service is: [0-89603-685-5/00 $10.00 + $00.25].

Printed in the United States of America. 10 9 8 7 6 5 4 3 2 1

Library of Congress Cataloging-in-Publication Data

Allergic diseases: diagnosis and treatment / edited by Phil Lieberman and
John A. Anderson -- 2nd ed.
    p. ; cm. -- (Current clinical practice)
  Includes bibliographical references and index.
  ISBN 0-89603-685-5 (alk. paper)
  1. Allergy. I. Lieberman, Phil L. II. Anderson, John A. (John Albert),
1935– III. Series. [DNLM: 1. Hypersensitivity--diagnosis. 2. Hypersensi-
tivity--therapy. WD 300 A43108 2000]
  RC584.A343 2000
  616.97--dc21
                                    00-020615

To Barbara
P. L.
and

To Nicole
J. A. A.

PREFACE

It hardly seems that three years have passed since the publication of the first edition of *Allergic Diseases: Diagnosis and Treatment*. We are gratified that it was enough of a success to warrant the second edition. As with the first, this edition is intended for the "front-line" physician who cares for the allergic patient. We have tried, once again, to make it as "user friendly" and clinically oriented as possible.

Our approach to the principles of pathophysiology is intended to allow them to be easily applied to the rationale for therapy. The major intent therefore is still to help the primary care physician deal with the day-to-day management of the allergic patient.

The arrangement of this text is similar to that of the first edition, with the major emphasis being on common allergic diseases and the pharmacologic tools we use to control them. To this end two new chapters have been added, one on antihistamines and the other on antileukotrienes. In addition, a new chapter has been added to help the physician deal with the child who experiences recurrent respiratory tract infections.

Many of the authors, because of the superb job they did with their first contributions, have been asked for an encore. However, to keep our approach fresh, some of these authors have been asked to write different chapters, and new contributors have been solicited.

Regardless of these changes, the thrust of the text remains the same—to disseminate the practical knowledge that we have accumulated in almost 70 years of practice and teaching in the field of allergy and immunology. As with the first edition of *Allergic Diseases: Diagnosis and Treatment*, our greatest hope is that the message has been delivered clearly, effectively, and in a manner to allow its easy application by the physician caring for those who suffer with allergic disease.

Phil Lieberman, MD
John A. Anderson, MD

CONTENTS

CONTRIBUTORS

JOHN A. ANDERSON, MD • *VIVRA Asthma and Allergy, Tucson, AZ*

LEONARD BIELORY, MD • *Division of Allergy, Immunology, and Rheumatology, UMDNJ–New Jersey Medical School, University Heights, Newark, NJ*

C. WARREN BIERMAN, MD • *Northwest Asthma and Allergy Center, Seattle, WA*

MICHAEL S. BLAISS, MD • *Clinical Professor of Pediatrics, Division of Clinical Immunology, University of Tennessee, Memphis, TN; Allergy and Asthma Care, Cordova, TN*

A. WESLEY BURKS, MD • *Department of Pediatrics, University of Arkansas for Medical Sciences, Little Rock, AR*

JONATHAN CORREN, MD • *Department of Medicine and Pediatrics, UCLA School of Medicine, Los Angeles, CA*

PEYTON A. EGGLESTON, MD • *Division of Allergy and Immunology, Department of Pediatrics, Johns Hopkins University School of Medicine, Baltimore, MD*

ELLIOT F. ELLIS, MD • *St. Petersburg, FL*

ALBERT F. FINN JR., MD • *National Allergy, Asthma, and Urticaria Centers of Charleston, Charleston, SC*

ROGER W. FOX, MD • *Division of Allergy and Immunology, Department of Internal Medicine, University of South Flordia College of Medicine, Tampa, FL*

CLIFTON T. FURUKAWA, MD • *Northwest Asthma and Allergy Center, University of Washington School of Medicine, Department of Pediatrics, Seattle, WA*

JERE D. GUIN, MD • *Professor Emeritus of Dermatology, University of Arkansas for Medical Sciences, Little Rock, AR*

RANDY J. HORWITZ, MD, PHD • *Madison, WI*

STACIE M. JONES, MD • *Arkansas Children's Hospital; Department of Pediatrics, University of Arkansas for Medical Sciences, Little Rock, AR*

LORI KAGY, MD • *Arkansas Allergy and Asthma Clinic, Little Rock, AR*

MICHAEL`A. KALINER, MD • *Institute for Asthma/Allergy at Washington Hospital Center, Washington, DC*

STEPHEN F. KEMP, MD • *Division of Allergy and Immunology, Departments of Medicine and Pediatrics, The University of Mississippi Medical Center School of Medicine, Jackson, MS*

DENNIS K. LEDFORD, MD • *Division of Allergy and Immunology, Department of Internal Medicine, University of South Florida and James A. Haley VA Hospital, Tampa, FL*

ROBERT F. LEMANSKE JR., MD • *Section of Allergy and Clinical Immunology, Departments of Pediatrics and Medicine, University of Wisconsin Medical School, Madison, WI*

PHIL LIEBERMAN, MD • *Allergy and Asthma Care, South, Cordova, TN*

RICHARD F. LOCKEY, MD • *University of South Florida, C/O VA Medical Center, Tampa, FL*

MARK H. MOSS, MD • *Section of Allergy and Clinical Immunology, University of Wisconsin Medical School, Madison, WI*

DENNIS R. OWNBY, MD • *Department of Pediatrics (Allergy and Immunology), Medical College of Georgia, Augusta, GA*

MARY E. PAUL, MD • *Department of Pediatrics (Allergy and Immunology), Texas Children's Hospital, Houston, TX*

GARY S. RACHELEFSKY, MD • *Department of Pediatrics, UCLA School of Medicine, Los Angeles, CA*

ROBERT E. REISMAN, MD • *Buffalo Medical Group, Williamsville, NY*

JUAN L. RODRIGUEZ, MD • *Division of Allergy and Clinical Immunology, Henry Ford Hospital, Detroit, MI*

GAIL G. SHAPIRO, MD • *Northwest Asthma and Allergy Center; Department of Pediatrics, University of Washington School of Medicine, Seattle, WA*

WILLIAM T. SHEARER, MD • *Department of Pediatrics, Division of Allergy and Immunology, Texas Children's Hospital, Houston, TX*

SCOTT H. SICHERER, MD • *Department of Pediatrics, Division of Allergy and Immunology, Mount Sinai School of Medicine, New York, NY*

JOSEPH D. SPAHN, MD • *Department of Pediatrics, Divisions of Clinical Pharmacology and Allergy and Clinical Immunology; Department of Pediatrics, National Jewish Medical and Research Center, Denver, CO*

SHELDON L. SPECTOR, MD • *California Allergy and Asthma, Los Angeles, CA*

STANLEY J. SZEFLER, MD • *Divisions of Clinical Pharmacology and Allergy and Clinical Immunology, National Jewish Medical Center; Departments of Pediatrics and Pharmacology, University of Colorado Health Sciences Center, Denver, CO*

ABBA I. TERR, MD • *San Francisco, CA*

FRANK S. VIRANT, MD • *Northwest Asthma and Allergy Center, Seattle, WA*

BRUCE L. WOLF, MD • *4230 Harding Road, Suite 307, Nashville, TN*

EDWARD M. ZORATTI, MD • *Division of Allergy and Clinical Immunology, Henry Ford Hospital, Detroit, MI*

1 Allergic Disease

Pathophysiology and Immunopathology

Mark H. Moss, MD, Randy J. Horwitz, MD, PhD, and Robert F. Lemanske, Jr., MD

CONTENTS

INTRODUCTION

Primary care physicians deal with allergic conditions far more often than they may suspect. Asthma, allergic rhinitis, and atopic dermatitis are some of the most common examples of these immunological diseases. On a daily basis, physicians obtain an allergy history before prescribing any antibiotic because of the high incidence of drug reactions in the population, illustrating one example of the importance of these disorders in clinical medicine.

With knowledge of the mechanisms mediating allergic reactions, a clinician can appreciate the pathophysiological changes brought about by introduction of a foreign antigen to a normally well balanced system. This knowledge of the underlying mechanisms of allergic disease enables the physician to recognize and even anticipate adverse reactions. Knowing that some asthmatics might experience a late-phase allergic response, for example, compels the physician to continue intensive therapy until the reaction has completely subsided.

From: *Current Clinical Practice: Allergic Diseases: Diagnosis and Treatment, 2nd Edition*
Edited by: P. Lieberman and J. Anderson © Humana Press Inc., Totowa, NJ

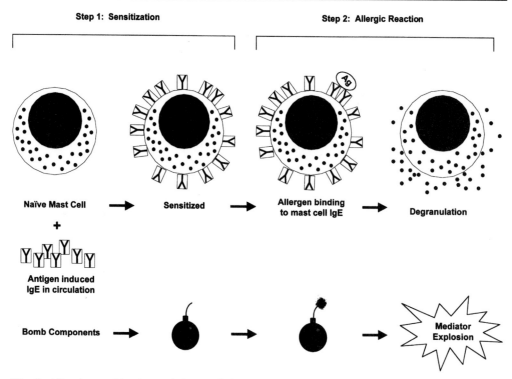

Fig. 1. Allergic sensitization and degranulation. The process of sensitization and degranulation in mast cells is analogous to the construction and detonation of a bomb. Initial binding of specific IgE to the naive mast cell surface "primes" the cell for activity, in effect building the bomb. Subsequent binding of allergen to the mast cell is akin to lighting the fuse of the bomb. Intracellular biochemical events lead to the ultimate "explosion"—a cellular degranulation leading to mediator release.

The development of allergies involving immunoglobulin E (IgE) antibody formation, also known as *atopy*, involves both complex genetic and environmental influences that are only now being elucidated. Put simply, based on simple mendelian inheritance patterns, we cannot predict which individuals will develop allergies and which will not. However, there does appear to be a higher incidence of allergies among children of allergic parents.

The two-step process by which one initially becomes "allergic" to a substance begins with *sensitization* and is outlined in Fig. 1. During the initial stage of sensitization, the individual develops significant amounts of IgE antibodies against an inhaled, ingested, or injected substance. Memory B-cells also appear that are capable of immediately producing more of this specific IgE antibody when stimulated. The second stage involves adherence of this newly formed IgE antibody to circulating blood basophils or to the mast cell located in the mucosal surfaces of the skin, the gastrointestinal tract, and the respiratory system. These tissue mast cells were previously coated with IgE antibodies directed specifically against other potentially allergenic substances. The new exposure simply added to the existing population. There are millions of IgE molecules of different specificities (directed against different allergens) on the surface of each mast cell and basophil. An individual is considered to be "sensitized" only after IgE antibodies against a certain substance have been produced and are bound to the surface of mast cells and basophils. The process of sensitization does not produce any of the symptoms that we equate with allergic disease—in fact, a person is usually unaware of these initial molecular and cellular changes. It is not until re-exposure to the allergen that allergic symptoms begin to appear.

The second step in the two-step process of becoming allergic involves the re-exposure of a sensitized person to the allergen, with the production of symptoms ranging from negligible rhinorrhea to sudden death. Most cases lie somewhere in between. The biochemical events that lead to allergic symptoms will be discussed in some detail later, using an anaphylactic reaction to an insect sting as an example. However, one should keep in mind that although the cellular and molecular events for all immediate hypersensitivity reactions are similar, differences in target organ responses ultimately dictate the clinical patterns of disease activity once a reaction has been induced.

THE ALLERGIC REACTION: *A SCENARIO*

A 6-yr-old boy was playing with toy trucks in his backyard, when he unwisely chose to bulldoze a yellow jacket nest. Fortunately, he escaped with a single sting on his ankle. While his mother was putting ice on the sting and wiping away her son's tears, yellow jacket antigens, which were injected at the time of the sting, were being filtered through the bloodstream and the lymphatics, with some lodging in regional lymph nodes. Here the antigens encountered T- and B-cells and were recognized as foreign proteins. The interaction with lymphocytes leads to IgE production in those genetically predisposed—allergic or atopic individuals. This IgE was specifically directed against the yellow jacket venom and circulated briefly through the bloodstream before binding to IgE receptors on tissue mast cells and blood basophils. These receptors bound the antibody at the F_c end of the molecule, leaving the F_{ab} (antigen binding) region exposed and free to bind circulating antigen. By this time the venom had long since been cleared by the reticuloendothelial system, producing only a mild local reaction at the site of the sting. The only evidence that the boy was ever stung was the presence of the specific antivenom IgE on his mast cells and the presence of a few memory B-cells capable of producing more antivenom IgE if they encounter it again.

Two years later, the boy was stung again by a yellow jacket while at a picnic. Within minutes, he developed wheezing and had difficulty breathing. He was gasping for air as paramedics were summoned and was cyanotic by the time they arrived. Fortunately, prompt treatment allowed him to recover. At a molecular level, the events responsible for the boy's problem began with the sensitization. From that point on, his immune system made him a living time bomb, ready to detonate when provoked by the yellow jacket antigen "trigger." Despite a 2-yr gap, the immune system never forgot its initial exposure to the venom. On his being stung for the second time, the yellow jacket venom again circulated through the bloodstream and lymphatics. This time, however, it flowed past the mast cells with IgE antivenom antibodies already situated on their surfaces. These IgE molecules acted like molecular hands and grabbed the venom as it passed by. Eventually, when the number of venom molecules bound to the IgE on the mast cell surface became high enough, some of the IgE antibodies crosslinked and a chain reaction began. The mast cells poured forth preformed chemicals that had until then been quiescent in intracellular granules—chemicals that cause bronchoconstriction, vasodilatation, and upper airway edema. In addition, the triggering and degranulation

---

The Allergic Process

- The familial tendency to be allergic by producing antigen-specific IgE is called atopy.
- Children born to allergic parents are born with the potential to be allergic, not with preformed specific allergies.
- Sensitization involves IgE antibody formation directed to specific allergens plus fixation to effector cells such as mast cells or basophils.
- Allergic reactions result from re-exposure to the allergen, allergen-IgE interaction at the cellular level, and release/formation of chemical mediators, which result in symptoms depending on the target organ in which these events occur.

---

of the mast cells led to the de novo production of other substances that also contributed to the reaction. The effect of the re-exposure to the venom in this boy's case is termed *anaphylaxis* and represents the most severe type of allergic reaction. Fortunately, such a reaction is rare and can often be prevented, or at least attenuated. We will now explore the pathophysiology of such a reaction in greater detail, starting with the effector cell in immediate hypersensitivity, the mast cell. We will also mention the basophil, a granulocyte that releases mediators similar to those of the mast cell.

ASPECTS OF IgE PRODUCTION

As noted above, the key intermediary in allergic conditions is the IgE antibody. It is an individual's propensity to produce IgE in response to an "allergic antigen" (also known as an allergen) that renders him or her atopic. The same allergen that would stimulate B-cells to produce IgG or IgM in a nonallergic individual may stimulate IgE antibody production in an atopic person.

What makes the body respond to allergen exposure by making IgE as opposed to other classes of antibodies? You may recall that antibody molecules consist of a variable region responsible for recognizing and binding the offending antigen, and a constant region whose purpose is to dictate the fate of the antigen-antibody complex. For example, a person may make both IgA and IgG antibodies against a virus. Both are capable of binding to that virus, but the IgA is found mainly in secretions (as in the nasal mucosa), whereas the IgG predominates in the bloodstream. Although all of the mechanisms by which a particular antigen favors the production of one class of antibody over another are not firmly established, several factors that may favor IgE formation are worth discussing.

All antigens initially elicit the production of IgM antibodies against an injected or inhaled allergen. With repeated exposure, the antigen may stimulate an event known as class switching, whereby the constant portion of the antibody will "switch" to another class (i.e., IgG, IgA, or IgE). The new antibody will still have the same antigen recognition region (against influenza virus, for example), but it will now be sitting on another constant region (IgG or IgA, for example). IgE production by B-cells as a result of class switching is regulated by other cells of the immune system (mainly T-cells and macrophages) and the *cytokines* they produce. Cytokines are small-molecular-weight

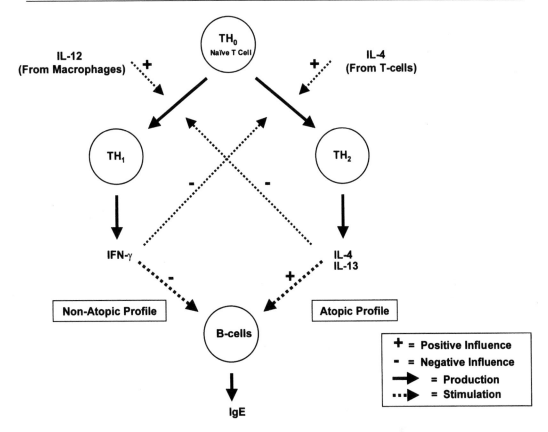

Fig. 2. The TH_1 and TH_2 paradigm. T helper cells uncommitted to an atopic or nonatopic cytokine profile (TH_0) receive stimulation from cytokines IL-4 and IL-12 to polarize to a TH_1 or TH_2 phenotype. The TH_1 profile is consistent with a nonatopic phenotype, whereas the TH_2 profile is consistent with an atopic phenotype. TH_1 cells produce IFN-γ, which inhibits IgE production from B-cells and TH_0 differentiation into TH_2 cells. TH_2 cells, on the contrary, produce IL-4 and IL-13, both potent stimulators of IgE production from B-cells. IL-4 also feeds back to inhibit TH_0 differentiation into TH_1 cells; it can also further self-promote TH_0 differentiation into TH_2 cells to perpetuate the cycle of an atopic cytokine response.

molecules that affect cell function at the local level. Two primary cytokines that favor IgE class switching are interleukin-4 (IL-4) and interleukin-13 (IL-13). IL-4 and IL-13 are produced by a subset of CD4+ T-cells that have a *T helper 2* (TH_2) cytokine profile. IL-4 is such an essential signal for IgE production that mice that have been genetically engineered to be devoid of IL-4 ("IL-4 knockout mice") are unable to synthesize IgE. In contrast, the primary cytokine that inhibits IgE class switching is called interferon-gamma (IFN-γ). IFN-γ is produced by a subset of T-cells that have a *T helper 1* (TH_1) cytokine profile. The cytokines produced by TH_1 and TH_2 cells reciprocally inhibit the other's development. These stimulatory and inhibitory interactions are outlined in Fig. 2. In atopic individuals the balance of TH_1 and TH_2 responses seems to favor the TH_2 response and IgE production. In nonatopic individuals, the balance between TH_1 and TH_2 favors a TH_1 dominant response.

The ability to produce polyclonal IgE antibody is present as early as 8–10 wk of gestation. Since IgE antibody cannot cross the placenta, any IgE present in cord blood

Table 1
Relative Distribution of the Two Predominant Human Mast Cell
Phenotypes in Immunologically Relevant Tissues and Cell Populations*

Organ	% MC_T Cells	% MC_{TC} Cells
Skin	5	95
Intestinal mucosa	80	20
Intestinal submucosa	30	70
Alveolar wall	95	5
Bronchial subepithelium	40	60
Dispersed lung mast cells	90	10
Tonsils	40	60
Nasal mucosa	65	35

*Adapted from Holgate and Church. *Allergy*, London: Gower Medical Publishing, London, 1993.

has been produced entirely by the fetus. During the first year of life, antigen-specific IgE antibody is directed primarily against food antigens; by age 2–3 yr, aeroallergen sensitivity begins to become more prevalent.

The biochemical structure of an antigen appears to play a role in determining the isotype response. A polysaccharide antigen, from the surface of Streptococcus, for instance, will prompt B-cells to produce IgG but not IgE antibodies. In contrast, certain proteins from parasites can cause the B-lymphocytes (with help from the T-cells and their IL-4) to cease production of IgG or IgM and, instead, to churn out vast quantities of IgE. However, exactly what it is about the structure of proteins that preferentially leads them to become allergens, thus stimulating IgE synthesis, remains unresolved.

THE MAST CELL

The mast cell was first described by Paul Erlich in 1877 while he was still a medical student. He chose the name Mastzellen ("well fed") based on the cell's characteristic cytoplasmic granules (he incorrectly thought that the mast cells were phagocytes and that the granules were ingested debris). We now recognize the central role that mast cells play in the immediate hypersensitivity response.

As with all hematopoietic cells, the mast cells are formed by the action of soluble factors on a pluripotent stem cell (progenitor cell) in the bone marrow. The cells emerge from the bone marrow and migrate to the connective tissues, where they mature, acquiring both cytoplasmic granules and a coating of high-affinity IgE receptors (called $F_c\epsilon RI$) on their cell surface. Despite gross morphological homogeneity, it is now apparent that mast cells are a heterogeneous cell population. Subtle histochemical differences are apparent when analyzing mast cell populations in different anatomical compartments. For example, mast cells isolated from the lung differ from those obtained from the skin. Most pulmonary mast cells primarily contain one neutral protease, called tryptase. Skin mast cells, on the other hand, contain large amounts of both tryptase and another protease, called chymase (described below). Mast cells in humans are divided and named on the basis of this biochemical difference and are termed MC_T (for mast cell containing tryptase) or MC_{TC} (for mast cell containing chymase). The tissue distribution of these subtypes of mast cells is shown in Table 1. The relative numbers of MC_T or MC_{TC} may change locally with tissue inflammation or fibrosis. It is thought that cytokine differences in the microenvironment of the tissues are responsible for this differentiation.

The most characteristic feature of the mast cell is undoubtedly the metachromatic granules, which account for over 50% of the cell volume and dry weight. These granules contain the preformed chemical mediators of allergic reactions, many of which are still unidentified. There are no accurate means of discerning from what tissue an isolated mast cell population is derived, since mixtures of both MC_T and MC_{TC} cells are found in all tissues. In other words, although a given tissue may display a predominance of one type of mast cell, the population is heterogeneous in all locations.

MEDIATORS OF THE ALLERGIC RESPONSE

The mediators released by mast cells and basophils can be grouped into two categories: preformed substances contained within granules and newly generated chemicals synthesized following cellular activation. These mediators comprise the effector function of the mast cell. Together they are able to increase vascular permeability, dilate vessels, cause bronchospasm, contract smooth muscle, and summon inflammatory cells, as summarized in Fig. 3. Few cells in the body produce compounds with such a large and varied spectrum of activity. Several representative mediators from each category will now be reviewed.

Histamine is a prominent preformed vasoactive amine contained within the mast cell granule. It is formed by the action of histidine decarboxylase on the amino acid histidine. Histamine is the only preformed mediator of the human mast cell with direct vasoactive and smooth muscle spasmogenic effects. It can increase mucous production from airway epithelial cells and contract airway smooth muscle, thus contributing to both mucous plugging and bronchospasm. Histamine also acts to increase vascular permeability as well as to promote vasodilatation, thus causing extravasation of fluid into the tissues. In extreme cases, such intravascular fluid shifts can lead to hypotension and shock. Similarly, localized vasoactive effects of histamine are seen in the wheal and flare reaction of a percutaneous allergen skin test.

Neutral proteases are compounds that catalyze the cleavage of certain peptide bonds in proteins, thereby facilitating protein degradation. Their activity is optimum at a neutral pH, hence the name. The two major proteases of human mast cells and basophils are *tryptase* and *chymase*. Tryptase is found in both the MC_T and MC_{TC} subtypes of mast cells, whereas chymase is restricted to the MC_{TC} cells. Basophils have negligible, although detectable, levels of these proteases. The potentially dangerous proteolytic activity of these compounds is controlled by maintaining the interior of the granules at an acidic pH, thus inhibiting protease activity.

There are other accessory molecules that have prominent roles in the allergic response. *Proteoglycans*, including heparin and chondroitin sulfate A, are important in mast cell and basophil biochemistry, respectively. Both histamine and the proteolytic enzymes are bound to proteoglycan compounds within the granules. It is the proteoglycans that give the granules their distinctive crystalline structure. Their exact function is unclear, although many believe that proteoglycans stabilize the enzymes to which they are bound until degranulation occurs.

MEDIATORS OF ALLERGIC REACTIONS		
Molecules released from activated mast cells and basophils account for many allergic symptoms. This list includes a sampling of those chemicals and some of their effects, which can be redundant.		

	CHEMICAL	**ACTIVITY**	**SYMPTOMS**
MEDIATORS FROM GRANULES	Histamine	Constricts bronchial airways	Wheezing; difficulty breathing
		Dilates blood vessels	Local redness at sites of allergen delivery· widespread dilation can contribute to potentially lethal hypotension (shock)
		Increases permeability of small blood vessels	Swelling of local tissue; if widespread, increased permeability can contribute to shock
		Stimulates nerve endings	Itching and pain in skin
		Stimulates secretion of mucus in airways	Congestion of airways
	Platelet-activating factor	Constricts bronchial airways	*Same as for histamine*
		Dilates blood vessels	*Same as for histamine*
LIPID MEDIATORS	Leukotrienes	Constricts bronchial airways	*Same as for histamine*
		Increase permeability of small blood vessels	*Same as for histamine*
	Prostaglandin D	Constricts bronchial airways	*Same as for histamine*

Fig. 3. Mast cell mediators and their effects (adapted from Lichtenstein L. Allergy and the immune system. *Sci Am* 1993;369:117–124, with permission).

Two predominant classes of mediators are synthesized de novo following activation of the mast cells and basophils: the lipid derivatives and the cytokines. The lipid derivatives include the *leukotrienes* and the *prostaglandins*. They represent byproducts of the metabolism of arachidonic acid formed upon activation of the mast cell. The mast cell is able to catabolize essential membrane components and convert them into biologically active mediators through a complex cascade of membrane-bound and soluble enzymes. The overall pathway is seen in Fig. 4. The leukotrienes, produced by the action of the 5-lipoxygenase system on arachidonic acid (which was generated by phospholipase A_2 acting on cell membrane constituents), demonstrate many different activities, of which the most prominent is immediate bronchoconstriction. They also can cause vasoconstriction in both the pulmonary and vascular beds. The primary

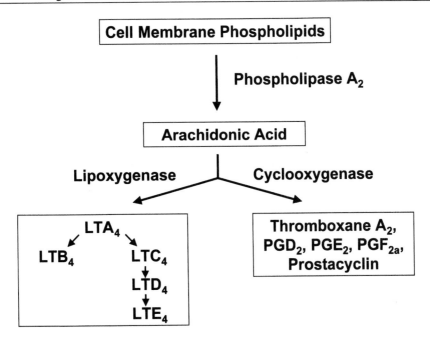

Fig. 4. Arachidonic acid metabolic pathways. Arachidonic acid, released as a result of phospholipase action on the cellular membrane, is broken down by two distinct biochemical pathways: The lipoxygenase pathway results in formation of the leukotrienes (LT), whereas the cyclooxygenase pathway generates prostacyclin, thromboxane, and the prostaglandins (PG).

leukotrienes made by human mast cells are B_4, C_4, D_4, and E_4. The leukotrienes, especially D_4, are greater than 10 times more potent than histamine.

Arachidonic acid is also broken down by the action of the cyclooxygenase pathway, resulting in the formation of *prostaglandins*, *prostacyclins*, and *thromboxane*. These compounds generally function as local hormones and produce many of the same symptoms as the leukotrienes, such as bronchoconstriction, cough, and vasodilatation. The main prostaglandin (PG) produced by human mast cells is PGD_2, a compound at least 30 times as potent as histamine in causing bronchoconstriction. Thromboxane A_2 and prostacyclin (PGI_2) produce bronchoconstriction and bronchodilatation, respectively. Together they function as a mechanism to maintain bronchial, as well as vascular, tone.

Platelet activating factor (PAF) is a phopholipid named after its discovery as a basophil-derived mediator of rabbit platelet activation. PAF is produced by mast cells (as well as macrophages, neutrophils, and eosinophils) and functions to activate platelets and neutrophils and vasoconstrict smooth muscle. Perhaps most importantly, PAF stimulates chemoattraction of eosinophils to endothelial surfaces and eosinophil release of other cell mediators. PAF is rapidly inactivated in vivo, suggesting that it serves as a trigger of inflammatory events rather than a major mediator itself.

The identification of the *cytokines* synthesized by mast cells and basophils is currently an area of intense investigation. Cytokines represent the primary mechanism by which cells can influence the activity and development of unrelated cells. In addition, many cells respond in an autocrine fashion to the cytokines they themselves secrete. Although most mast cell cytokine studies have been performed in rodent cells, several cytokines have been identified in human mast cells. We know that human mast cells produce IL-4 and interleukin-5 (IL-5) as well as tumor necrosis factor alpha (TNF-α). The IL-4 stimulates mast cell differentiation and promotes immunoglobulin class switching to the IgE isotype. Interleukin-5 is the most influential cytokine involved in eosinophil production and survival in humans. TNF-α increases vascular permeability and leukocyte migration.

Basophils have long been incorrectly viewed as the "blood-borne" equivalent of mast cells with analogous granules and functions. However, these cells represent a hematopoietic lineage distinct from mast cells, can also infiltrate tissues, and contain neither tryptase nor chymase. In addition, basophils seem to have a different role in the allergic reaction scenario. They tend to release abundant amounts of histamine, but little, if any, PGD_2. This finding has been cited as evidence of their contribution to late-phase allergic inflammatory events in the nose, skin, and lung. The presence of increased histamine, but undetectable PGD_2, during late responses implies that basophils are recruited to sites of allergic inflammation (see Early- and Late-Phase Responses).

ACTIVATION OF THE MAST CELL

The mechanism by which the external signal of IgE crosslinking is translated into cellular activation, granule release, and de novo synthesis of new molecules is a fascinating tale of cellular adaptation and biochemistry. Although immensely complex, a basic appreciation of the process will prove useful in understanding the nature of the allergic response. An overview of the reactions is illustrated in Fig. 5.

The process begins with the crosslinking of two or more IgE molecules on the mast cell surface. This requires a multivalent antigen (i.e., more than one IgE binding site on the same molecule); monovalent antigens will not trigger mast cell activation. It is important to remember that there are thousands of different IgE molecules on every mast cell—each of which is capable of binding to a different antigen. They float about freely on the mast cell surface, bound by the F_c portion of the IgE, until they bump into the appropriate antigen, at which point they bind tightly. Once bound by one IgE molecule, there is a strong possibility that other IgE molecules with similar specificities will also attach themselves to the antigen. Once the antigen is attached to the mast cell by more than one IgE molecule, a series of cytoplasmic signals occurs causing activation. This process is called *signal transduction* and is a method of cellular communication with the external environment. In this case the signal enters the cell via a conformational change in the $F_c\varepsilon RI$ receptor.

Once the antigen is bound to the mast cell via the IgE molecules, the cell begins a series of biochemical events that culminates in the release of its granules and the production of lipid mediators (arachidonic acid metabolites). A series of phosphorylation cascades begins the process. This is nature's way of conserving energy by using charged phosphate molecules that are transferred between different compounds (usually tyrosine or serine amino acids on proteins) using enzymes called kinases. Eventually a protein called phospholipase C becomes phosphorylated and moves from the cytosol to the membrane, where it assumes an active conformation. This protein catalyzes the release of inositol triphosphate (IP_3) and diacylglycerol (DAG) from the mast cell membrane. The IP_3 causes release of calcium from intracellular stores in the

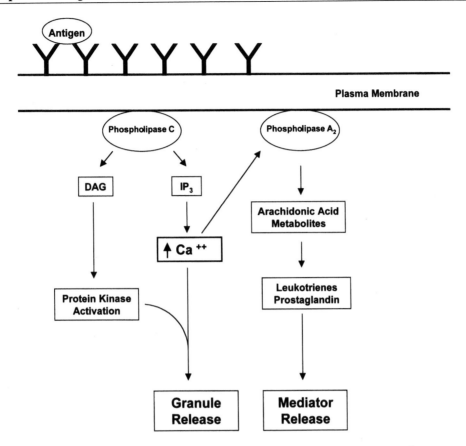

Fig. 5. Mast cell activation: biochemical reactions. Following IgE crosslinking by antigen, a series of protein kinase reactions culminate in the activation of phospholipase C, releasing diacylglycerol (DAG) and inositol triphosphate (IP_3) from the plasma membrane. The IP_3 releases calcium stores from the endoplasmic reticulum, which, along with DAG-stimulated kinases, leads to granule release. The intracellular calcium also activates phospholipase A_2, which generates arachidonic acid, a compound metabolized to form leukotrienes and prostaglandins.

endoplasmic reticulum, whereas DAG is used to activate proteins involved in granule release. The calcium serves two central functions: It is used as a cofactor for the release of the granules (with the DAG), and also it serves to activate a protein called phospholipase A_2 (PLA_2), the regulator of lipid mediator production. In summary, at this point we have the mast cell able to release granules, but the other effector function, that of prostaglandin and leukotriene production, is just beginning.

The production of the lipid mediators requires effective intracellular scavenging by the mast cell. The principle is to cannibalize lipids from the membrane and transform them into potent mediators. PLA_2, activated by the calcium released from the endoplasmic reticulum, starts degrading phosphatidyl choline, an integral membrane component. In turn, arachidonic acid is formed and metabolized via the two pathways mentioned earlier: the lipoxygenase pathway (which produces leukotrienes) and the cyclooxygenase pathway (which produces prostaglandins). As stated previously, the main prostaglandin produced by mast cells is PGD_2. Leukotrienes B_4 and C_4 are the primary leukotrienes made. Leukotriene C_4 is subsequently converted to active compounds LTD$_4$ and LTE$_4$. The activities of these lipid mediators are described elsewhere.

In summary, the mast cell needs to accomplish two functions following activation: to release its granules with their associated biologically active compounds and to synthesize additional mediators of the allergic reaction using its cell membrane constituents as precursors. These activities utilize a great deal of cellular energy, most of which is obtained from the high-energy phosphate bonds generated by the action of protein kinases. The initiation of these cascades depends on interaction of the mast cell with antigen. The prerequisite crosslinking of the IgE molecules probably evolved as a safety mechanism to prevent premature activation of the cell. A sufficient quantity of specific IgE must be bound to the mast cell to achieve a crosslink, which is possible only if sensitization had occurred previously.

Allergic (IgE-mediated) activation of the mast cell was summarized earlier, but there is an alternate, IgE-independent mechanism of mast cell degranulation that should be mentioned. This degranulation is the result of mast cell membrane perturbation at a molecular level, often requiring calcium influx. This nonimmunological degranulation may be triggered by opioids, anaphylatoxins (complement components), and radiological contrast dyes. In fact, the majority of patients who report a history of "allergic reactions" to contrast dyes have experienced non–IgE-mediated reactions.

EFFECTS OF MAST CELL MEDIATORS ON TARGET ORGANS

The examination of the mechanisms contributing to the release of mast cell mediators is only half the story of allergic pathophysiology. The spectrum of symptoms that prompts a visit to the allergist begins only after these substances are released from mast cells and interact with resident and infiltrating cells in various target organs. In the case involving the 6-yr-old boy sensitized and subsequently stung by a yellow jacket, these mediators combined to cause anaphylaxis. Histamine was liberated from the mast cell granules and was quickly dispersed through the bloodstream. Histamine receptors are located on many target organs, including the skin, the nasal mucosa, the smooth muscle of the lungs and gastrointestinal tract, and vascular epithelial cells. Once bound to its receptor, histamine causes such diverse effects as vasodilatation of small vessels with subsequent exudation of fluid into surrounding tissue; smooth muscle contraction, an effect of particular import when one is considering the muscles surrounding the bronchial airways; and increased glandular mucous secretion, an annoyance in the nasal mucosa but dangerous in the small bronchioles. Extremely high doses of histamine cause these effects to occur on a systemic level, possibly leading to hypotensive shock in the case of massive vasodilatation.

The lipid mediators cause symptoms that are very similar to histamine; however, their effects are more persistent. Histamine is rapidly degraded in the serum with a half-life 1 min, but the lipid mediators are slowly metabolized. As you recall, both leukotrienes and prostaglandins are synthesized only after an allergic reaction has begun, thus accounting for the delay in onset of action. Historically, leukotrienes were collectively termed the slow-reacting substance of anaphylaxis because of this delay in activity. Once released in the serum, the prostaglandins bind to specific receptors and lead to bronchial smooth muscle contraction in the lungs, vasodilatation in the skin, and nasal blockage. Leukotrienes are also highly potent bronchoconstrictors but utilize distinct receptors on the smooth muscle cells. They also increase permeability at postcapillary venules, leading to localized tissue edema.

ALLERGIC INFLAMMATION: *A TH$_2$-MEDIATED RESPONSE*

Just as IgE production and mast cell activation are key components to the initial allergic response, several other cells play a role in propogating this allergic inflammatory response. After the immediate release of mast cell mediators following allergen exposure, leukocytes influx into affected tissues. This occurs approximately 2–8 hr after allergen exposure and has been termed the late-phase reaction (LPR) or the late allergic response (LAR). It is explained in detail later. The primary cell types recruited to sites of LPR include basophils, eosinophils, neutrophils, lymphocytes, and macrophages. The main attractants for these cells are cytokines secreted by mast cells, T-cells, and epithelial cells. Cells present during the initial allergic response, such as mast cells, as well as cells that migrate into tissues following an increase in vascular permeability, such as lymphocytes, or cells present throughout the allergic response, such as epithelial cells, can generate cytokines. Many cytokines contribute to this influx; however, IL-4, IL-5, TNF-α, and chemotactic cytokines termed *chemokines* play major roles. TNF-α and IL-4 attract basophils. IL-5 is a potent eosinophil activator, and C-C chemokines such as RANTES (regulated on activation, normal T-cell expressed and secreted) promote eosinophil migration into tissues. These responses collectively parallel the TH$_2$ cytokine profile outlined earlier and shown in Fig. 2. It is interesting that IL-13, while a potent inducer of B-cell IgE production, is not an effective inflammatory mediator. IL-13, unlike IL-4, fails to induce TH$_2$ cell differentiation and in vitro inhibits pro-inflammatory cytokine and chemokine production. In cases of perennial allergic rhinitis, perennial asthma, and acute atopic dermatitis, T-cells isolated from the affected tissues (nose, lung, or skin, respectively) exhibit a predominantly TH$_2$ cytokine profile. However, it is important to remember that any T-cell population will express heterogeneity and not uniformly possess one cytokine profile.

EARLY- AND LATE-PHASE RESPONSES

An important aspect of allergic disease, with scientific as well as clinical implications, is the concept of the late-phase IgE-mediated reaction. The mast cell activation pathway (described above) occurs within minutes of allergen exposure. All mechanisms and components of the system are designed for almost instantaneous responses—from the signal transduction pathways to the presence of granules containing preformed, "ready-to-use" mediators. Once the initial surge of mediator release is completed, there is regeneration of the mast cell granules, although this process may take days to weeks to be completed. If one were to speculate that an allergic reaction represents an exaggerated host response to a foreign invader (or allergen), then it might make sense to have a backup system in place in case the immediate response is not completely successful. In the teleological sense, that is precisely what the late-phase response does.

The late-phase response is a delayed-in-time inflammatory response that occurs following mast cell activation. It may function to amplify an initial signal resulting from the first wave of allergen "attack." In response to a barrage of chemotactic and differentiative cytokines, multiple cell lineages (e.g., eosinophils, neutrophils) are

Early- vs Late-Phase Allergen Reactions	
Early	**Late**
Clinical response to stimuli within minutes and up to 2 h	Response to stimuli in 2–8 h, usually following an early reaction
Predominant effector cell: mast cell	Predominant effector cell(s): lymphocytes, eosinophils, and basophils
Predominant mediators include histamine, chemotactic agents, prostaglandins (PG), and leukotrienes	All mediators, except PGD_2 plus platelet activating factor (PAF)
Cellular response—sparse, if any	Cellular response marked— eosinophils neutrophils, and mononuclear cells

summoned to the site of this breach of the immune system. Together, these summoned cells constitute the inflammatory or late allergic response (LAR). The LAR lacks the speed of the immediate response, but it more than makes up for this in terms of magnitude. The LAR typically occurs 2–8 h after initial allergen exposure. As stated above, the LAR represents the inflammatory phase of an allergic reaction, no matter where in the body it occurs. Subtle differences in the nature and effect of the mediators involved in the LAR have been observed in each anatomical location where it has been described. We will consider three such environments: the skin, the nose, and the lungs.

The *cutaneous* early reactions are well described: A characteristic wheal and flare reaction is seen with a positive skin test in an atopic individual. It resembles a mosquito bite, in that it consists of a pale, circumscribed central area of edema, surrounded by an erythematous diffuse border. This typical early-phase reaction will peak in 15 min and resolve in 30–60 min. In some cases, however, the early-phase response will persist for hours and progress into a late-phase response that peaks at 6–8 h following allergen exposure and lasts up to 24 h. The cellular infiltrate observed 6–12 h after a cutaneous allergen challenge consists of a mixed population of neutrophils, eosinophils, and lymphocytes. Mediators produced in the cutaneous LAR reflect the nature of the cells summoned to the area and include various interleukins (IL-1, IL-4, IL-6).

The *nasal* late-phase response is characterized by a cellular infiltrate of eosinophils, mononuclear cells, and neutrophils and is often accompanied by fibrin deposition. The mediators produced in the nasal LAR are identical to those present in the early response with one exception: PGD_2 is absent. As mentioned earlier, the presence of histamine without PGD_2 suggests that basophils may play a prominent role in the nasal LAR, since in contrast to the mast cells, they characteristically produce negligible amounts of PGD_2 while maintaining a high histamine content. Nasal congestion is the predominant symptom associated with the nasal LAR (rhinorrhea and sneezing are generally associated with the early response).

The *pulmonary* LAR probably has received the most attention of all anatomical sites, probably owing to the increasing frequency and severity of asthma in the population. In the lung, the pattern response to different allergens is more variable, with numerous examples of solitary early responses and solitary late responses, as well as dual responses. The mediators released during an early allergic response summon more helper (CD4[+]) T-cells that, in turn, send out cytokine signals that attract other diverse cell types to the area. Among these cytokines are IL-4, which serves to increase IgE production, and IL-5 and granulocyte-macrophage colony-stimulating factor (GM-CSF), which increase eosinophil production and survival. In addition, other cytokines serve to increase the expression of specific leukocyte receptors on endothelial cells lining the pulmonary vasculature, thus facilitating transmigration of these cells from the bloodstream into the airway lumen.

Clinically, isolated immediate responses are those that cause airway obstruction (with wheezing, coughing, or shortness of breath) within minutes of allergen exposure. They typically resolve within 1 h. Late-phase reactions begin 3–4 h after allergen exposure and resolve within 24 h. The symptoms associated with the late response are similar to those of the immediate response, with dyspnea and cough predominating. The pulmonary dual response consists of both the early and late response, separated by an asymptomatic interval of normal baseline pulmonary function.

SUMMARY

In summary, it is evident that several generalities apply to all tissues in which an allergic reaction can occur. The early-phase response, the immediate result of an interaction between a sensitized mast cell and a specific allergen, results in the release of preformed mediators, which exhibit both local and distal target organ effects. The cellular effects of these mediators are similar in each tissue, but the clinical symptoms produced may differ. For example, increases in vascular permeability may present as angioedema in the skin or as congestion in the nose. The presence of a late-phase response is also seen in various tissues and represents the inflammatory response. Since the goal of the late-phase response is to attract inflammatory cells, the cytokine profile differs slightly from the immediate response.

How does all this relate to the 6-yr-old boy with allergies to yellow jackets? His primary care physician wisely sent him to a specialist, where he completed a course of immunotherapy, and has enjoyed carefree summers since then. As we will see in later chapters, there are many immunological and pharmacological interventions that may be useful in preventing both immediate and late-phase allergic reactions. An appreciation of the pathophysiology of the allergic reaction is essential to the proper use of these treatments.

SUGGESTED READING

Charlesworth EN. The skin as a model to study the pathogenesis of IgE-mediated acute and late phase responses. *J Allergy Clin Immunol* 1994;94:1240–1250.

Costa J, et al. The cells of the allergic response: Mast cells, basophils, and eosinophils. *JAMA* 1997;278:1815–1822.

De Vries J. The role of IL-13 and its receptor in allergy and inflammatory responses. *J Allergy Clin Immunol* 1998;102:165–169.

Galli SJ. New concepts about the mast cell. *N Engl J Med* 1993;328:257–265.

Kaliner MA, Lemanske R. Rhinitis and asthma. *JAMA* 1992;268:2807–2829.

Marshall JS, Bienenstock J. The role of mast cells in inflammatory reactions of the airways, skin and intestine. *Curr Opin Immunol* 1994;6:853–859.

Mosmann T, Sad S. The expanding universe of T-cell subsets: Th1, Th2, and more. *Immunol Today* 1996;17:138–146.

Peters SP, Zangrilli JG, Fish JE. In: Middleton E, Reed CE, et al., eds. *Late Phase Allergic Reactions in Allergy: Principles and Practice.* St. Louis; Mosby, 1998, pp. 342–365.

Wasserman S. Mast cells and airway inflammation in asthma. *Am J Respir Crit Care Med* 1994; 150:S39–S41.

White M. Mediators of inflammation and the inflammatory process. *J Allergy Clin Immunol* 1999; 103:S378–S381.

2 Approach to the Allergic Patient

Bruce L. Wolf, MD

CONTENTS

INTRODUCTION
HISTORY
PHYSICAL EXAMINATION
ALLERGY TESTING
DIAGNOSTIC STUDIES
CONFERENCE
SUGGESTED READING

INTRODUCTION

Although it often is remarked that everyone is allergic to something, in truth, only about 25–30% of the population are allergic to anything. Thus, the allergic patient is a common visitor in every medical setting. In addition, many disorders mimic allergy symptoms. Therefore, the differential diagnoses of various disease states must include allergy as a possibility.

Allergy can affect virtually any organ system. Common types of presentation include conjunctivitis (eyes), rhinitis (nose), urticaria and angioedema or atopic (allergic) dermatitis (skin), asthma (lungs), and anaphylaxis (multi-organ). Evaluation of suspected allergy must include a detailed medical history, comprehensive physical examination, and appropriate diagnostic tests.

HISTORY

The most important component of the evaluation of a possible allergic problem is the patient's history. It is from the history that salient physical examination and tests follow. An allergy history is made up of chief complaint, determination of seasonality or diurnal variation of symptoms, identification of triggers, occupational exposure, response to medication, family history, and other pertinent medical history. It may not be obvious to the patient what historical factors are important; thus, a questionnaire is recommended that screens for contributory factors (Fig. 1).

From: *Current Clinical Practice: Allergic Diseases: Diagnosis and Treatment, 2nd Edition*
Edited by: P. Lieberman and J. Anderson © Humana Press Inc., Totowa, NJ

Primary reason for coming to Allergy & Asthma Specialists:

_____

Check your main symptoms – those that prompted your visit here:

Head or Nose	Chest	Skin	Insect Stings
O Sneezing	O Cough	O Eczema	O Hives
O Runny Nose	O Wheezing	O Itching	O Swelling
O Postnasal drainage	O Shortness of Breath	O Swelling	O Shortness of Breath
O Nose Blocking	O Hoarseness	O Hives	O Itching
O Sinus Infections	O Chest Infections		O Dizziness
O Sore Throat	O Voice Loss		O Fainting
O Ear Blocking			
O Headache			
O Snoring			
O Nosebleeds			
O Eye Symptoms			

How many <u>years</u> have you suffered from the chief complaints of:

Head or Nose symptoms _____   Chest symptoms _____
Skin symptoms _____   Insect Sting reactions _____

Please indicate pattern of symptoms:

	Head / Nose	Chest
Year round, no seasonal change	_____	_____
Year round, worse seasonally	_____	_____
Seasonally only	_____	_____

If seasonal, list months: _____

Are your symptoms worse at night?   Yes O No O

Do you note increased symptoms from any of the following?

Allergens	Irritants	Ingestants	Weather
O Mown grass	O Perfumes	O Alcoholic Beverages	O Windy days
O Dead grass	O Soap	O Drugs	O Cold fronts
O Dead leaves	O Detergent	O Foods	O Temperature change
O Hay	O Cleaning agents	Other (list):	O Damp weather
O House dust	O Smoke	_____	
O Cats	O Paint	_____	
O Dogs	O Hair spray	_____	

Please check the ones that best describe your home:

O House (Age:_____)   O Apartment   O City   O Country
Do you have a basement?   O Yes   O No
Type of heating system: O Central   O Floor   O Electric   O Other: _____
Type of mattress: O Conventional   O Waterbed
Type of pillow: O Synthetic   O Down   Do you have stuffed animals?   O Yes O No
Do you have carpet in your home?   O Yes Type: _____   O No
Are your symptoms worse anywhere in your home?   O Yes Location:_____   O No
Do you have pets at home?   O Yes   What kind: _____   O No
Are your pets kept: O Inside   O Outside

Fig. 1. Screening for contributory factors.

Are your symptoms worse at your workplace / school? O Yes O No
Have your symptoms been so severe as to cause you to miss work or school? O Yes O No
       If so, how many days? _____
Has travel affected your symptoms? O Yes O No
Do you have hobbies that expose you to allergens or irritants? O Yes O No
       If yes, explain briefly: _____

List medicines you use for the relief of allergy symptoms (including nose drops or sprays):
_____
_____

List other drugs you take for any reason. (Include all over-the-counter drugs, creams, suppositories, eyedrops, etc.):
_____

Can you take aspirin? O Yes O No

Are you allergic to any medications? O Yes O No
       If yes, please list: _____
       What type of reaction occurs? _____

Have you ever taken hypo-sensitization shots (allergy shots) before? O Yes O No

Have you ever had a chest x-ray? O Yes O No If yes, when? _____
       Where? _____
Have you ever had a sinus x-ray? O Yes O No If yes, when? _____
       Where? _____
Do you smoke? O Yes O No
       If yes, how many packs per day? _____ How long? _____
Have you ever smoked? O Yes O No
       If yes, how many packs per day? _____ How long? _____
Does anyone you live with smoke? O Yes O No If yes, who? _____
Are you exposed to smoke at work or school? O Yes O No

Is there a history of any of the following in your family?
O Asthma   O Hay fever   O Nasal polyps   O Eczema   O Hives

If so, which family member? _____

Have you ever been treated in an emergency room? O Yes O No
       If yes, how many times? _____
       For what were you treated? _____
List all hospitalizations in order of most recent:
       Cause of Hospitalization   Age
       _____ _____
       _____ _____
       _____ _____
       _____ _____
       _____ _____

Circle any of the following that you might have had:
       Stomach ulcer   Diabetes   Glaucoma   High Blood Pressure
Circle any of the problems that you might have had with the following:
       Blood   Bones   Heart   Nervous system   Urinary tract
List any medical problems you have not noted above: _____

Fig. 1. *(continued)*

> The history is the most important element in the evaluation of allergy. Key features of the history are:
>
> - Worsening of symptoms on exposure to aeroallergens
> - Seasonal variation in symptoms related to pollination of trees, grasses, and weeds
> - A family history of atopic disease
> - An environmental history assessing exposure at workplace and home
> - The presence of associated allergic conditions

An allergy history seeks to define the patient's chief complaint(s) and focuses on the details concerning those complaints. If the chief complaint is narrow in scope, for instance, "I sneeze all the time," then the clinician may be tempted to direct the majority of the questions toward a given organ system. This approach should be avoided and the patient given ample opportunity to expound upon the extent of the complaint.

There is a lexicon common to patients with allergy complaints. Many state they have "sinus" or "hay fever." They describe a wide array of symptoms ranging from itchy nose, eyes, or palate to runny nose or postnasal drainage to nasal congestion. Sinus pressure and headache are frequently cited as symptoms. "Popping or fullness of the ears" implying eustachian tube dysfunction is an often-heard complaint. Asthma symptoms may be overt and present as wheezing, but descriptions may be more subtle such as cough, tightness in the chest, or inability to get a good breath or let all the air out of the lungs.

The history taker should be attuned to the patient's perspective as an (yet to be determined) allergy sufferer. Where and when do the symptoms occur? Do they interfere with daily activities, school or work, or exercise? Is there seasonal variation to the symptoms or are they of a perennial nature? Are the symptoms worse at a particular time of day? During sleep?

At first, questions searching for triggers should be open-ended. For instance, "What seems to trigger your symptoms?" rather than "Does this or that bother you?" If the patient is reticent or answers are not forthcoming, direct questions may be appropriate. In most cases, the patient will have a preference if symptoms are worse inside the house or outdoors.

Increasingly, indoor allergens are recognized as important triggers and sensitizers of the allergic patient. Type of home and the presence of a basement may be important. For example, a wet environment tends to promote growth of molds and dust mites. House dust mite is likely the most common allergen in our society. It is found in greatest abundance in bedding, pillows, carpet, and upholstered furniture. Therefore, kind of bedding and type of flooring may be relevant to understanding a given patient. Cockroach is another allergen increasingly implicated with public housing, inner city asthma, and allergic respiratory disorders. Particular attention should be given to any exposure to pets. Do the pets sleep in the bedroom or on the bed?

It is difficult to distinguish between an irritant and an allergen. Irritants are often misconstrued as allergens since they can cause the same cascade of symptoms.

Examples of irritants include cigaret smoke, perfume, cold air, strong odors, and cleaning solvents.

Outdoors, the allergic patient faces pollution (irritant) and pollens (allergens). Trees, grasses, and weeds can wreak havoc on an allergic sufferer. Likewise, different pollens may predominate in a particular region. For example, Bermuda grass may be prevalent in Florida but not Montana. Each allergen has its own season. One pollen season can overlap another; that is, grass pollination can coincide with pollination of ragweed. This is often important because one allergen can "prime" a person to have heightened sensitivity to another. Growing seasons may vary according to residential area. In summary, the history taker is always confronted with the puzzle of microcosm versus macrocosm. Although television pollen counts may report elm pollen, those same reports probably do not include what trees predominate outside a bedroom window or in a given neighborhood or in the courtyard where the patient takes a work break.

Occupational exposure must always be considered. If indicated, material safety data (MSD) information sheets may be requested to better overview what the patient may be in contact with. Day-care facilities can be an insidious source of recurrent viral and bacterial exposure for children.

Family history of an allergic diathesis should be sought. The genetics of allergy are not entirely understood, but each parent with atopy roughly doubles a patient's chance of being atopic; that is, risk of atopy is increased from 25% in the general population to about 75% when both parents are atopic. In one study, 90% of allergic asthmatic children had one or both parents who were atopic.

In asthma, objective measures such as spirometry and peak flow measurements paint only part of the picture. History should attempt to delineate the asthma as mild, moderate, or severe. Degree of severity will ultimately dictate choice and intensity of treatment. Emergency room visits or hospitalization for asthma in the past year or use of oral steroids in the last 6 mo identify the more severe asthmatic. Psychosocial problems, lower socioeconomic status, and history of previous intubation are potential risk factors for increased asthma morbidity and mortality.

Questions to determine the extent of asthma control include type and amount of inflammatory medication used, type of delivery system and quality of inhaler technique, frequency of respiratory symptoms and need for β-agonists, interference with daily activities or sleep, and diurnal peak flow variability if known. In some practices a quality-of-life survey is now employed to address subjective parameters that contribute to asthma severity.

Maskers and confounders of allergy must always be kept in mind. For instance, a history of recurrent use of antibiotics, frequent colds, or cough in a supine position may point to chronic sinusitis. Gastroesophageal reflux can present as cough and sometimes exacerbate asthma. Irritation of the skin presenting as pruritus or rash is frequently attributed to soaps that are too drying.

A good drug history is necessary. Frequent use of decongestant nasal spray can lead to rebound nasal congestion and rhinitis medicamentosa. Over-the-counter preparations (such as aspirin or nonsteroidal anti-inflammatory compounds, vitamins, and alternative remedies and herbal supplements), often not considered medication by the patient, may be causal factors in urticaria. Likewise, ace inhibitors and oral or ocular β-blockers may lead to cough or worsening of asthma.

> The physical examination may be entirely normal at the time of the examination, since allergy symptoms and signs are often evanescent. The examination should emphasize the organs involved with allergy symptoms.

PHYSICAL EXAMINATION

An allergic patient's history may direct the clinician's examination to a particular area or organ system. A specific allergic symptom, however, should not divert the examiner's attention from the patient as a whole. Each patient should be approached in a systematic way. Often, physical examination may not be unusual; lack of findings do not rule out allergy.

Vital signs are a starting point in any examination. Pulse rate and pulsus paradoxicus >10 mmHg are two of the most sensitive indicators of severe airways obstruction. Respiratory rate is important as well, but hyperventilation is more a reflection of minute ventilation (respiratory rate times tidal volume) than respiratory rate alone. Fever is an infrequent manifestation of allergy and points the differential elsewhere.

With the worldwide rise in the use of inhaled corticosteroids for the treatment of allergic respiratory disease, growth in children has been more closely scrutinized. Height and weight should be measured in children on a periodic, at least annual, basis. While growth in children may occur in spurts, change in growth velocity or decremental change in percentile should alert the physician to consider reasons for growth reduction with the knowledge that growth in atopic children is generally delayed.

Clues to allergic propensity are often seen in the patient's face. Discoloration of the infraorbital skin or "allergic shiners" may imply nasal congestion and subsequent lymph stasis. Extension of the mid-face or adenoid facies in children with adenoid hypertrophy, an infraorbital crease or so-called Dennie's line, and a transverse crease along the lower half of the nose are frequent but are not absolute indicators of underlying allergy.

The eye examination is concerned principally with the state of the tarsal (lower lids) or palpebral (upper lids) and bulbar conjunctivae. Degree of injection is noteworthy. In vernal conjunctivitis and giant papillary conjunctivitis, the superior palpebral conjunctivae show papillary hypertrophy or "cobblestoning" and may be accompanied by a stringy, fibrinous secretion. Trantas' dots, small white spots at the limbus, are sometimes seen in association with vernal conjunctivitis. Cataracts are found with increased incidence in atopic individuals; pingueculae are not.

Tympanic membranes should be visualized. Tympanosclerosis implies previous recurrent otitis and/or a history of myringotomy. If the light reflex is not well appreciated or history suggests eustachian tube dysfunction, then the tympanic membranes should be examined while the patient performs a Valsalva maneuver or with an insufflator to judge the functional patency of the eustachian tube. Sterile fluid behind the eardrum, a condition known as secretory otitis, is often seen.

The nose is best examined with an otoscope or head lamp with a nasal speculum or a fiberoptic rhinoscope. Special attention should be directed to the degree of congestion and color of the nasal turbinates. A blue tint strongly points toward allergic etiology. Also, the condition of the nasal septum must be ascertained, especially the presence of deviation, bowing, spurs, or perforation. The integrity of Kesselbach's plexus—the most common source of epistaxis—is often aggravated by intranasal steroids. The examiner should rule out nasal polyps, other masses, and discharge. Many times, it may be necessary to shrink the mucosa with topical decongestants, oxymetazoline, or dilute cocaine, to visualize the nasal passages adequately. Lastly, a history of anosmia calls for testing with various spices to assess function of the olfactory system.

The size and character of the tonsils should be noted. However, tonsils do not predict presence or hypertrophy of adenoids. The oropharynx should be scrutinized for drainage or raised islands of lymphoid tissue (lymphoid hyperplasia) often seen in smokers or profound atopics. Lastly, estimation of the depth and width of the pharynx may lead to suspicion of obstructive sleep apnea. For those patients taking inhaled corticosteroids, thrush on the tongue and soft palate should be excluded at each visit.

The neck must be palpated to search for adenopathy. At the same time, the thyroid gland should be assessed, as thyroid hormone imbalance can confound allergic symptoms. In patients with wheezing, the larynx should be auscultated to rule out stridor as an upper airway origin. Accessory muscle use of the sternocleidomastoid muscles should not be missed as it is another sign of marked airway obstruction.

Lung examination is particularly relevant in the asthmatic. Configuration of the chest wall should be noted; in particular, pectus excavatum, kyphosis, lordosis, and scoliosis should be ruled out by inspection. Restrictive airways disease must always be delineated from obstructive airways disease; intercostal retractions imply severe obstructive disease. Increased anterioposterior diameter may imply air trapping and hyperinflation. Wheezing should be listened for during basal breathing as well as on forced expiration, but absence of wheezing or a "silent chest" does not rule out bronchospasm. Extent of chest excursion and the inspiratory:expiratory ratio noted on presentation may represent important markers of change on serial examinations.

Lastly, the skin is commonly affected by allergy, although skin findings are often falsely attributed to allergic disorders. Xerosis is unrelated to allergy per se; however, individuals with atopic dermatitis have eczema and, in general, exceedingly dry skin. In addition, in subacute atopic dermatitis the skin may contain erythematous, scaling papules. In patients with chronic atopic dermatitis the skin is thickened with increased markings, known as lichenification. Both groups of patients may show signs of excoriation. Lesions of urticaria, or hives, are pruritic, raised, and erythematous, varying in size from pinpoint (cholinergic) to giant. They are protean: rounded or morbilliform or appearing as target lesions. Dermatographism, a transient wheal and flare reaction, occurs on scratching the skin. The lesions of angioedema are indurated and usually not as well demarcated as urticarial lesions.

ALLERGY TESTING

Skin testing is the most sensitive and cost-effective way to screen for existing allergic sensitivity. Biological extracts of aeroallergens including trees, weeds, dust mites, cockroaches, molds, and animal danders are available for testing (Fig. 2). The most accepted way to test is by placing a drop of antigen on the surface of the patient's skin and scratching or pricking the skin with a lancet or sharp plastic. If tests are not reactive, an intradermal 1:1000 dilution of the concentrate may be applied to rule out any minor sensitivity of a given antigen. Reactions are immediate, and scoring of the

ALLERGY & ASTHMA SPECIALISTS

ALLERGEN TESTING

Name:_____

Date:_____

_____MEDICATIONS   WHICH   MAY   AFFECT TESTING_____

Date of Birth:_____ Sex:_____

MEDICATION   DATE OF LAST DOSE

_____

Location of Test(s):_____

TREES	PRICK	ID
Boxelder – Maple		
Sycamore		
Hackberry		
Walnut		
Elm		
Oak Mix		
Pecan		
Willow		
Ash		
Beech		
Cottonwood		
Birch Mix		
Cedar, Mountain		
Pine Mix		

GRASS	PRICK	ID
** Bermuda		
* Rye		
Johnson		
* Timothy		
Bahia		
* Kentucky Blue		
* Redtop		
* Orchard		
* Meadow Fescue		
* Sweet Vernal		

*   STANDARDIZED - 100,000 BAU/ML
** STANDARDIZED - 10,000 BAU/ML

COMMENTS_____

WEEDS	PRICK	ID
Ragweed Mix		
English Plantain		
Russian Thistle		
Lambs Quarter		
Careless-Pigweed		
Marshelder-Poverty		
Dock, Sorrel		
Cocklebur		
Mugwort		

MOLDS	PRICK	ID
Alternaria		
Hormodendrum		
Helminthosporium		
Aspergillus Fumigatus		
Rhizopus		
Aspergillus Niger		
Fusarium		
Penicillium Notatum		

ENVIRONMENTALS	PRICK	ID
Dust Mite F.		
Dust Mite P.		
Cockroach		
Cat 1 (Hair)		
Cat 2 (Pelt)		
Dog		
Feathers		

Control – Positive – Histamine_____
Control – Negative_____

PRICKS_____ TIME_____
I.D.s _____ TIME_____
TIME_____
EMPLOYEE INITIALS _____

EXTRACTS - BAYER, INC.
HISTAMINE - CENTER LAB

TREES: GRASSES: WEEDS - 1:20
MOLDS: COCKROACH: DOG - 1:10
DUST MITE F.: DUST MITE P.: - 10,000 AU/ML
CAT (HAIR): CAT (PELT) - 10,000 BAU/Ml

Fig. 2. Allergen testing.

> The most important ancillary test to confirm the diagnosis of allergy is the skin test, which is the "gold standard" in this regard. The skin test results must be interpreted in light of the history to determine the importance of a positive test.

tests, based on size of the wheal and flare of a given test, is done in 15 min. Negative (saline) and positive (histamine) controls are placed at the same time, the latter to ensure that antihistamines are not present and blocking reactions.

Age and chief complaint will usually determine the number of tests applied. For instance, a child less than 4 yr (not a candidate for immunotherapy) would likely receive only a few skin tests (including dust mite and relevant animal danders) to see if he or she might be able to avoid or minimize exposure to an antigen.

Other types of testing are also available. Food testing (prick testing only) is infrequently indicated. Except for penicillin testing, skin testing to drugs is not well understood. This testing is usually done in a hospital setting when acceptable substitutes for penicillin cannot be found. Patients may also be skin tested to hymenoptera, or stinging insect, venom, to determine if anaphylactoid reactions are IgE mediated.

No matter how strong a history suggests allergy, testing must be done to confirm atopy. An important caveat is that a positive skin test does not prove that allergy is causing the patient's symptoms. A positive skin test must be correlated with the history to postulate cause and effect.

DIAGNOSTIC STUDIES

There are few blood abnormalities found in an allergic patient. Eosinophils are often associated with allergy, but are rarely increased in allergic rhinitis. More commonly, eosinophils are a peripheral marker of inflammation in nonallergic as well as allergic asthma. Eosinophils can be measured by means of a complete blood count or total eosinophil count. The number is considered abnormal if it is greater than 7% of the total white blood count or greater than $350/mm^3$.

Nasal smears may be helpful in distinguishing infectious process in the nose from an eosinophilic process. Predominance of segmented neutrophils implies underlying bacterial infection, >10 eosinophils/high power field as assessed by Wright's stain are frequent in allergic rhinitis. However, as in peripheral smears, eosinophils are not specific for allergy; they can also be seen in patients with nonallergic rhinitis with eosinophils (NARES).

IgE is the antibody that accounts for allergic reactions. IgE is measured in international units (1 IU = 2.4 ng IgE). Umbilical cord levels >1.0 IU are a good predictor of whether a newborn will develop allergic disease. Similarly, serum IgE levels greater than 20 IU/ml in infants predict allergic disease. On the other hand, total serum IgE is rarely helpful in children or adults, as roughly only 75% of atopic individuals have IgE levels greater than 100U/ml. Total IgE is useful in the diagnosis and treatment of ABPA. It is also elevated in active atopic dermatitis.

In vitro tests for specific IgE antibodies include the radioallergosorbent test (RAST) and other enzyme-linked immunosorbent assays. These tests are more expensive and less sensitive than skin tests. A disadvantage over skin tests is that their results are not immediately available to the clinician. Therefore, they are usually reserved for those patients with bad eczema or marked dermatographism that prohibits skin tests, patients who cannot forgo medications that block skin testing, or patients with a history of profound anaphylaxis when skin testing might be dangerous. These tests are usually scored on a class 0 (negative)–class 6 (highly positive) scale with 0–2 scores being considered indeterminant.

Sinusitis is one of the most underdiagnosed conditions in the patient suspected of allergy. In fact, allergy and sinusitis are often concomitants. Radiographic imaging may be useful in establishing the presence or absence of sinus infection. A simple screening Waters' view of the sinuses visualizes the maxillary and frontal sinuses fairly well. A Waters' view is inexpensive, but does not visualize the ethmoid and sphenoid sinuses with any certainty. Computed tomography is considered the gold standard for seeing all of the paranasal sinuses. Cost and x-ray exposure can be minimized with a limited scan, but this sometimes does not detect the patency of the osteomeatal complex.

CONFERENCE

Approach to the allergy patient has its culmination in the discussion of the findings with the patient. Effort should be made to express optimism that allergic conditions are almost always reversible and controllable. There is much myth and misconception among the general population concerning allergy. Adequate time should be allotted to explain in simple language the findings, plan, and prognosis for the patient.

Treatment of the allergic patient has three arms: avoidance of offending allergens, medication, and, when indicated, immunotherapy.

All medications and, in particular, inhalers should be explained. Terminology such as "opener" or "controller or healer" may help the patient accept and understand the difference between and need for bronchodilators and anti-inflammatory agents. Delivery systems for use in the nose and lungs must be demonstrated, and, in turn, the patient's technique observed. Side effects of drugs as well as risks and benefits to each treatment option, should be explained in simple terms.

It is fundamental and imperative that a patient understand the premise of the treatment plan before accepting and adhering to avoidance steps and medication regimens. Thus, there should be no shortcuts on education concerning the patient's condition or treatment plan. Questions should be welcomed, and an open foundation of dialogue between patient and clinician/staff established. The patient should leave the office comfortable that the clinician and staff are willing partners in his or her care.

SUGGESTED READING

Cockroft DW, Swystun VA. Asthma control versus asthma severity. *J Allergy Clin Immunol* 1996;98: 1016–1018.

Connell JT. Quantitative intranasal pollen challenge: II. Effect of daily pollen challenge, environmental pollen exposure, and placebo challenge on the nasal membrane. *J Allergy* 1968;41:123.

Demoly P, Michel FB, Bousquet J. In vivo methods for study of allergy skin tests, techniques, and interpretation. *In:* Middleton E, Reed CE, Ellis EF, et al, eds. *Allergy Principles and Practice*, 5th ed., 1998, St. Louis: Mosby, pp. 430–439.

Global Initiative for Asthma. National Heart, Lung, and Blood Institute, World Health Organization Workshop Reports. 1995. Bethesda, MD; National Institutes of Health. Publication No. 95-3659, pp. 1–76.

Platts-Mills TAE, et al. Indoor allergens and asthma: Report of the Third International Workshop. *J Allergy Clin Immunol* 1997;100:S1–S24.

Tovey E, Marks G. Methods and effectiveness of environmental control. *J Allergy Clin Immunol* 1999;103:179–191.

Van Cauwenberge PB, Ingels KJAO. Rhinitis: The spectrum of the disease. *In:* Busse WW, Holgate ST, eds. Asthma and Rhinitis, 1995, Skokie, IL: Rand McNally, pp. 7–12.

3 Diagnostic Tests in Allergy

Dennis R. Ownby, MD

INTRODUCTION

Many physicians have the mistaken impression that allergic diseases are diagnosed by allergy tests. Allergic diseases can be diagnosed only from the patient's history of symptoms and compatible physical findings. If the symptoms are typical of allergic disease and repeatedly associated with allergen exposure, a diagnosis of allergy is highly probable. A common clinical example is a patient who states that every time he or she is around cats, red, itchy eyes, sneezing, and nasal congestion develop. These typical allergic symptoms when associated with exposure to cats suggest that the patient is cat allergic. Two other important factors are the number of times the symptoms have been associated with allergen exposure and whether similar symptoms occur without allergen exposure. If the symptoms are exclusively related to cat exposure and have occurred on multiple occasions, the diagnosis is relatively certain. Finding superficial conjunctivitis, nasal congestion, and rhinitis on examination would help confirm the history. The final step for confirming a diagnosis of cat allergy would be to demonstrate that the patient has cat-specific IgE antibodies.

To further clarify the role of allergy tests in allergy diagnosis, it is useful to define a "gold standard" for diagnosis (see Table 1). The critical elements of the gold standard are demonstration that exposure to the allergen under double-blind, placebo-controlled conditions reproduces suspected symptoms. It is also necessary to demonstrate that the symptoms are the result of IgE-mediated release of mediators from mast cells or basophils. This stringent definition of allergic disease is rarely met, even in research studies, because of the difficulties of performing allergen challenges and measuring mediator release.

From: *Current Clinical Practice: Allergic Diseases: Diagnosis and Treatment, 2nd Edition*
Edited by: P. Lieberman and J. Anderson © Humana Press Inc., Totowa, NJ

Table 1
Criteria for Diagnosis of Allergic Disease

Absolute Criteria (The Gold Standard)
1. Reproducible symptoms occurring during double-blind, placebo-controlled, allergen exposure when the route, dose, and duration of allergen exposure are consistent with estimated or measured natural or occupational exposure.
2. The observed symptoms must be the direct result of the release of chemical mediators when the release of the mediators is triggered by the binding of IgE antibodies to the allergen.

Clinical Criteria
1. A history of signs and symptoms typical of allergic disease at a time and place when allergen exposure is probably occurring.
2. Demonstration that the patient has IgE antibodies specific for the allergen associated with the occurrence of symptoms.

Because of the difficulty in trying to satisfy the criteria of the gold standard, clinical criteria are usually accepted for diagnosis. Clinical criteria include a history of recurrent symptoms of allergic disease when allergen exposure is likely to be occurring and demonstration of corresponding allergen-specific IgE antibodies (Table 1). The application of clinical criteria must always be made in light of the potential risks and benefits of a diagnosis for the patient. Thus, allergy tests are only adjuncts to the clinical diagnosis of allergic disease.

Individuals with allergen-specific IgE antibodies may be asymptomatic. In fact, two studies of large, relatively unselected populations have shown that more than 90% of persons with IgE antibodies to stinging insect venoms have no history of allergic reactions from insect stings. It is important to remember that tests for allergen-specific IgE antibody, whether skin tests or in vitro tests, have little clinical value until they are interpreted within the context of the patient's history.

SKIN TESTING FOR DETECTION OF ALLERGEN-SPECIFIC IgE

Physiology of Skin Tests

Skin tests are performed by introducing a small quantity of allergen into the epidermis by pricking, puncturing, or scratching the skin or by intradermal injection. This is usually accomplished using a suitable concentration of an allergen extract. An allergen extract is an aqueous extract or solution of the allergen in question. Occasionally some materials may be used directly for testing, e.g., the fresh juice of fruit. The immediate wheal and flare response resulting from a skin test is the result of a complex series of interactions. After the allergen has been introduced into the skin, it diffuses through the skin where it may bind to IgE antibodies affixed to mast cells. When an allergen can crosslink two or more mast-cell–bound IgE antibodies, mediator release is initiated. Released mediators include preformed (histamine, tryptase, chymase, heparin) and newly synthesized (prostaglandins, leukotrienes, cytokines) cell products.

The central wheal of the skin response is princiflly due to histamine-induced vasopermeability and secondary edema. The central erythema results from histamine-induced arteriolar vasodilation, and the circumferential erythema results from the

---

Allergen Skin Testing Precautions

- The individual to be tested must be off usual conventional antihistamines for 24 h, loratadine and fexofenadine for 2–5 d, hydroxyzine and cetirizine for 5–7 d, and astemizole for 6–12 wk[a,b].
- Tricyclic antidepressant drugs often have profound "antihistamine effects" and usually preclude allergy skin testing.[a,b]
- Use of β-blocker drugs (e.g., for hypertension or migraine headache) increases the risk of a serious reaction if a reaction to an allergy skin test occurs.[a]
- Allergy skin testing should not be performed when the patient is acutely ill, including an acute asthma attack or with generalized skin rash.[a]

[a]Alternative in vitro IgE allergen-specific skin testing should be considered.
[b]Histime skin testing may be necessary prior to Allergen skin testing in questionable situations.

---

stimulation of nerve receptors and resulting axon reflex vasodilation. The wheal and flare responses are typically maximal at 15 min after introduction of the allergen. Most of the skin response can be blocked by an H_1 receptor antagonist (antihistamine), but complete inhibition requires both H_1 and H_2 antagonists.

Following the immediate skin response, and depending upon the dose of allergen and the sensitivity of the patient, there may be a late-phase reaction (LPR). These usually begin at 3–5 h, peak at 6–12 h, and resolve approximately 24 h, after the immediate response. Clinically, LPRs are characterized by pruritus and edema, often larger than the immediate reaction. Pathologically, LPRs are characterized by local infiltration of inflammatory cells, including neutrophils, monocytes, and eosinophils, into the involved site. Fibrin deposition also occurs. LPRs may follow immediate skin testing, especially if large reactions have occurred. Large local reactions following administration of allergen immunotherapy injections may also be LPRs.

Evaluation Prior to Skin Testing

Before skin testing is done, a patient must be examined by an experienced physician. Beyond establishing the likelihood of allergic disease, a patient's history and physical examination should alert the physician to any unusual risks of skin testing. Skin testing is generally safe, but there is always a small risk of inducing a systemic allergic reaction (anaphylaxis) that could be life threatening. Anything that might increase the risk of skin testing for a patient must be evaluated before skin testing is undertaken. A physician and emergency equipment for treatment of anaphylaxis must always be immediately available when a patients is skin tested. Since epinephrine is the drug of choice for treatment of major allergic reactions, drugs altering the response to epinephrine, such as β-blocking agents, should be discontinued prior to skin testing. Pregnancy is a relative contraindication to skin testing, because the fetus in utero may be highly vulnerable to hypoxia resulting from a systemic reaction in the mother. Patients with chronic medical problems, such as severe lung disease or unstable angina, should not normally be skin tested. Finally, patients with current, severe, allergic symptoms, especially unstable asthma, should not be skin tested until after their symptoms have been stabilized, because of a greater risk of systemic reactions.

In addition to general medical concerns, the physician supervising skin tests must be sure that the patient has an area of normal skin suitable for skin testing. Patients must not be taking antihistamines or drugs with antihistamine actions, such as tricyclic antidepressants, because these agents can block skin test responses. Patients with severe skin disease or with marked dermatographism cannot be reliably tested. Both the very young and the very old have less reactive skin, and criteria for grading skin test reactions need to be adjusted in these individuals. Following viral exanthems or sunburns the skin may not be normally reactive for several weeks, and skin testing should be postponed.

Epicutaneous Skin Tests

Percutaneous or epicutaneous tests may be performed using a variety of methods, but the most common are the prick and puncture techniques. The prick test is performed on previously cleansed skin by passing a small needle (e.g., 25- or 26-gage) through a drop of allergen extract at approximately a 45° angle to the surface of the skin. The needle is lightly pressed into the epidermis, and its tip lifted up, producing a pricking sensation. The skin pricks should not be deep enough to produce visible bleeding.

Another epicutaneous method is the puncture technique. A drop of allergen extract is placed on cleansed skin. A puncture device is then pushed into the skin through the drop of extract. Commonly used puncture devices are constructed to allow a small point to penetrate 1–1.5 mm into the skin. Further penetration is prevented by the instrument's shape. The bifurcated needle, originally designed for smallpox vaccination, can also be used for puncture testing; it is pressed firmly against the skin, through a drop of extract, and rocked back and forth or side to side.

A single needle or puncture device can be used for multiple-prick skin tests on the same patient, if all residual extract is cleaned from the needle between each drop of extract. Adequate cleaning can usually be accomplished by briefly swirling the device in a container of alcohol and wiping between tests. This method is falling out of favor because of the risk of puncture injuries to the person performing the tests. An alternative procedure is to use a new device to apply each test. After the tests on a patient are completed, the device(s) should be disposed of properly. Tests can be applied to any area of normal skin, but the most commonly used sites are the back, volar forearms, and top of the thighs. Each test should be placed a minimum of 4 cm or more from other tests, and care should be taken to avoid smearing or mixing of the extracts. Tests placed too close together may interact, leading to false-positive reactions.

Intradermal Tests

Intradermal tests are more sensitive than prick or puncture tests, but they are more difficult to perform properly. Intradermal tests are typically performed with 25-, 26-, or 27-gage needles. Some manufacturers provide needles with special intradermal bevels that help limit the depth of needle penetration. After drawing the allergen extract into the syringe, the tip of the needle is inserted into the superficial dermis and approximately

Type of Allergen Skin Testing in Different Conditions		
	Type of skin test	
Condition	E^a	ID^b
Allergic rhinitis and asthma	x	x
Food allergy	x	Not done
Penicillin allergy	x	x
Insect venom allergy	Not done	x (serial)
Latex allergy	Not validated (use in vitro test)	

[a]Epicutaneous: prick, scratch, puncture.
[b]Intradermal.

0.02–0.05 mL of extract is injected. If the injection is performed properly, a distinct bleb, 2–3 mm in diameter, will be produced. Extracts used for intradermal testing are normally diluted 1000-fold more than extracts used for epicutaneous tests. As with prick or puncture tests, intradermal tests should be placed at least 6 cm apart to prevent interactions leading to false-positive results.

The most common errors with intradermal tests are injecting too deeply, injecting too large a volume, and inducing excess bleeding. If extract is injected too deeply, little or no reaction will be visible on the surface of the skin. Injecting too large a volume may lead to false-positive reactions because of irritation, and a large volume increases the risk of a systemic reaction. Bleeding at the injection site may also cause false-positive reactions. Because of the risks, technical difficulties, and problems of interpretation, intradermal testing is usually best left to a specialist.

Positive and Negative Controls for Skin Testing

Because of the many variables present during skin testing, positive and negative controls must be included to allow accurate interpretation of test results, regardless whether the prick, puncture, or intradermal techniques are used. The negative control is either normal saline or the same buffer that has been used to dilute the allergen extracts. The negative control must be applied in the same fashion as in all of the other tests. There is a tendency to apply the negative control more lightly, since it is expected to be negative, thus diminishing its value.

Positive controls for skin testing are usually either histamine or a mast cell secretagogue, such as codeine. For epicutaneous tests, histamine is usually used at a concentration of 1 mg/mL, although a concentration of 10 mg/mL also has been recommended because some normal individuals do not respond to the 1 mg/mL concentration. For intradermal testing, histamine is most often used at a concentration of 0.01 mg/mL.

Recording and Scoring Skin Test Results

Skin test reactions to allergens are normally evaluated at 15 min after the tests are placed, when the reactions are typically maximal. Despite many years of use and many investigations, there is still great variation in the scoring and recording of skin test results. The most commonly used system grades both epicutaneous and intradermal tests on a 5-point scale in which 0 is a negative test and increasing degrees of reaction are graded from 1+ to 4+, according to the size of both the wheal and flare reactions. An alternative is to measure the diameters of the wheal and flare reactions in millimeters and to record these diameters. The advantage of measurements is that they can be evaluated by another physician or re-evaluated at a later time. In terms of patient management, the actual size or grade of the skin test reaction is less important than the physician's criteria for determining whether the test is positive or negative. Most allergists consider an epicutaneous test positive when the wheal of the test is 3 mm larger than the wheal produced by the negative control and the wheal is surrounded by an area of erythema clearly larger than the wheal. Similarly, a positive intradermal test should have a wheal at least 5–6 mm larger than that of the negative control with surrounding flare of 20 mm or more.

Quality Control of Skin Testing

As with all diagnostic tests, persons supervising and performing skin tests should observe certain standards and quality controls. Quality control of skin testing should include making sure that: the person performing the tests understands the testing procedure, the interoperator and intraoperator reproducibility is acceptable, the procedures are consistent, the extract quality is maintained, and the results are consistently recorded. The person performing the tests must be technically proficient in applying the tests and also understand factors that may affect the results of the tests, such as interfering drugs and skin abnormalities. Allergen extracts used for testing must be properly stored and discarded when their expiration date is reached.

Value of Epicutaneous vs Intradermal Skin Tests

Epicutaneous tests are adequate for most diagnostic work in allergy, but in some circumstances the higher sensitivity of intradermal tests is required, especially when dealing with those allergens associated with a high risk of death if sensitivity is missed, as with penicillin or hymenoptera allergy. The increased sensitivity of intradermal tests comes at the expense of an increased risk of false-positive results and an increased risk of inducing anaphylaxis. Considering these risks, intradermal testing is best left to an allergy specialist.

MEASUREMENT OF ALLERGEN-SPECIFIC IgE

Basic Methods

Most available assays for allergen-specific IgE antibodies utilize the principle of immunoabsorption illustrated in Fig. 1. The allergen of interest is first bound to a solid phase support such as a paper disk, plastic microtiter well, or cellulose sponge. The patient's serum is then incubated with the solid phase. If the patient has antibodies specific for the allergen, the antibodies will become bound to the allergen, and the remaining serum proteins, including unbound antibodies, can be washed away from the solid phase (this is immunoabsorption and separation). After washing, a labeled antihuman IgE antibody is incubated with the solid phase to allow binding of the anti-IgE to any IgE bound to the solid phase. After unbound anti-IgE is washed away, the quantity of anti-IgE bound to the solid phase is measured and converted either to units of specific IgE or to a class score. The initial test for IgE antibodies used radiolabeled

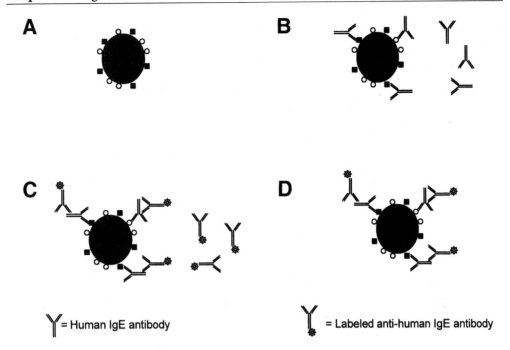

A

B

C

D

Y = Human IgE antibody   Y = Labeled anti-human IgE antibody

Fig. 1. Schematic presentation of an immunosorbent assay for allergen-specific IgE antibody. **(A)** Allergen represented by small circles and squares has been bound to solid phase. **(B)** Serum that may contain IgE antibodies specific for the allergen is incubated with the solid phase. Specific antibodies bind to the allergen, and nonbound antibodies are removed by washing. **(C)** Labeled antihuman IgE antibody is incubated with the solid phase, and the anti-IgE antibody binds to the immobilized IgE. Nonbound anti-IgE is washed away. **(D)** The amount of anti-IgE antibody on the solid phase is proportional to the concentration of allergen-specific IgE in the serum tested.

anti-IgE antibodies and was called the *radio allergo sorbent test* or RAST. Because of its initial market dominance the term RAST is often used as a generic term to mean any test for allergen-specific IgE antibodies. In recent years, other methods have become more widely available. The major modification in newer assays is the use of enzyme labels in place of radiolabels. Thus, newer assays are most commonly enzyme-linked immunosorbert assays (ELISA), although the term RAST is still commonly used. Both radiolabeled and enzyme-labeled assays are capable of detecting specific IgE at concentrations of nanograms per milliliter of serum.

Reporting Results of In Vitro Tests

Currently, there is no universally agreed upon standard for reporting the results of tests for allergen-specific IgE antibodies. The most commonly used method is class scores, usually ranging from 0 to 4–6. Class 0 indicated undetectable IgE, whereas classes 1–4 or 6 represented increasing quantities of IgE. Some laboratories also report a class 0/1 or indeterminate class. While some physicians would like to interpret this indeterminate class as a very weak positive, the correct interpretation is that samples in this class have an equal probability of being positive or negative and should therefore not be considered positive.

Many laboratories report results using what is known as modified RAST scoring. The modified scoring system produces an apparent increase in the sensitivity of the test

Table 2
Comparative Advantages of Skin Tests and In Vitro Tests in Allergy Diagnosis

Advantages of Skin Tests	Advantages of In Vitro Tests
Highest sensitivity	No risk of anaphylaxis
Results available in minutes	Medications do not affect results
Greater selection of allergens for testing	Not dependent upon skin condition
Less personnel and reagent expense per test	Better documentation of quality control
Minimal equipment required	May be more convenient for patients
Patient can see and feel the results of the test	Perceived as being more scientific

by reducing the level of reaction needed to call a test positive. This apparent increase in sensitivity comes at the expense of specificity, since only the scoring system and not the actual detection limit of the assay has been changed.

Some modern assays are calibrated in terms of actual mass units of IgE, i.e., nanograms or units of IgE per serum volume. The use of mass units allows a direct comparison of IgE levels between individuals or in the same individual over time. Calibration in mass units may also provide useful clinical information in some circumstances.

When one is interpreting the results of in vitro assays, it is important to remember that the sensitivity and specificity of an in vitro test can vary markedly from one allergen to another. While in vitro assays typically have sensitivities of 70–80% when compared to skin tests, much lower sensitivities are found with some allergens. It is important to remember that a test with a sensitivity of 75% will fail to detect 25% of truly sensitive individuals.

Advantages and Disadvantages of In Vitro and In Vivo Tests

Depending upon the clinical situation, either skin tests or in vitro tests may be used to detect allergen specific IgE. As listed in Table 2, there are certain advantages of each testing method. The most important advantage of skin testing is the high degree of sensitivity. When an intradermal skin test is properly performed, the risk of failing to detect allergic sensitization is extremely low. This degree of sensitivity is very important when the risk of failing to detect specific IgE may lead to the patient's death. While not as sensitive as intradermal tests, epicutaneous tests are very sensitive when properly performed with potent allergen extracts.

The most important advantage of in vitro tests is their safety. If an individual has had a life-threatening reaction to an allergen, an in vitro test offers the possibility of detecting specific IgE without the risk of inducing an allergic reaction in the patient. The patient should understand that if the in vitro test is positive and consistent with the patient's history, the diagnosis is relatively assured, but a negative in vitro test does not adequately exclude the possibility of sensitivity. In the face of a suggestive history and a negative in vitro test, the patient should still be skin tested before a final clinical judgment is made.

In routine allergy practice, skin testing has been found to be more cost-effective than in vitro testing. The cost-effectiveness is more pronounced as multiple allergens are tested. There are also advantages to the patient's being able to see the immediate

Table 3
Total Serum IgE Levels in Skin-Test–Negative Children and Adults

Age (yr)	N	Sex	Geometric Mean[a]	Mean + 2 s.d.[a]
6–14	69	M	40.9	2.0–824.1
	71	F	40.7	3.4–452.9
15–34	213	M	23.3	0.9–635.3
	201	F	16.5	0.8–349.1
35–54	145	M	20.4	0.9–443.6
	154	F	14.6	0.7–286.4
55–74	224	M	19.8	0.8–484.2
	348	F	10.7	0.6–198.6
75+	61	M	17.8	0.8–387.3
	83	F	8.9	0.4–208.9

From Klink M, Cline MG, Halonen M, et al: *J Allergy Clin Immunol* 1990;85:440.
[a]All values are International Units per milliliter.

allergic reaction on his or her skin and to having immediately available results. In comparison, in vitro tests offer the ability to test patients who do not have normal skin or who cannot discontinue certain medicaions. It may also be more convenient for both the patient and the physician to send blood samples to a reference laboratory for testing rather than for the patient to travel to another location, especially when testing is needed only for one or two allergens.

TOTAL SERUM IgE

Test Methods

Although a variety of assays have been used to measure the small concentrations of IgE normally present in human serum, the most frequently used method is a two-site immunometric assay using two different antihuman IgE antibodies. These assays are conceptually similar to the assays used for detection of allergen-specific IgE. The first antihuman IgE antibody is attached to a solid phase such as a plastic well in a microtiter plate. An appropriate dilution of the serum to be tested is then incubated with the solid-phase. IgE in the serum becomes bound to the solid-phase anti-IgE in proportion to the concentration of IgE in the serum sample. After unbound proteins are washed away, the quantity of IgE bound to the solid phase is determined by reacting the solid phase with the second, soluble, labeled anti-IgE antibody. After another wash to remove the unbound, labeled anti-IgE, the quantity of labeled IgE on the solid phase is measured and converted into units of IgE by comparison to a standard curve. A variety of commercial assays is available. Most are accurate to a concentration of less than 5 IU/mL (12 ng/mL) of IgE and reproducible within 10–15%.

Serum concentrations of IgE vary widely in normal individuals (Table 3). IgE levels are very low at birth and gradually increase, peaking in the second decade of life, and followed by a slow decline into old age. While the geometric mean values are relatively low, there is a very large 95% confidence interval at all ages (Table 3). Most laboratories report IgE concentrations as international units (IU) or nanograms (ng) per milliliter. 1 IU = 2.4 ng IgE. The Système International (SI) specifies that IgE be reported as micrograms per liter (μg/L) with two significant digits ($XX \times 10^n$). Values in IU/mL can be converted to μg/L by multiplying by 2.4.

Relationship of Total IgE to Allergic Disease

Many studies have shown that total serum IgE concentrations are higher in allergic adults and children when compared to nonallergic individuals of similar ages. There is, however, a relatively large overlap between serum IgE concentrations in allergic and nonallergic individuals, limiting the diagnostic value of total IgE measurements. When a high value of IgE is chosen to distinguish allergic from nonallergic individuals, the specificity of the test is often over 90% but the sensitivity is low at 30–50%. Lowering the threshold level increases the sensitivity but lowers the specificity. For adults, the optimal IgE concentration for distinguishing allergic from nonallergic individuals is approximately 100 IU/mL, while in children the threshold level varies with age.

Even though measurements of total serum IgE concentrations are not generally useful for diagnosis of allergic disease, total serum IgE measurements are valuable in the diagnosis and management of allergic fungal sinusitis (AFS) and allergic bronchopulmonary aspergillosis (ABPA). (The term *mycosis* is probably more appropriate than *aspergillosis* since organisms other than aspergillius may be responsible). Patients with ABPA and AFS typically have serum IgE levels greater than 500 IU/mL, often more than 1000 IU/mL. With adequate glucocorticoid therapy, total serum IgE levels fall. A sudden increase in serum IgE may herald disease exacerbation and allow time to alter therapy before symptoms increase or more lung damage occurs.

There are other conditions in which total serum levels of IgE may be abnormal. Among the more common nonallergic causes of elevated serum IgE are metazoan parasitic infections, smoking, and AIDS. IgE is grossly elevated in the rare cases of IgE myelomas that have been reported, but the levels of IgE may still be too low to be detected as a monoclonal spike on serum protein electrophoresis. IgE measurements are valuable in the evaluation of myelomas because IgE myelomas may be mistaken for light chain disease. The distinction between light chain disease and IgE myeloma is clinically important because the courses and responses to treatment differ. IgE is also elevated in patients with the hyper-IgE recurrent infection syndrome.

THE FUTURE OF ALLERGY TESTING

Currently, most allergy testing concentrates on IgE measurements, but some assays for the direct measurement of mediators are available, and more are likely to become clinically relevant. Histamine can be measured during or after allergic reactions, but because it is difficult to collect proper specimens, histamine measurements are usually limited to research studies. Eosinophil cationic protein (ECP) can be measured in sputum or serum and correlates with the activation of eosinophils. ECP may be useful for monitoring anti-inflammatory asthma therapy. Mast cell tryptase is elevated following massive release of mast cell mediators as during anaphylactic reactions. Tryptase levels usually peak 45–60 min after the onset of anaphylaxis and may remain elevated for several hours. Elevated tryptase measurements help document that a reaction resulted from mast cell mediator release. This distinction can be important during diagnostic evaluations and when counseling a patient about future risks. For as yet unknown reasons, tryptase does not appear to be increased during fatal or near-fatal anaphylactic reactions from foods in children. In the future, assays for histamine-releasing factor and other mediators may make the diagnosis of allergic disease easier and more precise.

SUGGESTED READING

Allergen skin testing. Position Statement. *J Allergy Clin Immunol* 1993;92:636–637.

Bernstein IL. The proceedings of the task force on guidelines for standardizing old and new technologies used for the diagnosis and treatment of allergic diseases. *J Allergy Clin Immunol* 1988;82:487–526.

Droste JHJ, Kerkhof M, de Monchy JGR, et al. Association of skin test reactivity, specific IgE, total IgE, and eosinophils with nasal symptoms in a community-based population study. *J Allergy Clin Immunol* 1996;97:922–932.

Gleeson M, Cripps AW, Hensley MJ. A clinical evaluation in children of the Pharmacia ImmunoCAP system for inhalant allergens. *Clin Exp Allergy* 1996;26:697–702.

Klink M, Cline MG, Halonen M, et al. Problems in defining normal limits for serum IgE. *J Allergy Clin Immunol* 1990;85:440–444.

Kristjánsson S, Shimizu T, Strannegård IL, Wennergren G. Eosinophil cationic protein, myeloperoxidase and tryptase in children with asthma and atopic dermatitis. *Pediatr Allergy Immunol* 1994;5:223–229.

Nelson HS, Rosloniec DM, McCAll LI, Ikle D. Comparative performance of five commercial prick skin test devices. *J Allergy Clin Immunol* 1993;92:750–756.

Reid MJ, Lockey RF, Turkeltaub, PC, et al. Survey of fatalities from skin testing and immunotherapy 1985–1989. *J Allergy Clin Immunol* 1993;79:6–15.

Schwartz J, Weiss ST. Relationship of skin test reactivity to decrements in pulmonary function in children with asthma or frequent wheezing. *Am J Respir Crit Care Med* 1995;152:2176–2180.

Sampson HA, Ho DG. Relationship between food-specific IgE concentrations and the risk of positive food challenges in children and adolescents. *J Allergy Clin Immunol* 1997;100:444–451.

Williams PB, Dolen WK, Koepke JW, et al. Immunoassay of specific IgE: Use of a single point calibration curve in the modified radioallergosorbent test. *Ann Allergy* 1992;69:48–52.

4 Environmental Allergens

Scott H. Sicherer, MD
and Peyton A. Eggleston, MD

CONTENTS

INTRODUCTION

Allergens are low-molecular-weight proteins capable of inducing IgE antibody and triggering an allergic response. For those with an atopic predisposition, exposure to these environmental allergens causes not only the immunological sensitization required for the development of atopic disease but also the provocation of acute symptoms and the maintenance of chronic symptoms. Several allergenic proteins usually are derived from any specific allergenic source (e.g., several proteins derived from grass pollen are allergenic). When a particular protein is recognized by IgE antibody from more than half of individuals allergic to the source, it is termed a major allergen. The major allergens are named with the first three letters of the genus and then the first letter of the species name followed by a group designation. Examples include Amb a 1 (*Ambrosia artemisiifolia*—ragweed), Lol p 1 (*Lolium perenne*—ryegrass); and Fel d 1 (*Felis domesticus*—domestic cat). For many allergenic proteins, DNA sequences are known and allergenic epitopes—sites on the protein binding IgE antibody and/or T cell receptors—have been delineated. It has become evident that allergic sensitization to particular proteins is not only related to environmental exposure but also, in part, dependent upon individual human leukocyte antigen (HLA) molecules that play a role in processing these allergens and presenting them to the immune system.

In our outdoor and indoor milieu, these allergenic proteins (along with a larger number of nonallergenic proteins) are carried on vectors, such as pollen grains or housedust particles, which may become airborne. Although there are many allergenic proteins on a variety of vectors in the environment, an understanding of just a few classes of the major outdoor allergens that cause seasonal symptoms and indoor

From: *Current Clinical Practice: Allergic Diseases: Diagnosis and Treatment, 2nd Edition*
Edited by: P. Lieberman and J. Anderson © Humana Press Inc., Totowa, NJ

Environmental Allergen Exposure

Intermittently, outdoors
- Seasonal plant pollens
- Mold spores

Continuously, in the house
- House dust mites
- Cats, dogs, birds, small animals
- Mold spores
- Cockroach

---

allergens responsible for perennial symptoms furnishes the physician with practical tools for the care of allergic individuals.

OUTDOOR ALLERGENS

To be clinically relevant, outdoor allergens, carried most often on plant pollens and mold spores, must reach a high airborne concentration. The level of exposure to these particles is determined by the vicinity of the flora to the patient, the density of production of the pollen or spores by its source, the seasonal and diurnal timing of pollen or spore release, weather conditions, and the aerodynamic characteristics of the vector carrying the allergenic proteins. Flora that are present in great numbers and produce large pollen or spore burdens tend to be the most significant allergenically. Exposure to pollens and mold spores occurs in seasonal patterns that will be detailed in the appropriate sections.

Weather conditions greatly influence the airborne concentrations of these particles. Pollination and mold sporulation require warmth and are highest at midday and on warm days. Particle concentration increases with increasing wind speed, but in gusty winds these particles may be swept into the upper atmosphere, reducing ground exposure. In the cool, calm evening hours, these particles may resettle toward the ground, increasing exposure. Surprisingly, the brisk rainfall caused by thunderstorms does not reduce the airborne pollen and spore levels, while long periods of rainfall can act to scour these particles and reduce exposure.

The aerodynamic characteristics of these particles play an important role in the degree and manner of exposure. Smaller particles remain airborne for longer periods, increasing exposure levels. Larger particles will settle more quickly, except in high winds. Particle size also determines the manner in which allergen exposure occurs. Particles that are larger than about 5 μm in diameter are deposited largely in the nose and are unlikely to penetrate to the lung. Despite the fact that most mold and pollen spores are 20–60 μm in diameter and impact mostly the eyes and nasal mucosa, lower airway symptoms can still be elicited by the allergenic proteins carried by these particles. These particles may exert their influence on the lung by reflexes elicited by nasopharyngeal stimulation or by hematogenous spread after the allergenic protein is eluted from vectors at mucosal surfaces, or the allergenic protein may become associated with smaller respirable particles in the environment, such as pollen fragments.

Pollen

About 60 families of higher plants in North America are implicated in pollinosis. Pollen contains the male genetic material of a plant and is released from mature

---

Plant Pollens

- The type of pollens responsible for seasonal allergies tend to be small, light, and windblown. They are dispersed in large numbers from plants that have small, nondiscrete flowers.
- The specific "pollinating seasons" for different tree, grass, or weed plant species vary within different areas of the country.
- Airborne concentration of pollens depends on the weather. Levels tend to be highest at midday during warm, slightly windy conditions.

---

anthers during specific weeks of a year. The pollen wall is composed of an outer exine, a middle layer termed the intine, and an inner protoplast. The exine has many micropores, but also larger pores or furrows through which the pollen tube emerges during successful pollination. Allergenic proteins dissolve through these pores onto mucosal surfaces allowing hypersensitivity reactions. The overall shape of the pollen grain and the geometry and configuration of the pores make speciation under light microscopy possible.

Pollens are dispersed in different ways by different species of plants. Wind-dispersed (anemophilous) pollens achieve high airborne concentrations and are primarily responsible for clinical allergy. These plants tend to have small, nonaromatic flowers, little or no nectar, and produce large numbers of pollen grains that have aerodynamic properties to improve buoyancy. The majority of flowering plants, however, rely on animal or insect vectors for pollination (entomophilous), and these species—with their large, aromatic, colorful flowers—are generally not clinically relevant because their pollens are not airborne.

The aerobiology of pollens is of great public health interest. Pollens are counted after collection in a standardized fashion using machines that trap the pollen either actively with rotating arms coated with adhesive substances or by passive wind and gravitational force. After identification of the particular pollens to which the individual is sensitized, the published pollen counts can be a helpful guide in directing patients toward allergen avoidance and efficacious medication usage. However, the interpretation of these counts and their relevance to the individual patient must be considered. For example, daily variation may be extreme, making interpretation for daily symptom predictions difficult. In addition, symptom intensity depends on many factors, so reporting of a doubling in pollen count, for example, may not be clinically relevant to an individual whose threshold level of allergen that causes symptoms has not been reached. In any event, knowing the patient's particular sensitivities, the yearly timing of symptoms, the seasonal timing of pollination, and the characteristics of local fauna will help to guide patient care.

POLLEN SEASONS

In temperate regions, pollen seasons are traditionally grouped as trees, grasses, and weeds. In general, trees pollinate from late winter to late spring, grasses from late spring to midsummer, and weeds from midsummer to autumn. However, this delineation may vary widely, depending on the yearly weather pattern and geographic location. Fig. 1 shows the timing of pollination of allergenically significant trees, grasses, and weeds by region in North America.

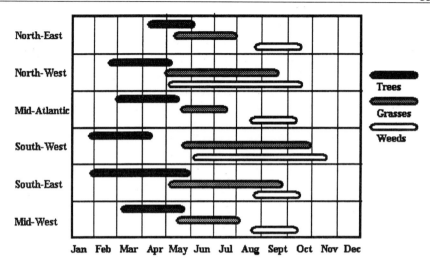

Fig. 1. Pollen seasons by region in the continental United States.

TREE POLLEN

Tree pollination heralds the beginning of the allergy season in most climates in North America, beginning in late February and lasting through April in Northern regions. In general, the greatest variety and concentration of tree pollens occur in March through May with the season ending in June. However, the tree pollen season may begin as early as December or January in areas of Arkansas, south Florida, and Texas and is caused by pollen of cedar trees. Some examples of species that pollinate earlier in the tree season include red cedar and elm; midseason pollinating species include poplar, birch, ash, and willow; and late-season species include sycamore, oak, and mulberry. Table 1 shows five allergenically significant trees in each region of North America in the sequence in which they bloom. Trees on this list were selected to illustrate both significant species and the breadth of pollens that contribute to the span of the tree season in each area.

GRASS POLLEN

In most areas of North America the grass pollen season overlaps and follows the close of the tree pollen season and runs from May through July, but there is much variation. Prominent grasses in temperate regions include orchard, timothy, ryegrass and bluegrass. There is a significant allergenic overlap among the proteins of these regional species, and skin test reactivity will often overlap. Because of this crossallergenicity, differences in exposure to specific temperate grass species are not clinically significant, as they are for tree or weed pollens. In the southern states and subtropical regions, Bermuda, Bahia, and Johnson grasses play a larger role in pollinosis. The allergens in these southern grass pollens are distinct. In some subtropical areas, Bermuda grass and other species may produce almost perennial pollination. Table 1 shows examples of allergenically significant grasses by region in North America.

WEED POLLEN

Weed pollination typically occurs in the late summer through October in most regions of North America. There are a tremendous variety of weeds, but ragweed species

Table 1
Selected Trees and Weeds of Allergenic Significance[a]

Region	Trees	Grasses	Weeds
Northeast (New England, New York, Pennsylvania, New Jersey)	Birch Elm Maple Poplar Oak	Orchard Timothy June Sweet vernal Bluegrass	Sheep sorrel Plantain Russian thistle Giant Ragweed Short Ragweed
Mid-Atlantic (Delaware, Maryland, District of Columbia, Virginia, North Carolina, South Carolina)	Birch Elm Maple Hickory Oak	Orchard Timothy Bluegrass June Bermuda	Plantain Dock Sage Short Ragweed Giant Ragweed
North Central (Ohio, Kentucky, Wisconsin, Michigan, North Missouri, Iowa, Wisconsin)	Ash Elm Maple Willow Box Elder	Orchard Timothy Blugrass June	Plantain Dock Russian Thistle Short Ragweed Giant Ragweed
Pacific Northwest (Washington, Nevada, Northern California, Oregon)	Alder Birch Maple Oak Walnut	Timothy Blugrass Fescue Rye Redtop	Dock Plantain Russian Thistle Nettle Sage Brush
Plains (Nebraska, Kansas, Minnesota, Eastern Montana, Dakotas)	Elm Oak Box Elder Willow Maple	Timothy Orchard Blugrass Bermuda Redtop	Marsh Elder Russian Thistle Western Hemp Short Ragweed Giant Ragweed
Rocky Mountains (Idaho, Wyoming, Colorado, Utah, Western Montana)	Cedar Elm Ash Birch Oak	Timothy Orchard Fescue Redtop June	Sagebrush Russian Thistle Short Ragweed Giant Ragweed
Southern (Florida, Georgia, Texas, Arkansas, Southern Missouri)	Cedar Elm Mulberry Poplar Oak	Bermuda Orchard Timothy Saltgrass	Dock Pigweed Russian Thistle Giant Ragweed Short Ragweed
Southwest (Western Texas, New Mexico, Arizona)	Cedar Ash Mulberry Oak Olive	Bermuda Johnson	Sagebrush Russian Thistle Saltbush Kochia Short Ragweed
Southern California	Ash Walnut Elm Oak Olive	Bermuda Saltgrass Brome	Nettle Bur Ragweed Russian Thistle Sage Western Ragweed

[a]Plants are shown in the order of bloom for each region. Grasses are listed by prevalence in each region.

Mold Spores

- Mold growth requires moisture.
- Mold spores can be found in the air outside year-round, but tend to peak in the spring, late summer, and fall with wet weather.
- Mold growth can also be a problem in the house, especially in the basement, bathrooms, and other areas that are damp.

(Ambrosia) are responsible for the greatest amount of seasonal symptoms. Many species of ragweed have crossallergenicity, so sensitized individuals may experience symptoms "out of season" when visiting some regions where ragweed pollinates either perennially or outside of the usual mid-August to early October ragweed season, such as Coastal ragweed, which is prevalent in winter months in southern Florida. Among other weeds responsible for significant regional allergy are pigweed, amaranth, marsh elder, dock, sorrel, plantain, and Russian thistle. Allergenically significant weeds are listed by region in the order of bloom within the weed pollen season in Table 1.

Fungi

Fungal spores (the term *molds* refers to fungi that lack macroscopic reproductive structures, but may produce visible colonies) are responsible for both seasonal and perennial allergic symptoms. Despite being able to survive a variety of extremes in temperature and humidity, most fungal forms grow best on a moist substrate. Outdoor varieties include *Cladosporium, Alternaria, Aspergillus, Penicillium*, and *Botrytis*. Allergenic proteins are found in the spores and in other fungal elements that may become airborne. Many of the allergenic proteins produced by these fungi have been characterized at the molecular level, such as Alt a 1 (*Alternaria alternata*) and Cla h 2 (*Cladosporium herbarium*).

Alternaria species are more prevalent in dry, warm climates while *Cladosporium* dominates temperate regions. Outdoor fungal particle levels peak seasonally, particularly in the midsummer in temperate regions, but this is variable. Fungal spore exposure may also increase in the spring when melting snow uncovers decaying vegetation, as well as immediately after rains. Patients may experience symptoms attributable to fungus exposure during outdoor activities that stir vegetation such as leaf raking, farming activities, grass cutting, or hiking. Although grass pollen, insect emanations, and other allergens can be stirred by these activities, the role of fungal allergens should not be overlooked.

INDOOR ALLERGENS

The house dust found in the indoor environment is a complex mixture that includes various levels of outdoor and indoor allergens (Table 2). Many atopic individuals experience perennial symptoms, such as rhinitis or asthma, because of allergens in the indoor environment. Frequently, even perennial symptoms may wax and wane, making physician detective work and diligent history taking imperative. For example, a patient allergic to dogs may experience an increase in symptoms during the winter months when an outdoor pet spends more time indoors. Similarly, although pollen is typically thought of as an outdoor allergen, open windows and passive transfer on clothing

Table 2
Selected Allergens Found in House Dust

Dust mites
Fungi
Furred pets
Cockroach
Furred pests (e.g., mouse, rat)
Pollens (from outdoors)
Miscellaneous debris (plant, food, etc.)

and pets can result in significant levels of pollen exposure in the indoor environment. Indoor allergens have attracted much attention since epidemiological studies have linked elevated concentrations of house dust mites and cockroach with asthma severity in sensitized subjects.

Just as it is possible to count pollens by morphological characteristics, the measurement of indoor allergen concentrations is also possible, but requires different methods. Determining the concentration of these indoor allergens is often helpful clinically, since exposure levels are less predictable than seasonal outdoor allergens. Molds may be measured by colony counts, and dust mite numbers can be counted in measured dust samples using a light microscope. Monoclonal antibody assays to major allergens of dust mites, cat, dog, and cockroach among others have made analysis of exposure levels to a number of relevant allergens possible. This work provides data to support the notion that there is a threshold level of a particular allergen that predisposes susceptible individuals to become sensitized and that there is a higher threshold level above which symptoms may be elicited. Thus, steps taken to reduce levels of relevant indoor allergens may help to prevent the development of specific allergic sensitization as well as reduction of symptoms. This work has also helped to elucidate the aerobiological properties of these allergens and the steps needed to reduce exposure to them.

Fungi

Examples of common indoor fungi include *Penicillium, Aspergillus, Rhizopus*, and *Cladosporium*. Fungal colonies may be visible as darkly stained growths or may be detected by a "musty" odor in some cases. *Penicillium*, for example, forms the greenish growth in damp areas and *Rhizopus* is the fluffy black growth seen on old bread. Damp basements, soiled upholstery, garbage containers, various wet bathroom items, and damp food or clothing storage areas are excellent sources for mold growth. Humidifiers that use a cold water reservoir and duct systems that have become damp may also disperse fungal allergens. Since molds are ubiquitous, trying to culture them from a patient's home environment may not be as helpful as correlating symptoms, exposure risks, and skin test or RAST results in diagnosing their role in an individual's symptoms. Like pollens, outdoor airborne fungal allergens can become significant indoor allergens by virtue of entry through doors and windows.

Dust Mites

The almost ubiquitous domestic house dust mites, the most prominent of which are *Dermatophagoides pteronyssinus* and *D. farinae*, are in the same family as scabies.

They are microscopic (approximately 0.3 mm in length), eight-legged, and feed on human skin scales. They rely upon ambient humidity for water that they absorb through a hygroscopic substance on their legs. They grow best at a relative humidity in excess of 75%—which may be easily achieved in, for example, a mattress, even when ambient humidity is lower. This requirement for humidity also results in a lower concentration of mites in surface dust as opposed to deeper areas as in blankets, pillows, and furred toys. The optimal temperature for their growth is 18.3–26.7°C. These requirements for growth explain why they are not as prevalent in cold, dry areas such as northern Sweden and central Canada or at high altitudes as in Colorado.

The major source of mite allergen is derived from fecal particles that are 10–35 µm in diameter (similar to the size of pollen grains). The fecal particles can become airborne with disturbance but settle rapidly. The particles are surrounded by a membrane that allows contained allergen to elute when in contact with wet surfaces such as mucous membranes. Although a patient may give a history that is suggestive of dust mite allergy, for example, acute symptoms occurring upon going to bed, frequently the role of this allergen may be more in the realm of chronic inflammation and chronic symptoms.

Animal Danders

An estimated 100 million domestic animals reside in the United States; one third to one half of homes have a pet, the most popular being cats and dogs. Animal dander carrying the allergenic proteins derive from emanations that include skin scales, urine, feces, and saliva. Exposure to a pet may elicit acute symptoms, but more often animal allergen in the home is responsible for chronic symptoms, often making the suspicion of an allergy to a household pet more difficult to diagnose. Lastly, it must be remembered that pets may act as a vector for bringing outdoor allergens, such as pollen, into the home environment.

CATS

Cats are among the most common household pet in urban areas, and survey data indicate that 20–40% of the atopic population has sensitivity to cat allergen and about one third of these people live with cats. The major allergen responsible for cat allergy is Fel d 1, although reactivity to other proteins, including cat albumin, play a role. All breeds, both long and short hair, produce Fel d 1 to varying extents, and males produce more than females. Even "big cats" produce this allergen. The allergen is found in both saliva and sebaceous glands and is distributed by licking and grooming. The size of vectors that carry the allergen are generally less than 25 µm, and 10–30% are smaller than 2.5 µm. These small particles remain airborne for long periods and are not readily cleared by the nasopharynx. This ability of the particles to reach the lower airway may explain the sudden asthma symptoms some sensitive individuals experience upon entering a home with cats. Cat allergen has been found in low levels even in homes without cats or in schools; presumably the allergen is brought in by passive transport from cat owners since these particles are adherent. In fact, cat allergen is tenacious in that it has been detected not only in settled dust but also on walls and fabrics, and can remain for months after a cat is removed from the home.

DOGS

The prevalence of sensitivity to dog allergen is about half of that seen with cat sensitivity. The major dog allergen, Can f 1, is detected on the coat and in saliva. The amount produced by different breeds varies, but all breeds produce the major allergen so there is not truly an allergen-free breed. Some breeds do, however, produce breed-specific allergens, but the clinical relevance of this is not well understood. The airborne characteristics of dog allergen are not well described, but the allergenic proteins are carried on a variety of particle sizes, including small particles that can potentially reach the lower airways directly. Like cat allergen, the major dog allergen can be detected in homes without dogs or in schools, showing that passive transport and persistence of allergen are possible.

BIRDS

IgE-mediated sensitivity to feathers has been found in canary fanciers and other bird breeders, but the incidence of sensitization is not known. Positive skin tests to feather extract may be due to contamination of the extract with dust mite allergen, leading to false estimates of the incidence of sensitivity. Similarly, feather pillows may induce symptoms because of the growth of dust mites or mold in them rather than any avian proteins associated with the feathers. Specific disease caused by bird exposure is, however, seen in pigeon breeders and in budgerigar, canary, and other bird fanciers, who may develop hypersensitivity pneumonitis. IgG antibody responses toward the avian serum γ-globulin is seen in these patients, although IgE-mediated sensitivity has also been demonstrated in some individuals with this disease.

OTHER FURRED ANIMALS

Furred animals are found in homes, schools, farms, and the workplaces. Furred pets found in homes or schools include hamsters, gerbils, guinea pigs, rabbits, and many exotic pets. The allergens from these animals may be found in their fur, urine, and saliva. Farm animals such as pigs, cattle, and horses are also responsible for allergic disease, although little is known about the prevalence of disease activity from these sources in the United States. Sensitivity to these farm animals is a more common problem in northern Europe, presumably because of the proximity of these animals to the homes of their keepers.

Furred pests, such as mice and rats, should also be considered a potential source of allergen. Mouse allergen (Mus m 1) has also been detected in air samples from urban dwellings, but the role in atopic disease in that setting is not well characterized. Among laboratory workers exposed to animals, 11–30% show sensitivity, and most of these become sensitive to more than one species. Studies with laboratory workers handling rats have shown that rat allergen (Rat n 1) levels vary widely according to the type of disturbance—cleaning cages, sacrificing—the animals are undergoing, and this may play a role in sensitization and the production of symptoms.

Insects

Aside from the allergic reactions that occur from insect stings, the fine wing scales, fecal pellets, and other emanations from moths, locusts, various beetles, flies, and other insects may be a source of inhalant allergens. The mayfly, for example, is responsible for allergic symptoms, especially in the area around the western end of Lake Erie. The allergen from the mayfly is carried on particles that are fragments of the insect's pellicle shed during molting.

Among the various insects that have been implicated in allergy, the cockroach is best studied. Three species of cockroach inhabit buildings: *Blattella germanica, Periplaneta americana*, and *B. orientalis*. *B. germanica* is the most prevalent in crowded North American cities. Its major allergens, Bla g 1 and Bla g 2, derive principally from the saliva and fecal material. The larger American cockroach produces the allergen Per a 1, which crossreacts with Bla g 1. Sensitivity to cockroach allergen has been shown to be associated with exposure levels, is more prevalent in urban than suburban areas, and has been associated as a risk factor for emergency room visits for asthma in the inner city. Although concentrated in kitchen and bathrooms, allergen is detectable in all areas of the home.

Other Indoor Allergens

A number of other potential allergens are detectable in the indoor environment, but their role in disease is not well understood. These include indoor plant material, bacteria, protozoa, algae, food debris, and low-molecular-weight chemicals. Indoor plants do not usually produce pollen, but some may be allergenic, e.g., the airborne leaf particles of *Ficus benjamina* (weeping fig). Other plant materials such as latex, and dust from cotton, coffee, and flour are probably relevant only in the industrial setting. Products such as enzymes secreted from bacteria and protozoa have been implicated in allergic disease, but the exact pathophysiology or epidemiology is not completely understood. Clinically relevant concentrations of food allergens may become aerosolized during cooking (especially egg, fish, and shellfish), or when consumed in small spaces (e.g., roasted peanuts on airplanes), or in industrial settings.

Low-molecular-weight chemicals, such as anhydrides, isocyanates, azodyes, and ethylenediamide, have been reported to cause allergic reactions in industrial settings. These chemicals are too small to evoke immune reactions unless they complex with proteins. Most exposures occur in industrial settings and not in domestic settings unless acrylic paints or glues are used without ventilation. Some of these chemicals may act as irritants rather than allergens. Again, the exposure history is important in considering these agents, and their significance in nonindustrial settings is unclear.

SUGGESTED READING

Bollinger ME, Eggleston PA, Flanagan E, Wood RA. Cat antigen in homes with and without cats may induce allergic symptoms. *J Allergy Clin Immunol* 1996;97:907–914.

Burge HA. Fungus allergens. *Clin Rev Allergy* 1985;3:319–329.

Custovic A, Green R, Fletcher A, Smith A, Pickering CA, Chapman MD, et al. Aerodynamic properties of the major dog allergen Can f 1: Distribution in homes, concentration, and particle size of allergen in the air. *Am J Respir Crit Care Med* 1997;155:94–98.

Einarsson R, Aukrust, L. Allergens of the Fungi Imperfecti. *Clin Rev Allergy* 1992;10:165–190.

Hamilton RG, Eggleston P. Environmental allergen analyses. *Methods* 1997;13:53–60.

Knox RB. Grass pollen, thunderstorms and asthma. *Clin Exp Allergy* 1993;23:354–359.

Ledford D. Indoor allergens. *J Allergy Clin Immunol* 1994;94:327–334.

Lewis WH, Vinay P, Zenger VE. *Airborne and Allergenic Pollen of North America*. Baltimore, Johns Hopkins University Press, 1983.

Mathews KP. Inhalant insect-derived allergens. *Immunol Allergy Clin North Am* 1989;9:321–338.

Platts-Mills TAE, Ward GW, Sporik R, Gelber LE, Chapman MD, Heymann PW. Epidemiology of the relationship between exposure to indoor allergens and asthma. *Int Arch Allergy Appl Immunol* 1991;94:339–345.

Pope AM, Patterson R, Burge H, eds. *Indoor allergens: Assessing and controlling adverse health effects.* Report of the Committee on the Health Effects of Indoor Allergens, Division of Health Promotion and Disease Prevention, Institute of Medicine. Washington, DC, National Academy Press, 1993.

Smith EG. *Sampling and Identifying Allergenic Pollens and Molds.* San Antonio, Bluestone Press, 1990.

Stewart GA, Thompson PJ. The biochemistry of common aeroallergens. *Clin Exp Allergy* 1996; 26:1020–1044.

Weber R, Nelson H. Pollen allergens and their interrelationships. *Clin Rev Allergy* 1985;3:291–318.

5 Anaphylaxis

Lori Kagy, MD and Michael S. Blaiss, MD

CONTENTS

INTRODUCTION

Anaphylaxis and anaphylactoid reactions are true emergencies in clinical allergy. Unless immediate treatment is instituted, the possibility of fatal outcome exists. Two French physicians, Charles Richet and Paul Portier, coined the term *anaphylaxis* in 1902. They described the phenomenon that occurred when they injected dogs with venom from the sea anemone. Several days later, when they gave a second nonlethal dose of the venom to the dogs, they quickly died. They called this reaction anaphylaxis as the opposite of prophylaxis or protection. The list of agents that can trigger these life-threatening reactions in the population continues to grow. Common causes of anaphylaxis and anaphylactoid reactions are medications, foods, insect venoms, vaccines, and even latex. The incidence of anaphylaxis is not clearly known, though one study in Munich in 1995 from emergency rescue teams found the rate of cases to be 9.79/100,000 population. Release of potent pharmacological mediators from tissue mast cells and peripheral blood basophils is the basis for the clinical manifestations seen in anaphylaxis and anaphylactoid reactions. Anaphylaxis and anaphylactoid reactions differ in that true anaphylaxis involves antigen response to IgE antibody, while IgE is not involved in anaphylactoid reactions.

From: *Current Clinical Practice: Allergic Diseases: Diagnosis and Treatment, 2nd Edition*
Edited by: P. Lieberman and J. Anderson © Humana Press Inc., Totowa, NJ

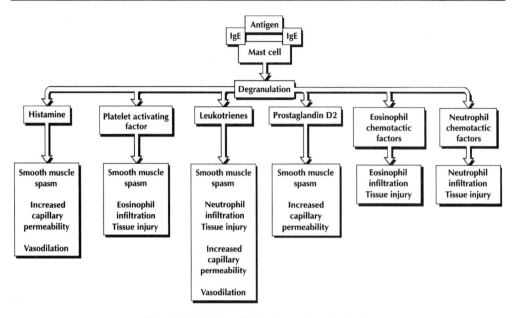

Fig. 1. Clinical manifestations of anaphylaxis.

PATHOPHYSIOLOGY

Anaphylaxis is a generalized, immediate IgE-mediated hypersensitivity reaction to a foreign antigen such as a protein, a hapten, or a polysaccharide. In susceptible persons, initial exposure to an antigen results in formation of specific IgE antibodies to that antigen. These antibodies attach to receptors on the surface of mast cells and basophils, which leads to changes in the cell membrane with degranulation and release of preformed chemical mediators and generation of new potent mediators. It is these mediators that produce the clinical symptoms of anaphylaxis (Fig. 1).

Mast cells are marrow-derived, tissue-resident cells that are essential for IgE-mediated inflammatory reactions. These cells are scattered in connective tissues throughout the body, but are found in especially large numbers beneath mucosal and cutaneous surfaces such as the skin, the lung alveoli, the gastrointestinal mucosa, and the nasal mucous membranes. Mast cells express on their surfaces large numbers of high-affinity Fc receptors for IgE. Therefore, the surface of each mast cell is coated with IgE molecules that have been absorbed from the circulation and serve as receptors for specific antigens. When antigens bind to the mast cell's surface IgE molecules, it undergoes activation that leads to its subsequent degranulation and release of granule contents into the surrounding tissues. The granules contain large amounts of histamine and other inflammatory mediators.

Histamine is a major mediator of anaphylaxis, and histamine infusion has been shown to reproduce the majority of the manifestations of anaphylaxis. The activities of histamine are shown in detail in Table 1. The actions of histamine are mediated through three receptor types (H_1, H_2, and H_3). Two of these, the H_1 and H_2 receptors, are active in producing the symptoms of anaphylaxis. The overall effect of histamine on the vascular bed is to produce vasodilation. This causes flushing and lowering of peripheral resistance, thus resulting in a fall in systolic pressure. Vascular permeability

Table 1
Actions of Histamine Pertinent to Anaphylaxis Mediated Through H_1 and H_2

H_1	H_2	Requires H_1 and H_2 for Maximum Effect

Smooth muscle contraction	Cardiac effects
	    Positive chronotropic
	    Positive inotropic
	    Decreased fibrillation
	        threshold
		Vasodilatation
		Hypotension
		Headache
		Flush

Vascular permeability	Vasodilation	Increased amount mucous gland secretion

Stimulation of nerve endings
    Pruritus
    Vagal irritant receptors
Vasodilation
    Nitric oxide
    Direct effect
Cardiac effects
    Increased rate of depolarization
        of SA node coronary artery
    Vasospasm
Increased viscosity mucous
    gland secretion
	Mucous glycoprotein
	    Secretion from goblet cells
	    and bronchial glands	

also occurs, owing to a separation of endothelial cells at the postcapillary venule level. Both H_1 and H_2 receptors are operative in the production of vasodilation.

Cardiac effects of histamine are mediated primarily through the H_2 receptor. H_2-receptor stimulation causes an increase in rate and force of atrial and ventricular contraction and decreases the fibrillation threshold. H_1-receptor stimulation can cause coronary artery vasospasm and an increased rate of depolarization of the SA node. Histamine leads to constriction of smooth muscle in the bronchial tree, uterus, and gastrointestinal tract. Both H_1 and H_2 stimulation increase glandular secretion.

Like mast cells, basophils also bear high-affinity Fc receptors for IgE and contain histamine-rich cytoplasmic granules. The basophil participates in IgE-mediated reactions in a manner similar to that of the mast cell. Other chemical mediators involved in the IgE-mediated anaphylactic reaction include arachidonic acid metabolites, such as leukotrienes (LTC_4, D_4, E_4) and the prostaglandins (PGD_2, PGF_{2a}), as well as thromboxane A_2 (TXA_2). These substances can cause contraction of airway smooth muscle, increased vascular permeability, goblet and mucosal gland secretion, and peripheral vasodilation. Platelet activating factor also contracts smooth muscle and enhances vascular permeability. Thus, histamine, arachidonic metabolites, and platelet activation factor produce smooth muscle spasm, enhance vascular permeability, cause vasodilation. Also, these mediators stimulate sensory nerves, thus activating vagal effector pathways, and alter myocardial function. The results of these events are the classic symptoms of flushing, urticaria and angioedema, wheezing, hypotension and shock, myocardial ischemia, and gastrointestinal smooth muscle contraction with nausea, vomiting, and diarrhea. Other mediators such as tryptase, chymase,

> **Clinical Manifestation**
>
> - Risk of anaphylaxis is higher if an agent is given by injection than orally.
> - In general, the more rapid the onset of anaphylaxis after the inciting event, the more severe the manifestations in the patient.
> - Patients with a significant anaphylactic episode should be observed in a hospital setting overnight for the possibility of biphasic anaphylaxis.

mast cell kininogen, and basophil kallikrein are involved and can activate secondary inflammatory pathways.

Recently the role of nitric oxide as a mediator of anaphylaxis has been described. It can cause smooth muscle dilation and increased vascular permeability leading to hypotension. On the other hand, the relaxation of the smooth muscle by nitric oxide can lead to improvement of bronchospasm and myocardial ischemia. In anaphylaxis, it appears that the harmful effects of nitric oxide outweigh its benefit.

It is also important to note that chemotactic factors are released from mast cells and basophils. These factors recruit other cells, which then degranulate and release a second wave of mediators. This second wave of mediators is thought to account for relapses of anaphylaxis that can occur after initial symptoms have resolved. These are termed late-phase reactions. In addition, these chemotactic mediators can result in protracted or prolonged episodes of anaphylaxis that persist long after the initial degranulation of mast cells and basophils.

Several mechanisms can lead to anaphylactoid reactions. One is activation of the complement system, resulting in formation of the potent anaphylatoxins, C3a and C5a. These proteins can directly trigger mast cell and basophil degranulation, releasing the same potent mediators. Another mechanism is the direct action of certain agents on mast cells and basophils, stimulating the release of mediators. This mechanism is independent of IgE and complement. Anaphylactoid reactions can also occur in situations in which the mechanism is not clearly understood. These include systemic reactions initiated by exercise, aspirin, nonsteroidal anti-inflammatory drugs, and synthetic steroid hormones.

CLINICAL MANIFESTATIONS

The signs and symptoms of anaphylaxis vary greatly in onset, presentation, and course. The skin, the upper and lower airways, the cardiovascular system, and the gastrointestinal tract may be affected solely or in any combination (Fig. 2). Symptoms of anaphylaxis usually begin within 5–30 min after exposure to the inciting agent. However, symptoms may be delayed for up to an hour or more.

The clinical signs and symptoms of anaphylaxis have been compiled in a review of 266 cases. The most commonly affected organ is the skin. Urticaria and angioedema were the most prevalent skin manifestations, occurring in 90% of the subjects. Flushing was seen in 28%, whereas only 4% had generalized pruritus without a rash. The

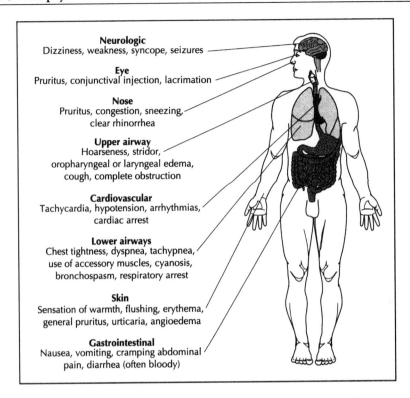

Neurologic
Dizziness, weakness, syncope, seizures

Eye
Pruritus, conjunctival injection, lacrimation

Nose
Pruritus, congestion, sneezing,
clear rhinorrhea

Upper airway
Hoarseness, stridor,
oropharyngeal or laryngeal edema,
cough, complete obstruction

Cardiovascular
Tachycardia, hypotension, arrhythmias,
cardiac arrest

Lower airways
Chest tightness, dyspnea, tachypnea,
use of accessory muscles, cyanosis,
bronchospasm, respiratory arrest

Skin
Sensation of warmth, flushing, erythema,
general pruritus, urticaria, angioedema

Gastrointestinal
Nausea, vomiting, cramping abdominal
pain, diarrhea (often bloody)

Fig. 2. Major chemical mediators of anaphylaxis and their actions.

respiratory tract, involving both the upper and the lower airways, was the next most generally involved system, with 60% experiencing shortness of breath, dyspnea, and wheezing. Upper airway symptoms were documented in 24% and included laryngeal edema, tongue swelling, choking, dysphonia, and dysphagia.

Symptoms of hypotension or documented hypotension were frequent and were seen in 49% of the patients. The gastrointestinal tract was also regularly involved. Diarrhea, abdominal cramps, nausea, and emesis developed in 46% of the patients. Less frequent symptoms included headache, blurred vision, transient blindness, and seizures.

It is thought that there is a direct correlation between the immediacy of the onset of the symptoms after exposure to the triggering agent and the severity of the anaphylactic episode: the more rapid the onset, the more severe the event. In some patients, the episode may appear to resolve, and then the symptoms recur after several hours. This is called biphasic anaphylaxis. It can occur despite appropriate treatment of the initial event. It is therefore recommended that patients who have a significant anaphylactic event be hospitalized for overnight observation.

Death due to anaphylaxis usually occurs as a result of respiratory obstruction and/or cardiovascular shock. In patients who die of anaphylaxis, the prominent pathological features are acute pulmonary hyperinflation, laryngeal edema, pulmonary edema, intra-alveolar hemorrhage, visceral congestion, urticaria, and angioedema. In some instances, death occurs without any gross pathological change and is presumed to be the result of profound cardiovascular collapse. Sudden vascular collapse is usually attributed to vasodilation or cardiac arrhythmia. Myocardial damage may occur in up to 80% of fatal cases.

> **Etiology**
>
> Drugs and foods are probably the most common causes of ana-
> phylaxis. In children, peanuts are probably the most common cause
> of fatal reactions. In adults, shellfish, nuts, fish, and peanuts are
> the most frequent foods implicated as the cause of anaphylactic
> episodes.

RISK FACTORS

There are many factors that increase the risk of anaphylaxis in the population. Patients with atopy are at a higher risk of anaphylaxis from antigens administered by the mucosa route, such as food, compared to parenterally administered agents, such as vaccines. The longer the interval between doses for certain antigens, the less likely a recurrence of anaphylaxis. Interruption of therapy may lead to predisposition to anaphylactic reactions, as has been documented with insulin treatment. Route of administration appears to be a risk factor with a higher likelihood of anaphylaxis when an agent is given by injection than orally. Gender and age have been evaluated as potential risk factors. Women have a higher incidence of anaphylaxis in general compared to men as well as to latex, muscle relaxants, and aspirin. Men have a higher rate of anaphylaxis to insects than females. These higher rates based on gender may be more related to exposure than to a genetic difference. Adults tend to have a higher incidence of anaphylaxis to radiocontrast media, insects, plasma expanders, and anesthetics than children do. Again, this may be due to more exposure to these agents in adults than in children.

ETIOLOGY

Although any substance has the potential to cause anaphylaxis, the most common causes of IgE-mediated anaphylaxis are medications, foods, insect bites and stings, and latex. Table 2 lists the etiological and pathophysiological classification of anaphylaxis and anaphylactoid reactions. The following discussion is a review of some of the more common factors known to produce anaphylaxis.

Medications

Hundreds of agents have been documented as causes of anaphylaxis, and medications comprise one of the largest groups (Table 3). Penicillin and its derivatives make up one of the most common causes of anaphylaxis to medication. Penicillin has been reported to cause fatal anaphylaxis at the rate of 0.002% in the general population, or 1/7.5 million injections. Estimates of nonfatal anaphylaxis vary, ranging from 0.7–10%. Crossreactivity exists between the various penicillins. All β-lactam antibiotics (penicillins, cephalosporins, monobactams, carbapenems, oxacephems, clavams, carbacephems) contain the main four-member β-lactam ring linked to a second five- or six-member ring, except for the monobactams, which lack the second ring. Table 4 is a list of β-lactam antibiotics. There is much crossreactivity with ampicillin, but only minimal crossreactivity with methicillin and oxacillin. Cephalosporins also crossreact in approximately 30% of patients with allergy to penicillin. Aztreonam, a β-lactam

Table 2
Etiological and Pathophysiological Classification of Anaphylaxis and Anaphylactoid Reactions

Anaphylaxis-IgE-mediated reactions
    Drugs
    Food
    Insect bites and stings
    Latex
    Exercise (some cases)
Anaphylactoid
    Disturbances in arachidonic acid metabolism
    Aspirin
    Nonsteroidal anti-inflammatory drugs
Immune aggregates
    γ-globulin
    IgG-anti-IgA
    Possibly protamine, dextran, and albumin
Director release of mediators from mast cells and basophils
    Drugs
    Idiopathic
    Exercise
    Physical factors (cold or sunlight)
Miscellaneous and multimediator activity
    Nonantigen-antibody-mediated complement activation
        Radiocontrast material
        Possibly some cases of protamine reactions
        Dialysis membranes
Activation of contact system
    Dialysis membranes
    Radiocontrast material

with a monobactam structure, can be used safely in patients with penicillin allergy. Anaphylaxis can occur from parenteral, oral, or topical drug administration, although the highest incidence is from parenteral administration.

Aspirin and other nonsteroidal anti-inflammatory drugs are important causes of anaphylactoid events. These reactions are not IgE mediated. They apparently produce anaphylactoid reactions through the aberrant mechanism of arachidonicacid, with inhibition of cyclooxygenase and subsequent increased production of leukotrienes. However, some episodes may be caused by the direct degranulation of mast cells. In sensitive individuals, adverse reactions to aspirin typically include urticaria, angioedema, asthma, chronic rhinosinusitis, and nasal polyps. Because the sensitivity persists for life, management entails strict avoidance. Acetaminophen is the alternative recommended drug. Salsalate, choline salicylate, magnesium salicylate, and propoxyphene hydrochloride are the other drugs that can be used.

All nonsteroidal anti-inflammatory drugs may crossreact with aspirin to varying degrees. Even the new cyclooxygenase-2 inhibitors, such as celecoxib, crossreact with aspirin and should be avoided in aspirin-sensitive patients. Desensitization can be considered in aspirin-sensitive patients with respiratory disease.

Table 3
Medicinal Agents Causing Anaphylaxis

Antibiotics	Chemotherapeutic agents	Miscellaneous
Penicillin and derivatives	Asparaginase	Aspirin
Cephalosporins	Vincristine	Nonsteroidal anti-inflammatory drugs
Tetracycline	Cyclosporine	Allergy extracts
Sulfonamides	Methotrexate	Human γ-globulin
Ciprofloxacin	5-Fluorouracil	Insulin
Nitrofurantion		Radiocontrast material
Vancomycin		Heparin
		Vaccines, (tetanus, measles, influenza, mumps)
		Dextran
		Opiates
		Protamine
		Local anesthetics
		Glucocorticosteroids
		Antithymocyte globulin

Foods

Any food has the potential to cause anaphylaxis, but some foods are more allergenic than others. The most frequent causes of food anaphylaxis include crustaceans, legumes, fish, seeds, nuts, berries, egg whites, and dairy products.

Table 5 is a representative listing of foods reported to cause anaphylaxis. The incidence of anaphylactic reactions to foods is unknown, but may be more common than stinging insect anaphylaxis. A review of patients with a history of food-related anaphylaxis who had been instructed in epinephrine self-administration demonstrated that these patients required injections at a rate of 0.97 times per year, which was three times higher than that required in insect-allergic individuals. It appears that certain foods cause anaphylaxis more frequently in children than in adults and vice versa. The most common offender in adults is probably shellfish, while in children the most common are milk, eggs, and peanuts.

The peanut is responsible for allergic reactions in both children and adults. Peanut allergy is probably the most common cause of death due to food anaphylaxis in the United States. Peanut allergy, unlike other food allergies, is rarely outgrown. Once a diagnosis has been made, there should be strict lifelong avoidance of peanuts. Patients with peanut allergy should be warned of "hidden" peanuts in many foods, including candy, chili, spaghetti sauce, and egg rolls.

If it is not apparent from the patient's history what food triggered anaphylaxis, then skin testing with different food extracts may help in isolation of the cause. Though rare, it is important to note that prick skin testing with foods can itself cause an anaphylactic reaction. Therefore, an in vitro test such as the radioallergosorbent (RAST) test, although less sensitive in determining the allergen, may be safer in verifying a particular food as the etiological agent when the history suggested a severe anaphylactic reaction to that food.

Table 4
β-Lactam Antibiotics

Penicillins	Cephalosporins
Penicillin G	Cefazolin
Penicillin V	Cephalexin
Methicillin	Cefadroxil
Oxacillin	Cephalothin
Carbenicillin	Cefamandole
Ticarcillin	Cefuroxime
Mezlocillin	Cefonicid
Piperacillin	Cefpodoxime proxetil
Cloxacillin	Cefaclor
Nafcillin	Cephalexin
Ampicillin	Cefotetan
Clavams	
Clavulanic Acid	Cefotaxime
Monobactams	Ceftriaxone
Aztreonam	Cefoperazone
Carbapenems	Ceftazidime
Imipenem	Cefixime
Meropenem	Cefprozil
Carbacephems	**Oxaceophems**
Loracarbef	Moxalactam

Table 5
Foods Causing Anaphylaxis

Legumes	Peanuts, beans, peas, soybeans
Shellfish	Shrimp, lobster, crab, crawfish
Milk	
Eggs	
Wheat	
Fish	
Nuts	Cashews, almonds, pecans, walnuts
Seeds	Sesame, sunflower, poppy, cottonseed
Spices	Cinnamon, nutmeg, mustard, sage
Fruits	Apples, bananas, peaches, oranges, melons
Chocolate	
Potato	
Corn	

Insect Bites and Stings

Anaphylaxis occurs from stings of Hymenoptera, including bees (honeybee, bumblebee, and sweatbee), vespids (wasps, yellow jackets, and hornets), and imported fire ants. The importance of each of these insects as a cause of anaphylaxis varies according to the geographic region. Bees and yellow jacket stings cause the most problems in the northern portions of the United States, with the wasps and fire ants causing most problems in the southern half of the United States. Compared with Hymenoptera stings, anaphylaxis from insect bites is rare. Bites from kissing bugs and deer flies have been documented as causes of IgE-mediated anaphylaxis.

Skin testing with insect venoms is warranted in adults in whom there is only skin manifestation of anaphylaxis or involvement of any other organ system. In contrast, it is only recommended to skin test children to insect venoms if they have skin manifestations along with involvement of one other organ system. Studies suggest those children with just skin reactions such as urticaria and angioedema after venom sting do not worsen on repeated stings and lose their sensitivity over time. If positive, appropriate venom immunotherapy should be instituted. In addition to venom immunotherapy, the individual should carry an auto injector of epinephrine, wear a medical identification bracelet, and practice insect avoidance procedures.

Latex

The incidence of latex allergy has increased dramatically in the past 10–15 years with the universal increased use of latex gloves as a precaution against AIDS and other infections. Latex is now a significant cause of anaphylaxis, with more than 1000 cases of latex anaphylaxis reported to the Food and Drug Administration between 1988 and 1992. Three groups appear to be at high risk for development of anaphylaxis to latex: health care workers, people with a history of pruritus from exposure to latex objects, and patients with spina bifida.

Many different latex proteins have been demonstrated to be allergenic. Some allergens have been isolated from natural latex, and others are produced from the processing of the rubber compound. Exposure to latex can be topical, inhalational, mucosal (from surgical and dental procedures), and intravenous. Patients with latex allergy also have a high incidence of anaphylaxis to certain foods, including bananas, kiwi fruit, chestnuts, and avocados. They should therefore be counseled regarding these foods.

Exercise-Induced Anaphylaxis

Exercise has been documented as a source of severe anaphylactoid reactions. Symptoms include angioedema, urticaria, abdominal cramping, diarrhea, laryngeal edema, bronchospasm, and respiratory distress. The reaction typically begins during exercise or shortly after exercise is completed. A special group of patients with exercise-induced anaphylaxis have symptoms only when they exercise within 2–4 hours of eating. This entity is called food-dependent exercise-induced anaphylaxis. Some patients with this condition have symptoms with exercise only after eating certain foods, such as celery, wheat, shellfish, and oysters. Others have symptoms in association with any food and exercise. All individuals with these conditions should exercise with a companion capable of administering epinephrine. Individuals with food-dependent exercise-induced anaphylaxis should not exercise within 2–4 hours of eating. About two thirds of individuals with exercise-induced anaphylaxis have a family history of atopy, and about one half have a personal history of atopy. The exact mechanism is unknown, and it has been speculated that the release of endogenous opioid peptides with vigorous exercise may release mediators in susceptible individuals. There is also evidence for mast cell activation in skin biopsy from patients with exercise-induced anaphylaxis.

Plasma Exchange

Patients undergoing plasma exchange can experience anaphylaxis from multiple causes. The reported incidence is as high as 12%. Reactions can be from the plasma or the apparatus used during the plasmapheresis procedure. Changing the plasmapheresis equipment may help to prevent subsequent reactions. Pretreatment with prednisone and diphenhydramine can also be helpful.

Hemodialysis

Anaphylaxis and anaphylactoid reactions during hemodialysis have been attributed to a number of different factors. Ethylene oxide used for sterilization can produce an IgE-mediated event. Other reactions have been related to the procedure used in processing the hemodialyzer. The type of hemodialysis membrane can be important. Severe reactions have been reported with the use of hollow-fiber membranes made of cuprammonium cellulose. The use of ACE inhibitors during dialysis seems to predispose to anaphylactoid events. When a patient experiences anaphylaxis during hemodialysis, the type of membrane should be changed, no reprocessed membrane should be used, and ACE inhibitors and β-blockers should be discontinued if possible.

Insulin

Reactions to insulin include local or systemic responses and insulin resistance. Although human recombinant DNA insulin appears to be less antigenic than bovine-type insulin, it can cause allergic reactions. Local reactions are the most common and are generally encountered during the first 1–4 weeks of therapy. They are usually IgE mediated and consist of mild erythema, swelling, burning, and pruritus at the injection site. These local reactions usually disappear in 3–4 weeks with continued administration of insulin. Dividing the insulin dose into two or more sites or switching to a different preparation is generally helpful. If not, antihistamines may be given until the reaction disappears. Local reactions may precede anaphylactic reactions. Therefore, epinephrine should be available to these patients. Systemic reactions include urticaria, angioedema, bronchospasm, and hypotension. Most of these reactions occur upon restarting insulin therapy after an interruption. In treatment of systemic reactions it is very important that the insulin therapy not be discontinued. If the last dose is given within 24 hours, the subsequent dose should be decreased by one third and then subsequently increased slowly by 2–5 units until the desired dose is reached. If it has been more than 24 hours since the onset of anaphylaxis, a serious reaction with readministration of insulin is more likely to occur. The least allergenic insulin is selected by skin testing, using several different preparations of insulin. Desensitization of a patient with a history of a systemic reaction to insulin should be carried out in an intensive care unit setting.

Radiocontrast Media

Generalized reactions to radiocontrast media that occur immediately after administration are encountered in 0.5–3% of patients who receive the substance. The majority of patients who experience a reaction have urticaria. Reactions to radiocontrast media are not IgE mediated but probably involve mast cell activation with release of histamine and other mediators. Use of non-ionic, lower osmolarity agents reduces the risk of

---

Differential Diagnosis

The most common condition mimicking anaphylaxis is the vasodepressor (vasovagal) reaction. It is distinguished from anaphylaxis by its lack of urticaria, pruritus, angioedema, tachycardia, and bronchospasm.

---

a reaction. Unfortunately, their use is limited because of higher expense. In patients who receive β-adrenergic blocking agents, the reactions may be more severe and less responsive to treatment. There is no association between reaction to radiocontrast media and topical iodine solution or shellfish allergy.

he risk of subsequent reactions is substantially reduced by pretreatment regimens of corticosteroids, antihistamines, and adrenergic agents or by use of low-osmolarity non-ionic radiocontrast material.

Local Anesthetics

IgE-mediated reactions to local anesthetics are extremely rare. The adverse reactions most commonly seen with these agents are vasovagal or hyperventilation episodes, toxic reactions, or epinephrine side effects. The preservatives in local anesthetics, which include sulfites and parabens, may be responsible for allergy-type reactions. Skin-prick testing can be done with a local anesthetic that does not contain epinephrine. If the result of the test is negative, graded subcutaneous injections of diluted and full-strength doses of that local anesthetic are given at 15-min intervals. If the patient tolerates that local anesthetic, it may be used for future procedures.

Idiopathic Anaphylaxis

Frequently, no identifiable factor can be found for the patient's anaphylaxis, a situation labeled idiopathic anaphylaxis. Patients who are victims of frequent and life-threatening episodes of idiopathic anaphylaxis may need prophylactic treatment with oral H_1 antihistamines and prednisone.

DIFFERENTIAL DIAGNOSIS

The differential diagnosis of anaphylaxis and anaphylactoid events is listed in Table 6. The most common condition mimicking anaphylaxis is the vasodepressor (vasovagal) reaction. Most of these events precede emotional trauma or a threatening event. Hypotension, pallor, diaphoresis, weakness, nausea, vomiting, and bradycardia are classically seen in these reactions. Patients lack the urticaria, pruritus, angioedema, tachycardia, and bronchospasm that are commonly seen in anaphylaxis. Symptoms are almost immediately reversed by recumbency and leg elevation. Other forms of shock such as hemorrhagic, cardiogenic, and endotoxic must be included in the differential diagnosis of anaphylaxis. These forms of shock, however, are usually not difficult to distinguish from anaphylaxis.

A number of reactions involving the "restaurant syndromes" have been observed that can mimic anaphylaxis. These include reactions to monosodium glutamate (MSG), sulfites, and saurine. MSG ingestion can cause chest pain, facial burning, flushing,

Table 6
Differential Diagnosis of Anaphylaxis

Vasodepressor reactions	Excess Endogenous Production of Histamine
Other Forms of Shock	Syndromes
Hemorrhagic shock	Systemic mastocytosis
Cardiogenic shock	Urticaria pigmentosa
Endotoxic shock	Basophilic leukemia
Adrenal insufficiency	Acute promyelocytic leukemia
"Restaurant Syndromes"	(tretinoin treatment)
MSG	Hydatid cyst
Sulfites	Nonorganic Diseases
Saurine (scombroidosis)	Panic attacks
Flush Syndromes	Munchausen's stridor
Carcinoid flush	VCD syndrome
Postmenopausal flush	Globus hystericus
Chlorpropamide/alcohol-induced flush	Miscellaneous Conditions
Medullary carcinoma of the thyroid	Hereditary angioedema
Autonomic epilepsy	"Progesterone anaphylaxis"
Idiopathic flush	Urticarial vasculitis
	Pheochromocytoma
	Hyperimmunoglobulin E, urticaria syndrome
	Neurological (seizures, stroke)
	Pseudoanaphylaxis
	"Red man syndrome"
	Recurrent syncope of unknown cause

sweating, dizziness, paresthesias, headaches, palpitations, nausea, and vomiting. In children, screaming, chills, irritability, and delirium have been reported. Symptoms typically begin no later than 1 h after ingestion, although they can be delayed in some instances for up to 14 h. The exact mechanism is unknown; however, it has been postulated that transient acetylcholinosis occurs. Approximately 15–20% of the population is thought to be susceptible to MSG reactions; however, these reactions can occur in anyone if the dose is large enough.

In some individuals the ingestion of sulfites can produce a reaction that can be confused with anaphylaxis. Sulfites can be found in many foods, including dried fruits, gelatin, wine, sausage, shellfish, and pickles. After ingestion of a food containing sulfites, certain patients may experience flushing, hypotension, and bronchospasm. Bronchospasm is typically the most prominent symptom of this syndrome, and it can be very severe.

Ingestion of saurine, which is contained in spoiled fish, can result in scombroidosis. Saurine is a histamine-like chemical that is produced by bacterial decarboxylation of histidine. Symptoms of scombroidosis can be very similar to those seen in true anaphylactic events, and at times can be difficult to distinguish unless a careful history is taken. Symptoms typically include, flushing, urticaria and angioedema, pruritus, headache, nausea, and vomiting. A helpful clue in distinguishing scombroidosis from a true anaphylactic event is that usually everyone who ate the spoiled fish in sufficient quantities will also have symptoms of scombroidosis. Patients who are taking isoniazid seem to be particularly susceptible to this reaction.

> **Differential Diagnosis**
>
> A helpful clue in distinguishing scombroidosis from a true anaphylactic event is that usually everyone who ate the spoiled fish in sufficient quantities will also have symptoms of scombroidosis.

There are several syndromes that produce flushing that can mistaken for anaphylaxis. These include carcinoid tumors, postmenopausal flush, chlorpropamide/alcohol-induced flush, medullary carcinoma of the thyroid, autonomic epilepsy, and idiopathic flush. Individuals with carcinoid tumors can have symptoms similar to those seen during anaphylaxis. These tumors can secrete histamine, neuropeptides, kallikrein, and prostaglandins, in addition to 5-hydroxytryptamine (serotonin). As a result of these substances, patients with carcinoid tumors can exhibit flushing, abdominal pain, diarrhea, and occasionally wheezing. Postmenopausal flush typically occurs over the face, neck, upper chest, and breasts. The flush may last anywhere from 3–5 min and can occur several times throughout the day. Stress and alcohol can aggravate it. There is no associated urticaria, angioedema, hypotension, or gastrointestinal involvement. The ingestion of alcohol with chlorpropamide (a sulfonylurea agent) can cause flushing with hypoglycemia and its associated symptomatology. The flush usually begins 3–5 min after alcohol ingestion and peaks in about 15 min. Patients with medullary carcinoma of the thyroid can have a protracted flush of the face and upper extremities. These patients typically have telangiectasias, mucosal neuromas, and a family history of the disease. These thyroid tumors can secrete histamine, prostaglandins, substance P, and serotonin. Autonomic epilepsy is a rare disorder caused by the release of paroxysmal autonomic discharges. Individuals with this disorder may have tachycardia, flush, and syncope, as well as hypotension or hypertension.

Idiopathic flush occurs primarily in women. It can be associated with diarrhea, syncope, palpitations, and hypotension. Bronchospasm, urticaria, and angioedema are absent from this disorder. Several syndromes are characterized by excessive endogenous production of histamine. These include systemic mastocytosis, urticaria pigmentosa, basophilic leukemia, acute promyelocytic leukemia, and hydatid cyst. Anaphylactic events can occur in such patients. Patients with systemic mastocytosis can experience anaphylactic episodes after the ingestion of opiates. Patients with promyelocytic leukemia can experience episodes after treatment with tretinoin. Human infection with the larval stage of the canine tapeworm *Echinococcus granulosus* causes hydatid cysts. If the hydatid cyst ruptures, the contents are released and an IgE-mediated anaphylactic reaction can occur.

Patients with emotional disturbances can have episodes that may be confused with anaphylaxis. Flushing, tachycardia, gastrointestinal symptoms, and shortness of breath often accompany panic attacks. Two other conditions that can sometimes be confused with anaphylaxis are Munchausen's stridor and vocal cord dysfunction. Their presentations are similar; however, one is consciously self-induced, and the other is involuntary. Vocal cord dysfunction is caused by involuntary adduction of the vocal cords, which produces obstruction in both expiration and inspiration. The patient is not aware of the process and is unable to reproduce the event. In Munchausen's stridor, the laryngeal spasm is self-induced. In both, the patients will have symptoms mimicking

---

Differential Diagnosis

Measuring the serum mast cell tryptase level is more useful than measuring serum histamine levels in diagnosing anaphylaxis because of its longer half-life, approximately 2 h.

Prevention

- A complete history taken from the patient about reactions to medication is paramount in preventing prescription of a crossreacting drug.
- All patients with food and insect anaphylaxis should carry an autoinjector of epinephrine on their body and not leave it in their car or at home.
- All patients who receive an in-office parenteral injection should remain for observation at least 20–30 min for the possibility of anaphylaxis.

---

laryngeal edema with stridor. However, these patients will lack urticaria, angioedema, or other cutaneous symptoms.

Several other miscellaneous conditions can be included in the differential diagnosis of anaphylaxis: hereditary angioedema, urticarial vasculitis, pheochromocytoma, and "red man syndrome." Hereditary angioedema is an autosomal dominant disorder that can be mistaken for anaphylaxis. This condition is associated with painful swellings, laryngeal edema, and abdominal pain. It usually has a slower onset, lacks urticaria and hypotension, and often is accompanied by a family history of similar reactions. Obtaining a C_4 level, which is decreased in this condition, can confirm the diagnosis.

At times it may not be clear whether or not a patient has had an anaphylactic reaction. The reaction may be verified by measuring the serum mast cell tryptase level. Unlike plasma histamine, which usually declines within 30 min of the anaphylactic reaction, the mast cell tryptase level peaks at 60–90 min and then declines, with a half-life of approximately 2 h.

PREVENTION

Once the diagnosis of anaphylaxis has been established and a cause has been identified, prevention of future episodes by avoidance is the cornerstone of therapy. Table 7 lists measures to reduce the incidence of anaphylaxis and anaphylactic deaths. In the case of drug or food allergy, the offending agent as well as those agents that may crossreact must be avoided. If an individual has a history of an allergic reaction to a drug such as penicillin, a drug that does not crossreact with the penicillin family should be used. When medications must be given, oral administration is preferable to parenteral administration because reactions are usually less severe after oral administration. If in-office parenteral administration of a drug is required, the patient should remain for observation for at least 20–30 min. period. Patients allergic to insects should avoid flowers, garbage, mowing the lawn, and walking barefoot outdoors. Latex-allergic individuals should avoid contact with all latex products and should use only nonlatex

Table 7
Measures to Reduce the Incidence of Anaphylaxis

Steps for the Physician
  Take a detailed medical history noting past anaphylactic reactions
  Mark all medical records regarding past anaphylactic reactions
  Require clear indication of a drug's use
  Avoid drugs with immunological or biochemical crossreactivity with any agents to which
    the patient is sensitive
  Administer medication orally if possible
  Keep patient in office 20–30 min after injections
  Be prepared to treat anaphylaxis
  Have emergency equipment available
  Use pretreatment and desensitization protocols when indicated
Specific Measures for Patients at Risk
  Patients should be instructed on self-administration of epinephrine
  Patients should avoid β-blocker agents, ACE inhibitors, and monoamine oxidase inhibitors
  Patients should discard all unused medications
  Patients with food-induced anaphylaxis need to check all labels for the offending agent

gloves. If these patients require surgery or dental procedures, the procedures should be performed only in a latex-free area.

Patients at risk for anaphylaxis should carry appropriate identification, such as a Medic Alert bracelet or necklace and/or an identification card in their wallet or purse. All patients should carry a preloaded syringe of epinephrine or an auto-injector of epinephrine (EpiPen®) at all times and should be instructed in its use. Any individual who has had an anaphylactic reaction should not take β-adrenergic blocking agents, angiotensin converting enzyme inhibitors, monoamine oxidase inhibitors, or certain tricyclic antidepressants such as amitriptyline. β-Blockers inhibit the therapeutic action of epinephrine and can also increase the severity of an attack. Angiotensin converting enzyme inhibitors prevent the conversion of angiotensin I to angiotensin II. This is turn prevents a compensatory response to hypotension. Monoamine oxidase inhibitors and some tricyclic antidepressants are dangerous in some situations because they interfere with the degradation of epinephrine.

MANAGEMENT

Anaphylaxis has a highly variable presentation; therefore, rapid recognition with immediate treatment is essential. The treatment of anaphylaxis should follow established principles for emergency resuscitation (Table 8). This approach is required to counteract the effects of mediator release, prevent further release of mediators, and to support vital functions. The drugs used in the treatment of anaphylaxis are shown in Table 9.

At the first sign of anaphylaxis, epinephrine should be administered. Simultaneously a rapid assessment of the patient's airway status and state of consciousness should be assessed. An airway should be secured immediately if there is any compromise. The patient should be placed in a recumbent position and pulse and blood pressure should be assessed, and then reassessed frequently throughout the treatment period. The position may need to be modified if the patient is wheezing, since lying supine

Table 8
Initial Management of Anaphylaxis

Immediate Action
Assessment
Secure and maintain airway
Rapid assessment of level of consciousness
Vital signs
Treatment
Epinephrine 1:1000;0.01 mL/kg up to 0.3 mL sc; repeat every 15 min as necessary
Supine position, legs elevated
Oxygen
Tourniquet proximal to injection site
H_1 antihistamine (diphenhydramine 1–2 mg/kg im or iv up to 50 mg/kg every 4–6 h
Corticosteroids (hydrocortisone 5–10 mg/kg up to 500 mg iv every 4–6 h)
H_2 antihistamine (ranitidine 12.5–50 mg iv every 6–8 h)
Monitor vital signs frequently
Peripheral iv fluids
If hypotension persists, norepinephrine bitartrate, 208 mg/min, or dopamine, 2–10 mg/kg/min, to maintain BP
If hypotension caused by β-blocker, administer glucagon, 1–5 mg iv over 1 min, and begin continuous infusion 1–5 mg/h
Administer specific antiarrhythmic agents if indicated
For persistent bronchospasm, administer aminophylline, 6 mg/kg over 20 min, then continue iv aminophylline drip at 0.9 mg/lg/h; aerosolized β-2 agonist as needed
Keep patient in observation for at least 24 h when following a protracted course

Table 9
Equipment for Treatment of Anaphylaxis

Medications
Epinephrine 1:1000 for SC, IM
Epinephrine 1:100,000 for IV
Corticosteroids (methylprednisolone, hydrocortisone)
H_1 antihistamines (diphenhydramine, hydroxyzine)
H_2 antihistamines (cimetidine, ranitidine)
$β_2$ agonists (albuterol)
Aminophylline
Glucagon
Dopamine
Norepinephrine bitartrate
Oxygen, face mask, nasal cannula
IV fluids (normal saline, albumin)
Airway kit, Ambu bag, laryngoscope, scalpel and 11-gauge needle for cricothyroidotomy
Electrocardiograph
Sphygmomanometer and stethoscopes
Tourniquets

SC, subcutaneous; IM, intramuscular; IV, intravenous.

> **Treatment**
>
> Epinephrine is the drug of choice in the treatment of anaphylaxis. Delaying or failing to administer epinephrine can result in a fatal outcome.

increases the work of breathing. The Trendelenburg position can increase intrathoracic pressure and reduce the pressure gradient between the right atrium and the inferior vena cava, thus limiting the benefit of increased venous return. Supplemental oxygen should be administered if there is any question about the cardiopulmonary status.

Epinephrine is the most single important agent in the treatment of anaphylaxis. Delaying administration or failure to administer the drug can result in a fatal outcome. The dose and route of administration of epinephrine depend on the severity of the reaction. In most instances, the intramuscular or the subcutaneous route is preferred. The dose for an adult is 0.3–0.5 mL (0.3–0.5 mg) of 1:1000 preparation, while the dose for a child is based on body weight (0.01 mL/kg). The initial dose may be repeated every 15 min as needed up to a maximum of three doses. Rarely, severe refractory anaphylaxis might require intravenous epinephrine. The amount administered depends on the severity of the episode. Generally a 1:10,000 aqueous preparation can be prepared by diluting 1.0 mL of a 1:1000 aqueous epinephrine solution in 9 mL normal saline. This 1:10,000 solution can then be administered in doses of 0.1 to 0.2 mL every 5–15 min, depending on the response of the patient. Of course, lower doses may be needed for patients with underlying cardiac disease.

If the reaction is from an injection or an insect sting a tourniquet should be placed proximal to the site of the injection or sting. The tourniquet should then be released every 10 min for 1 to 2 min. If anaphylaxis resulted from an injection or sting, as long as the sting is not in the head, neck, hands, or feet, a second injection of epinephrine can be given at the site of the injection or sting to reduce the antigen absorption.

Other medications can be given to supplement the effect of epinephrine. Antihistamines can be used after administration of epinephrine; however, they should not be used as the sole form of therapy. Diphenhydramine may be administered intravenously or intramuscularly. The dose in adults is 25–50 mg and in children 1–2 mg/kg. The dose of diphenhydramine may be continued thereafter every 6 h for 48 h to help reduce the risk of recurrence. Other rapidly absorbed antihistamines may be substituted, as well as the addition of H_2 antagonists to the previous therapy. Ranitidine is administered in a dose of 1 mg/kg iv. The dose of cimetidine is 4 mg/kg iv. H_2 antagonists should be administered slowly, since rapid administration of these agents has been associated with hypotension.

If the patient does not respond to the above measures and remains symptomatic with either hypotension or persistent respiratory distress, admission to the intensive care unit is essential. In these instances, intravenous fluids and vasopressors should be considered for administration. Intubation and tracheostomy may be necessary if upper airway obstruction is severe enough to impair adequate ventilation. Corticosteroids are not helpful in the acute management of anaphylaxis; however, they should be administered in moderate or severe reactions to prevent protracted or recurrent anaphylaxis. Hydrocortisone can be administered in a dose of 5 mg/kg up to 1 g im or

iv. Methylprednisolone may also be used at a dose of 80–125 mg iv in adults and 40 mg iv in children. For milder episodes, oral prednisone may be given at a dose of 60 mg in adults and 30 mg in children. Glucagon may be given to patients who are taking β-adrenergic blocking agents, because of its positive inotropic and chrontropic effects on the heart. The dose is administered as an iv bolus of 1–5 mg followed by a 5–15 μg/min titration. Atropine may also be beneficial if the patient has bradycardia. The dose is 0.3–0.5 mg subcutaneously, repeated every 10 min to a maximum of 2 mg. Wheezing unresponsive to epinephrine can be managed with an aerosolized β-adrenergic agent. An example is albuterol, 0.5 mL of 0.5% solution in 2.5 mL normal saline. When a compressor nebulizer is not available, a metered-dose inhaler is acceptable.

SUGGESTED READING

Dykewicz MS, Fineman S, et al. The diagnosis and management of anaphylaxis. Joint Task Force on Practice Parameters, American Academy of Allergy, Asthma and Immunology, American College of Allergy, Asthma and Immunology, and the Joint Council of Allergy, Asthma and Immunology. *J Allergy Clin Immunol* 1998;101(6 Pt 2):S465–S528.

Freeman TM. Anaphylaxis: diagnosis and treatment. *Prim Care* 1998;25:809–817.

Kemp SF, Lockey RF, Wolf BL, Lieberman P. Anaphylaxis: A review of 266 cases. *Arch Intern Med* 1995;155:1749–1754.

Lieberman P. Anaphylaxis and anaphylactoid reactions. In: Middleton E, Reed C, Ellis E, eds. *Allergy Principles and Practice*. St. Louis; Mosby, 1998 pp. 1079–1090.

Lieberman P. Anaphylaxis: How to quickly narrow the differential. *J Resp Dis* 1999;20:221–231.

6

Insect Sting Allergy

Robert E. Reisman, MD

CONTENTS

INTRODUCTION

Allergic reactions to insect stings are very common, and occasionally, a serious medical problem. The incidence of anaphylaxis in the general population has been estimated to range from 0.3 to 3%. Vital statistic registry data document at least 40 deaths/yr as a result of insect sting anaphylaxis with the likelihood that other episodes of unexplained sudden death are also the result of insect stings. Individuals at risk are often very anxious about further stings and, as a result, make significant changes in their life-styles.

In recent years, particularly since the availability of purified venoms for diagnosis and therapy, major advances have occurred. The natural history of insect sting allergy is now understood, and tools are available for appropriate diagnosis and for treatment of individuals at risk for insect sting anaphylaxis. For many individuals, this is a self-limited disease, and for others, treatment results in a permanent "cure."

INSECTS

The stinging insects are members of the order Hymenoptera of the class Insecta. They may be broadly divided into two families: the vespids, which include the yellow jacket, hornet, and wasp, and the apids, which include the honeybee and bumblebee. People may be allergic to one or all of the stinging insects. The identification of the

From: *Current Clinical Practice: Allergic Diseases: Diagnosis and Treatment, 2nd Edition*
Edited by: P. Lieberman and J. Anderson © Humana Press Inc., Totowa, NJ

> • Insects most commonly responsible for allergic reactions are
>   yellow jackets, wasps, hornets, bees, and fire ants.
> • Estimates of the incidence of anaphylaxis to insect stings range
>   as high as 3% of the general population.
> • The test of choice to identify individuals at risk of a repeat reaction
>   and the species of insect responsible for previous reactions is the
>   allergy skin test.

culprit insect responsible for reactions is thus important in terms of specific advice and specific venom immunotherapy discussed later.

The presence of the different stinging insects varies in different parts of the country. For example, the wasp is most common in Texas, and honeybees may be more common in farm areas where they are used for plant fertilization.

The yellow jacket is the most common cause for allergic reactions resulting from insect stings. These insects primarily nest in the ground and are easily disturbed by activity such as lawn mowing and gardening. They are also attracted to food and thus are commonly found around garbage and picnic areas. Yellow jackets are particularly noted in the late summer and fall. Hornets, which are closely related to the yellow jacket, nest in shrubs and are easily provoked by activities such as hedge clipping. Wasps are found in nests, usually hanging from eaves. In general, there are few wasps per nest, and thus stings are relatively uncommon in most of the country. The honeybee hive may contain thousands of honeybees. As a rule, these insects are quite docile, as exemplified by the common picture of the beekeeper handling thousands of bees on the face or other parts of the body. However, if the honeybee hive is disturbed, multiple stings may occur. The bumblebee, which is a solitary bee, is a rare cause for a sting reaction.

The problem of multiple insect stings has recently been intensified by the introduction of the "Africanized" honeybee, the so-called killer bee, into the southwestern United States. The African honeybee was introduced into Brazil in 1956 for the purpose of providing a more productive bee in tropical climates. These bees are much more aggressive than domesticated European honeybees that are found throughout the United States. The African honeybee has interbred with the European honeybee, but unfortunately the aggressive characteristics have persisted. These bees are extremely aggressive, and massive stinging incidents have occurred, resulting in death from venom toxicity. The Africanized honeybees entered South Texas in 1990 and are now present in Arizona and California. It is anticipated that these bees will continue to spread throughout the southern United States. They are unable to survive in colder climates, but may make periodic forays into the northern United States during the summer months.

The fire ant, which is a non-winged stinging insect, is found in the southeastern and south central United States, primarily near the Gulf coast. These insects are gradually spreading northward and westward, and it is anticipated the will extend as far north as Virginia and eventually as far west as Arizona, New Mexico, and California. The fire ant is increasingly responsible for allergic reactions. It attaches itself by biting with its jaws. It then pivots around its head and stings at multiple sites in a circular pattern. Within 24 h a sterile pustule develops that is diagnostic of the fire ant sting.

In contrast to stinging insects, biting insects, such as the mosquito, rarely cause serious allergic reactions. These insects deposit salivary gland secretions, which have no relationship to the venom deposited by stinging insects. Anaphylaxis has occurred from bites of the deerfly, kissing bug, and bedbug. Isolated reports also suggest that on rare occasions mosquito bites have caused anaphylaxis. It is much more common, however, for insect bites to cause large local reactions, which may have an immune pathogenesis.

REACTIONS TO INSECT STINGS

Normal Reaction

Insect stings, in contrast to insect bites, always cause pain at the sting site. The usual or "normal" reaction is this localized pain, swelling, and redness. This reaction usually subsides within a few hours. Little treatment is needed other than analgesics and cold compresses.

Large Local Reactions

Extensive swelling and erythema, extending from the sting site over a large area, are fairly common. The swelling usually peaks in 24–48 h and may last 7–10 d; a sting on the hand may cause swelling extending as far as the elbow. On occasion, when the reaction is severe, fatigue, nausea, and malaise may be present. If mild, a large local reaction can be treated with aspirin and antihistamines. When a reaction is severe or disabling, steroids such as prednisone, 40 mg d for 2–3 d, are very helpful in diminishing the swelling. There is no documentation that application of papain (meat tenderizer) or "mud" alleviates local swelling. These large local reactions have been confused with infection and cellulitis. Insect sting sites are rarely infected and antibiotic therapy rarely indicated. Tetanus prophylaxis is unnecessary.

The natural history of reactions that occur following subsequent re-stings in individuals who have had large local reactions has been well studied. After subsequent stings, large local reactions tend to recur in about 80% of individuals. The risk for subsequent insect anaphylaxis is very low, <5% Thus, individuals who have had large local reactions are not considered candidates for venom immunotherapy (discussed later) and do not require venom skin tests.

ANAPHYLAXIS

There are no clinical criteria or risk factors that identify individuals at potential risk for insect sting anaphylaxis other than a history of a prior anaphylactic reaction. The clinical features of anaphylaxis following an insect sting are similar to anaphylaxis from other causes. The most common symptoms are dermal, generalized urticaria, flushing, and angioedema. The most severe symptoms, which may be life threatening, include respiratory distress due to asthma and upper airway swelling, circulatory collapse, and shock. Other symptoms include nausea, bowel cramps, diarrhea, rarely uterine cramps, and a feeling of "impending doom." Anaphylactic symptoms usually start immediately after a sting, within 10–30 min. On rare occasions, reactions have started after a longer interval.

Estimates of the incidence of anaphylaxis in the general population range as high as 3%. The majority of reactions have occurred in individuals under the age of 20 yr, with a 2:1 male to female ratio. These data probably reflect exposure rather than any specific age or sex predilection for anaphylaxis. Although the majority of insect sting reactions occur in younger individuals, severe anaphylaxis may occur at any age. Most deaths have occurred in older individuals, many of whom had cardiovascular disease.

The natural history of insect sting anaphylaxis has been the subject of fairly intense investigation. In individuals who have had insect sting anaphylaxis, the recurrence rate after subsequent stings is approximately 60%. Viewed from a different perspective, not all individuals presumed to be at risk react to re-stings. The incidence of these re-sting reactions is influenced by age and severity of the initial anaphylactic reaction. In general, children are less likely than adults to have re-sting reactions. The more severe the anaphylactic reaction, the more likely it is to recur. For example, children who have had dermal symptoms as the only manifestation of anaphylaxis have a remarkably low re-sting reaction rate. On the other hand, in individuals of any age who have had severe anaphylaxis the likelihood of repeat reactions is approximately 80%. When anaphylaxis does recur, the severity of the reaction tends to be similar to the initial reaction. No relationship has been found between the occurrence and degree of anaphylaxis and the intensity of venom skin test reactions.

Unusual Reactions

Serum sickness-type reactions, characterized by urticaria, joint pain, and fever, have occurred approximately 7 d after an insect sting. Individuals who have this reaction are subsequently at risk for acute anaphylaxis after repeat stings and thus are considered candidates for venom immunotherapy.

There have been isolated reports of other reactions, such as vasculitis, nephritis, neuritis, and encephalitis, occurring in a temporal relationship to an insect sting. The specific etiology for these reactions has not been established, and in general venom immunotherapy is not indicated.

Toxic Reactions

Many simultaneous insect stings, for example, 100 or more, may lead to toxic reactions due to venom constituents. The clinical symptoms that characterize these reactions are primarily cardiovascular and respiratory in nature. Immediate treatment is directed to cardiovascular and respiratory support. Following toxic reactions, individuals may develop IgE antibody and may then be at risk for subsequent allergic sting reactions. Thus, individuals who have had toxic reactions should be tested for the possibility of potential sensitization and need for specific therapy. The frequency of these toxic reactions has increased because of the Africanized honeybees.

ALLERGY TESTS

Acute allergic reactions from insect stings are due to IgE antibodies reacting with insect venoms. These antibodies are best detected by the immediate skin test reaction. Individual insect venoms—yellow jacket, honeybee, white-faced hornet, yellow hornet, and wasp—are commercially available for diagnostic skin tests. A positive skin test is defined as an immediate wheal and flare reaction occurring within 10 min after an intradermal skin test with venom doses up to 0.1–1.0 µg/mL. Higher venom doses

> • Patients at risk of a future systemic (anaphylactic) reaction should carry epinephrine, be instructed in avoidance techniques, and receive immunotherapy.
> • Patients who are candidates for immunotherapy are adults with any form of anaphylactic reaction and children whose previous anaphylactic episode extended beyond cutaneous manifestations only.
> • The success rate of venom immunotherapy is better than 98%.

cause nonspecific irritative reactions. IgE antibodies in the serum can also be measured by the radioallergosorbent test (RAST). This in vitro test is more expensive and generally much less sensitive than the simple immediate skin test. It is estimated that approximately 20% of individuals with positive venom skin tests will not have a positive RAST. Thus, the RAST is not recommended for routine diagnosis unless a skin test cannot be performed.

At the present time, fire ant venom is not available. The commercial whole-body fire ant extract is reasonably reliable for skin test diagnosis and immunotherapy for fire ant allergic individuals.

THERAPY

Acute Reaction

The immediate medical treatment for acute anaphylaxis due to insect stings is the same as that for anaphylaxis from any other cause. This treatment is detailed in Chapter 5.

If the insect stinger remains in the skin, it should be gently flicked off, with care being taken not to squeeze the sac. Unfortunately, the majority of the venom is deposited very quickly after the sting, and removal of the sac will be helpful only if done immediately.

Prophylaxis

Individuals who have had insect sting anaphylaxis and have positive venom skin tests are at risk for further reactions after re-stings. Prophylactic measures include advice to minimize potential exposure, available medication for immediate treatment of anaphylaxis, and consideration of venom immunotherapy.

Measures that might minimize insect stings include wearing protective clothing when outside, such as shoes, slacks, long sleeves, and gloves. Cosmetics, perfumes, and black or drab clothing, which attract insects, should be avoided. Great care should be taken when eating outdoors, since food and garbage attract insects.

The primary medication for treatment of anaphylaxis is epinephrine. Individuals at potential risk should be given epinephrine, available in preloaded syringes, (Ana-Kit, Bayer Laboratories, Spokane, WA; Epi-Pen, Center Laboratories, Port Washington, NY). Antihistamines, such as diphenhydramine, are also recommended and may be helpful for treatment of hives and edema.

Table 1
Indications for Venom Immunotherapy in Patients with Positive Venom Skin Tests[a]

Table 1
Indications for Venom Immunotherapy in Patients with Positive Venom Skin Tests[a]

Insect Sting Reaction	Venom Immunotherapy
"Normal"—transient pain, swelling	No
Extensive local swelling	No
Anaphylaxis	
Severe	Yes
Moderate	Yes[b]
Mild; dermal only	
Children	No
Adults	Yes[b]
Serum sickness	Yes
Toxic	Yes

[a]Venom immunotherapy is not indicated for individuals with negative venom skin tests.
[b]Patients in these groups might be managed without immunotherapy. See text.

VENOM IMMUNOTHERAPY

Injection of purified venoms (venom immunotherapy) is extremely effective treatment for individuals at risk for venom anaphylaxis. The overall success rate in preventing subsequent anaphylaxis is over 98%. Venom immunotherapy reduces the risk for anaphylaxis from approximately 50–60% in untreated individuals to about 10% after 2 yr of therapy and to about 2% after 3–5 yr of treatment. The guidelines for selection of individuals for treatment and venom immunotherapy dosing are now well established and are outlined in Tables 1–3.

Selection of Individuals (Table 1)

All individuals with severe symptoms of anaphylaxis and positive venom skin tests should receive venom immunotherapy. Children who have had very mild reactions with dermal symptoms only do not require therapy. Their families should be advised to keep epinephrine and antihistamines available. Adults with similar mild anaphylaxis can probably be treated in a similar fashion, but there is less evidence to support this practice in adults than in children. Currently, venom immunotherapy is still recommended for these adults. Those individuals who have had reactions of moderate intensity such as mild asthma, nausea, and urticaria, without serious life-threatening reactions, might also be treated without immunotherapy and with the availability of emergency medication. They are likely to have similar moderate reactions to subsequent stings. This decision is influenced by other factors, such as risk of a exposure, other disease processes such as cardiac disease, and medication use.

Following serum sickness reactions, individuals usually have positive skin tests and are then at risk for subsequent anaphylaxis. These observations are similar to the classic horse-serum–induced serum sickness. If skin tests are positive, these individuals should then receive immunotherapy. Because venom is a highly sensitizing agent, individuals who have had toxic reactions may develop IgE antibody and then are at potential risk for anaphylaxis. In that situation, immunotherapy is indicated. As

Table 2
General Venom Immunotherapy Dosing Guidelines

Initial dose	.01–0.1 µg, depending upon degree of skin test reaction
Incremental doses	Schedules vary from "rush" therapy administering multiple venom injections over several days to traditional once-weekly injections
Maintenance dose	50–100 µ/g of single venoms 300 µg of mixed vespid venom
Maintenance interval	4 wk 1st yr 6 wk 2nd yr 8 wk 3rd yr
Duration of therapy	Stop if skin test becomes negative finite time; 3–5 yr (see text)

already noted, individuals with large local reactions are not candidates for venom immunotherapy.

Venom Selection

The product brochure, which has not changed since the availability of commercial venoms in 1979, recommends venom immunotherapy with each venom that elicits a positive skin test reaction. Studies of venom antigenic crossreactivity explain the common observation of multiple positive venom skin tests despite only one insect sting reaction. For example, an individual who has had an allergic reaction following a yellow jacket sting will almost always have a positive skin test to hornet venom and possibly a positive skin test to wasp venom. Awareness of this crossreactivity allows more selective venom treatment. The selection of venom for therapy is based on a history of the culprit insect responsible for the reaction and the degree of skin test reactivity. This approach utilizing single venoms despite multiple positive skin tests is less expensive, requires fewer injections, and is therapeutically as effective.

Dosing Schedule (Tables 2 and 3)

Venom immunotherapy is initiated with injection of small doses of venom and followed by increasing doses until the recommended maintenance dose has been reached. The initial dose of venom is based upon the degree of skin test reactivity, not the severity of the anaphylactic reaction. Incremental doses are given according to a number of schedules, ranging from single doses once weekly to rush immunotherapy, which utilizes multiple doses over a 2- to 3-d period. A typical dose schedule is shown in Table 3. Maintenance doses of 100 µ/g of single venoms or 300 µ/g of a mixed vespid preparation (yellow jacket, white-faced hornet, yellow hornet) are the traditional recommendation. Recent studies indicate that top doses of 50 µ/g of individual venoms are effective. Once the maintenance dose is reached, injections are usually given at 4-wk intervals through the first year and then 6- and 8-wk intervals after the second and third year, respectively.

Table 3
Representative Examples of Venom Immunotherapy Dosing Schedules[a]

Traditional		Modified Rush	Rush	
Day				
1	0.1	0.1	0.1[c]	3.0
		0.3	0.3	5.0
		0.6	0.6	10
			1.0	
2			20	
			35	
			50[b]	
			75	
3			100	
Week				
1	0.3	1.0		
		3.0		
2	1.0	5.0	100	
		10	Repeat every 4 wk	
3	3.0	20		
4	5.0	35		
5	10	50[b]		
6	20	65		
7	35	80		
8	50[b]	100		
9	65			
10	80	100		
11	100	Repeat every 4 wk		
12				
13	100			
	Repeat every 4 wk			

[a]Starting dose may vary depending on patient's skin test sensitivity. Subsequent doses modified by local or systemic reactions. Doses expressed in micrograms.
[b]50 µg may be used as top dose.
[c]Sequential venom doses administered on same day at 20- to 30-min intervals.

Reactions to Venom Immunotherapy

SYSTEMIC ALLERGIC REACTIONS

Systemic allergic reactions due to venom immunotherapy are relatively uncommon, compared to reactions that follow other types of allergen immunotherapy. However, because of the possibility of such reactions, it is important that venom immunotherapy, as with other allergenic extracts, should be administered only in the setting in which personnel and equipment are available for treatment of an anaphylactic reaction. Following such a reaction the venom dose is usually decreased about 25–33% and subsequent doses given at lesser increasing increments. If the patient is receiving several different venoms, it is prudent to give only one venom at each treatment time or to separate the time of dosing. Inability to ultimately tolerate a maintenance venom dose is rare.

LOCAL REACTIONS

Large local reactions following venom immunotherapy are more common. When other types of allergenic extracts are administered, doses are decreased and a smaller dose might be maintained to avoid such reactions. In the case of venom, however, it is necessary to administer a maintenance dose (50–100 µg) to assure protection from insect stings. Measures to minimize these local reactions include splitting the venom dose into two injection sites and addition of a small amount of epinephrine, such as 0.05–0.1 mL, with the venom, a commonly used procedure although its efficacy has never been documented. When these local reactions are extensive and particularly somewhat delayed in onset, there may be accompanying nausea and fatigue. Addition of a small amount of steroid, such as betamethasone 0.05–0.1 mL, to the venom may markedly reduce such reactions.

FATIGUE, MALAISE

Fatigue, nausea, malaise, and even fever are unusual symptoms that have been reported after venom injections and also after injection of other types of allergenic solutions such as dust and mold. of These symptoms usually start several hours after the venom injection and may last 1–2 d. Concomitant administration of aspirin with the venom injection and then further doses of aspirin for the next 24 h may eliminate these reactions. If the reactions persist despite aspirin, then a small dose of oral steroids, such as prednisone 20 mg, given with the venom dose and repeated once in 6–8 h has been very helpful.

LONG-TERM THERAPY

There have been no reported adverse reactions from long-term venom immunotherapy.

PREGNANCY

Venom injections appear to be safe for use during pregnancy.

Monitoring During Venom Immunotherapy

VENOM SKIN TESTS

In a small minority of venom-treated patients the venom skin test does become negative. The loss of skin test reactivity indicates that venom-specific IgE is not present, and thus the need for continued venom treatment is unnecessary (discussed later). As a general rule, it is reasonable to retest individuals with venom every 1–2 yr to examine this possibility.

MEASUREMENT OF SERUM–VENOM-SPECIFIC IgG

Venom-specific IgG has been associated with immunity to insect stings. During the course of venom immunotherapy, venom-specific IgG is stimulated. It has been suggested that individuals receiving venom immunotherapy should have serial monitoring of this antibody titer, and those individuals who have failed to develop adequate titers should have a modification in dosing. In my opinion, careful review of these data does not support that recommendation. As venom immunotherapy is 98% effective in preventing subsequent sting reactions, it does not seem reasonable to monitor any type of immune parameter looking for possible treatment failures. In addition, published

- Conversion to a negative venom test reaction is an absolute criterion to stop venom immunotherapy.
- When venom skin test reactions remain positive, 3–5 yr of venom immunotherapy is sufficient for patients who have had mild to moderate anaphylaxis. Venom immunotherapy for an indefinite time is probably advisable for patients who have had severe anaphylaxis.

data do not indicate that for an individual patient there is that close a correlation between absolute antibody titers and the success of venom immunotherapy.

Treatment Failures

Persistent allergic reactions following insect stings in individuals receiving venom immunotherapy are most uncommon. As noted previously, the success rate of venom immunotherapy is better than 98%. When these reactions do occur, it is first necessary to determine whether the patient has been treated with the correct venom. This might require reassessment by history and repeat skin tests. If other insects are suspect, then venom immunotherapy should be modified. If it appears that the patient is receiving the correct venom, then the dose of the venom must be increased. For example, if the individual is receiving 100 μ/g of venom, the dose should be increased to 150–200 μ/g.

Cessation of Venom Immunotherapy

Definitive criteria for safe cessation of venom immunotherapy are being evolved. These include immunological criteria and a specific period of treatment unrelated to the persistence of IgE antibody.

CONVERSION TO A NEGATIVE SKIN TEST

Conversion to a negative skin test is an absolute criterion for cessation of therapy, indicating that the IgE antibody, the immune mediator of this reaction, is no longer present. In my experience, there will be conversion to a negative skin test in approximately 20% of individuals after 3–5 yr of therapy.

SPECIFIC TIME PERIOD

Three to five years of venom immunotherapy appear adequate for the large majority of individuals who have had mild to moderate anaphylactic reactions despite persistence of a positive venom skin test. The re-sting reaction rate after cessation of venom immunotherapy is low, generally in the range of 5–10%. Individuals who have had severe anaphylactic symptoms such as hypotension, laryngeal edema, or loss of consciousness have a higher risk of a repeat severe systemic reaction if therapy is discontinued. For this reason, I currently recommend that individuals who have had severe symptoms and retain positive venom skin tests receive immunotherapy indefinitely, which at this point can be administered every 8–12 wk. Other factors that have been associated with the occurrence of re-sting reactions after cessation of venom immunotherapy include systemic reactions to venom immunotherapy, persistence of significant skin test reactivity, and honeybee venom allergy as compared to vespid venom allergy. These decisions regarding cessation of therapy should include consideration of other medical problems, concomitant medication, patient life-style, and patient preference.

CONCLUSION

In summary, while problems remain, such as prediction or selection of individuals at potential risk for initial anaphylaxis and issues regarding duration of treatment, the understanding and approach to treatment of individuals with insect sting allergy have been defined, and for the majority of individuals, effective treatment is available.

SUGGESTED READING

American Academy of Allergy, Asthma and Immunology Position Statement. Report from the Committee on Insects. *J Allergy Clin Immunol* 1998;101:573–575.

DeShazo RD, Butcher BT, Banks WA. Reactions to the stings of the imported fire ant. *N Engl J Med* 1990;313:462–466.

Golden DBK, Kwiterovich KA, Kagey-Sobotka A, Lichtenstein LM. Discontinuing venom immunotherapy: Extended observations. *J Allergy Clin Immunol* 1998;101:298–305.

Lerch E, Müller UR. Long-term protection after stopping venom immunotherapy; Results of re-stings in 200 patients. *J Allergy Clin Immunol* 1998;101:606–612.

Lockey RF, Turkeltaub PC, Bair-Warren IA, et al. The Hymenoptera venom study I, 1979–1982: Demographics and history sting data. *J Allergy Clin Immunol* 1988;82:370–381.

Mauriello PM, Barde SH, Georgitis JW, Reisman RE. Natural history of large location reactions from stinging insects. *J Allergy Clin Immunol* 1984;74:494–498.

McKenna WR. Killer bees: what the allergist should know. *Pediatr Asthma Allergy Immunol* 1992; 4:275–285.

Reisman RE. Natural history of insect sting allergy: Relationship of severity of symptoms of initial sting anaphylaxis to re-sting reactions. *J Allergy Clin Immunol* 1992;90:335–339.

Reisman RE. Venom hypersensitivity *J Allergy Clin Immunol* 1994;94:651–658.

Reisman RE, Livingston A. Venom immunotherapy; 10 years of experience with administration of single venoms and 50 mcg maintenance doses. *J Allergy Clin Immunol* 1992;89:1189–1195.

Valentine MD, Schuberth KC, Kagey-Sobotka A, et al. The value of immunotherapy with venom in children with allergy to insect stings. *N Engl J Med* 1991;323:1601–1603.

van Halteren HK, van der Linden PWG, Burgers JA, Bartelink AKM. Discontinuation of yellow jacket venom immunotherapy. Follow up of 75 patients by means of deliberate sting challenge. *J Allergy Clin Immunol* 1997;100:767–770.

7 The Child with Asthma
Evaluation and Treatment

Gail G. Shapiro, MD, C. Warren Bierman, MD, and Frank S. Virant, MD

INTRODUCTION

Asthma is a pulmonary disorder characterized by reversible periods of airway obstruction, bronchial hyperresponsiveness, and associated airway inflammation. A comprehensive approach to asthma therapy in children should include assessment of disease severity and scrutiny for exacerbating factors, followed by appropriate environmental modifications as well as pharmacotherapy. Long-term successful management is clearly linked to education of patients and their parents about asthma, proper use of medication, and a plan of action for periods of exacerbation.

In a child with a history of chronic cough or wheezing, a thorough history and directed physical examination should reduce the differential diagnoses to only a few considerations (Table 1). Historically, the appearance of symptoms shortly after birth, such as vascular rings, laryngeal webs, tracheostenosis, or bronchiostenosis, greatly

From: *Current Clinical Practice: Allergic Diseases: Diagnosis and Treatment, 2nd Edition*
Edited by: P. Lieberman and J. Anderson © Humana Press Inc., Totowa, NJ

Table 1
Differential Diagnosis of Asthma[a]

α_1-antitrypsin deficiency
Asthma
Bronchiectasis
Bronchiolitis
Bronchopulmonary dysplasia
Congenital anomalies
Cystic fibrosis
Foreign body (nasal, tracheal, bronchial)
Gastroesophageal reflux
Laryngotracheomalacia
Laryngotracheobronchitis
Laryngeal webs
Pertussis
Pulmonary hypersensitivity diseases (e.g., mold, fibers)
Pulmonary eosinophilia
Pulmonary hemosiderosis
Pulmonary interstitial emphysema
Stenosis (tracheal, bronchial)
Toxic inhalations
Tracheoesophageal fistula
Tumor

[a]From Virant FS, Shapiro GG. Treatment of asthma in children. In Gershwin ME, Halpern GM, eds. *Bronchial Asthma: Principles of Diagnosis and Treatment*, Totowa, NJ, Humana Press, 1994, pp. 273–298.

increases the likelihood of a congenital abnormality as their source. The abrupt onset of coughing or wheezing in a young child, often associated with eating and in the absence of concurrent airway infection, should be considered secondary to foreign body aspiration until proven otherwise. Gastroesophageal reflux (GER) should be considered in any infant with postprandial vomiting or nocturnal cough or in an older child who has associated complaints of dysphagia or heartburn. The combination of recurrent sinobronchitis, failure to thrive, and chronic malabsorption associated with chronic cough and wheezing suggests the possibility of cystic fibrosis.

The probability of asthma as the diagnosis is greatly increased with a positive family history for atopy or other family members with asthma. In a child with obvious asthma, signs of atopy, including eczema, episodic urticaria, recurrent middle ear effusion, and rhinitis, increase the probability that allergy plays a significant role in chronic airway symptoms. It is also useful to ask about possible exacerbating factors for symptoms including allergens, irritants, drugs, cold air, and exercise.

There are three important elements in the evaluation of asthma: the history, the physical examination, and measurement of pulmonary function.

HISTORY

The history should uncover the evolution of symptoms over days, months, or years, specific days of the week, and time of day, with an eye toward associations such as

---

Key Features of Asthma

- Reversible airway obstruction
- Bronchial hyperresponsiveness
- Airway inflammation
- Familial tendency
- Association with allergy: children more than 2 yr of age: 80%; adults: 50%

---

seasonality, visits to homes with pets, times of respiratory infections, and physical activity. Is the problem episodic or continual? If episodic, how often are the episodes, and are they truly isolated or rather acute bursts connected by more subtle symptoms of disease? Are there specific cause-and-effect associations or trigger factors? These should be clarified so that their avoidance can be incorporated in a management plan. Have there been emergency room visits, hospitalizations, need for intubation and assisted ventilation? Have these problems occurred in the face of appropriate medication, or has the patient been undertreated?

Symptoms vary with age. The infant and young child may have histories of recurrent bronchitis or pneumonia, persistent coughing with colds, recurrent "croup," or just a chronic "chest rattle." Older children and adolescents often develop "tight" chests with colds, recurrent "chest congestion," "bronchitis," or persistent coughing or wheezing. Respiratory symptoms may be precipitated or exacerbated also by exposure to animals, moldy or dusty areas, tobacco smoke, or cold air or by exercise.

The past medical history and review of systems often clarify the clinical picture. If the patient had food allergy and eczema in infancy, allergy will probably remain an important factor. One needs to inquire about such allergic manifestations as gastrointestinal problems, including vomiting or diarrhea; skin conditions, such as atopic dermatitis or hives; and the presence or absence of factors such as perennial or seasonal nasal obstruction, frequent respiratory and ear infections, and exercise intolerance. One needs to ask specifically about factors that may aggravate symptoms such as exposure to house dust, animals, grass cuttings, and irritants such as aerosol sprays and cigaret smoke, or reactions to outdoor pollutants. Drug reactions are particularly important, especially idiosyncratic or allergic reactions to antibiotics, aspirin and other nonsteroidal antiinflammatory drugs, bronchodilators, or antihistamines. One should also inquire about unusual reactions to insect stings and about hospitalizations. Details about whether the patient had previously had an allergy-related workup with studies for specific IgE identification and immunotherapy (hyposensitization), and lung function assessment should be recorded.

The environmental history is a unique and important element in the patient with suspected asthma, since many of the symptoms may be exacerbated by factors found in the surroundings, whether home, school, day-care, work, or play. The environmental history is of importance primarily because it provides information on potential allergens to which the patient is exposed, and it is the cornerstone of therapy in terms of avoidance of specific factors that may be identified by allergy testing. In patients of all ages, it is very important to ask about cigaret smoking or exposure to second-hand tobacco smoke.

PHYSICAL EXAMINATION

The physical examination may be dramatic or unrevealing. It begins with an overall visual impression and should include at least an assessment of the head, neck, chest, and skin, but other systems as well, if indicated by the history. If the patient is experiencing an acute episode of airway obstruction, it is common to note anxiety, dyspnea, and increased respiratory rate. There may be audible wheezing and cough. None of this is apparent between acute episodes. If chronic obstruction has been long-standing, one may see a bowing of the ribs and increased anterior-posterior diameter, since growth and bony remodeling will accommodate chronic pulmonary hyperinflation. On auscultation, one may notice increased expiratory phase of respiration. There may be wheezing on expiration or on both inspiration and expiration; coarse wheezes may take on the quality of rhonchi. Rales typically indicate parenchymal disease; however, they may also be present if there is localized atelectasis, not uncommon with asthma. Sudden deterioration and absence of breath sounds suggests the rare complication of pneumothorax. More common is crepitus and extrapulmonary dissection of air with apparent edema extending upward from the chest into the neck and face because of dissecting pneumomediastinum, usually a spontaneously resolving event, but one that suggests severe obstruction.

The head and neck examination is often abnormal in patients with asthma. Children may show evidence of middle-ear disease that may be a complication of allergic rhinitis: middle-ear fluid, otitis, or ventilating tubes. In both children and adults, the eyes may show conjunctival edema and injection compatible with allergic disease. There may be periorbital edema and discoloration due to the venous and lymphatic stasis that may accompany allergic rhinitis (so-called allergic shiners). The nose may show the pallor, edema, and clear secretions of allergic rhinitis or erythema and purulent secretion from infectious rhinitis or sinusitis. The presence of nasal polyps in children suggests cystic fibrosis, while in the adolescent and adult it suggests nonallergic eosinophilic disease (possibly with aspirin sensitivity) that may involve the upper and lower airway. Since sinusitis and viral upper respiratory infections both exacerbate asthma, it is important to diagnose and treat those problems that are likely to be bacterial. Skin manifestations of atopy such as the lichenification and flexor crease rash of atopic dermatitis (eczema) frequently precede the onset of chronic asthma.

LABORATORY EVALUATION (TABLE 2)

Lung Function Tests

Lung function tests are objective, noninvasive, and cost effective in diagnosing and following the patient with asthma. A simple mechanical spirometer and peak flow meter (pediatric meters are available for younger children) are useful in office practice. Failure to use these objective measures will lead to underdiagnosis and incomplete understanding of disease fluctuations. Children as young as four years old can be taught to perform pulmonary function maneuvers with birthday party favors that make whistle sounds to reinforce forced expiration. Results can be compared with normal standards.

Table 2
Laboratory Tests in Asthma[a]

Tests	Possible Abnormalities in Asthma	Comments
Complete blood count	Leukocytosis (occasionally)	Induced by infection, epinephrine, administration, "stress"
	Eosinophilia (frequently)	Varies with medication, time of day adrenal function; not necessarily related to "allergy." (Often higher in "intrinsic" than "extrinsic" asthma)
Sputum examination	Eosinophils	In both "intrinsic" and "extrinsic" asthma
White or "clear" and small yellow plugs	Charcot-Leyden crystals	Derived from eosinophils
	Creola bodies	Clusters of epithelial cells
	Curschmann spirals	Threads of glycoprotein.
Nasal smear	Eosinophils	Suggests probably concomitant nasal allergy
	Lymphocytes, PMNs, macrophages	Sometimes replace eosinophils in upper respiratory infections.
	PMNs with ingested bacteria	Bacterial rhinitis or sinusitis
Serum tests	IgG IgA, IgM	Often normal. May be abnormal— various patterns seen
	IgE	Sometimes elevated in "allergic" asthma; markedly elevated in active bronchopulmonary aspergillosis. Often normal
	Aspergillus-precipitating antibody	Suggestive, not diagnostic of broncho-pulmonary aspergillosis
Sweat test	Normal in asthma	Cystic fibrosis and asthma can coexist
	Perform to rule out cystic fibrosis.	
Chest x-ray	Hyperinflation, infiltrates, pneumo-mediastinum, pneumothorax.	Indicated once in all patients with asthma; should be considered on hospitalization for asthma
Lung function tests	FEV_1, $FEF_{25-75\%}$, PEFR; FEV_1/FVC	Useful for following course of disease, response to treatment
Response to bronchodilators	> 15% improvement FEV_1, PEFR	Safest diagnostic test for asthma
Exercise tests	Decreased lung function after 6 min of exercise.	Useful to diagnose asthma. Often abnormal when resting lung function is normal
	PEFR and FEV_1 >15% $FEF_{25-75\%}$ > 25%	
Methacholine inhalation test (mecholyl test); histamine inhalation test	20% fall in lung function with dose tolerated by "normal" subjects	Should be performed by specialists only
Antigen inhalation test	20% fall in lung function immediately after challenge; may cause delayed response 6–8 h later	Potentially dangerous; should be performed by specialist only
Allergy skin tests	Identifies allergic factors that might be causative factors	Test likely factors only—select by history
Serological tests for IgE antibody (e.g. RAST)	Same significance as skin tests	More expensive than skin tests

[a]From Bierman CW, Shapiro GG, Carr DO, Bush RK, Busse WW. Evaluation and treatment of the patient with asthma. In: Bierman CW, Pearlman DS, Shapiro GG, Busse WW, eds. *Allergic Diseases from Infancy to Adulthood*, ed. 3. Philadelphia, WB Saunders, 1996.

Confirmation of Asthma Diagnosis

- Difficult to confirm below the age of 2 yr because of "wheezing/congestion" associated with viral infection.
- Asthma is a chronic condition; documentation of repeated clinical episodes of respiratory distress, which responds to bronchodilators, is helpful information.
- Office pulmonary function test results are helpful objective information after the age of 5 yr.
- Response to bronchodilators, which document reversible pulmonary obstruction: FEV_1: 15–20%; FEF_{25-75}: 20–25%.
- Exercise tolerance in some cases, and methacholine/histamine challenges in select cases by a specialist may be necessary to confirm diagnosis.

Spirometry involves certain pitfalls, but adequate results generally can be obtained from children over 5 yr of age. The best of three forced expiratory tracings should be used as the best estimate of a patient's pulmonary function. Coaching and teaching are required for the patient to achieve good technique. If the curves that are generated do not fit the clinical picture, one must look at the quality of data entry and technique before assuming that there is lung disease. Spirometry may be expressed with flow-volume curves rather than time-volume curves. Flow-volume loops include a tracing for inspiratory flow. This is helpful for distinguishing extrathoracic from intrathoracic obstruction. When patients are uncooperative or unable to learn proper spirometric technique, body plethysmography can be used, generally available in hospital pulmonary function laboratories.

Response to Bronchodilators

A straighforward diagnostic test for asthma is to look for an improvement in lung function before and after administration of bronchodilators, preferably β-2 agonists (inhalation of two actuations of albuterol or equivalent by pressurized metered-dose inhaler or 0.1–0.15 mg/kg aerosol solution of albuterol [5 mg maximum], or epinephrine injections [epinephrine hydrochloride 1:1000], 0.01 mL/kg up to a maximum dosage 0.3 mL subcutaneously). A greater than 15% improvement in forced expiratory volume in 1 s (FEV_1) is virtually diagnostic of asthma. If there is a lack of improvement in FEV_1, it does not necessarily rule out asthma. With severe airway inflammation, a 1–2 wk course of oral corticosteroids may be necessary to demonstrate a reversible component to airflow obstruction. With mild disease, lung function will be normal unless the patient is experiencing an exacerbation.

Exercise Tolerance Tests

In older children and adolescents, a free-running exercise tolerance test is simple to perform and requires little equipment. One may also use a treadmill in a pulmonary function laboratory. A fall of greater than 15% in FEV_1 and in peak expiratory flow rate (PEFR) or greater than 25% in forced expiratory flow of 25–75% ($FEF_{25-75\%}$) is diagnostic of exercise-induced asthma.

Chemical Challenge Tests

Chemical challenges are valuable for the patients with presumptive asthma and/or chronic cough when baseline pulmonary function is normal and therapeutic trials with anti-asthma medications are inconclusive. Patients with asthma have airways that are overly sensitive to bronchoconstrictors. Methacholine and histamine challenges can be performed with standardized protocols that have high specificity and sensitivity for airway hyperresponsiveness and asthma. Patients inhale increasing concentrations of either of these chemical irritants according to a standardized protocol and perform spirometry after inhaling each concentration of the drug. The challenge is complete when FEV_1 has dropped 20% or more from baseline or when one completes inhalation of a dosage of 25 mg/mL. A decline in FEV_1 of 20% indicates bronchial hyperresponsiveness. When this information is melded with a supporting clinical history, the diagnosis of asthma becomes likely. (On the other hand, a negative challenge usually excludes asthma).

Distilled water inhalation, eucapneic hyperventilation of cold air, and hypertonic water inhalation are alternative challenge procedures. These are less well standardized than methacholine and exercise challenge. Inhalation challenge of specific antigens would seem to offer valuable diagnostic information regarding asthma triggers; however, in practice, antigen challenge has severe limitations. Antigen inhalation may produce bronchospasm in the laboratory while only rhinitis occurs after natural inhalation. Also, late phase reactions are common that may occur after the patient leaves the laboratory. All bronchial challenge tests are potentially dangerous. They should be performed only by specialists who have had special training in their use.

Nasal Cytology

These studies may be helpful in evaluation. The patient blows the nose or coughs into plastic wrap, the secretions are applied to a glass slide, heat fixed, and stained with Hansel's stain, an eosin-methylene blue combination that stains eosinophils distinctively. Alternatively, a tiny nasal brush or rhinoprobe device can be used to obtain a specimen from the wall of the nasal vault. The presence of greater than 5–10% eosinophils indicates probable allergic inflammatory disease but not necessarily asthma. The presence of large numbers of neutrophils and bacteria suggests infection. If the problem has been long-standing, the possibility of subacute or chronic sinusitis that serves to aggravate bronchial hyperresponsiveness should be considered.

Total Serum IgE

Total serum IgE determination may be helpful at times; approximately 80% of children with allergen-induced asthma will have a total serum IgE greater than two standard deviations from the nonallergic population mean. More helpful, however, is evaluation of antigen-specific IgE.

Chest X-Ray Examinations

All patients with asthma should have chest x-ray examinations at some time to rule out parenchymal disease, congenital anomaly, and foreign body. A chest x-ray study should be considered for every patient admitted to a hospital with asthma, depending on the presentation and severity of asthma and any suspicion of complications, such

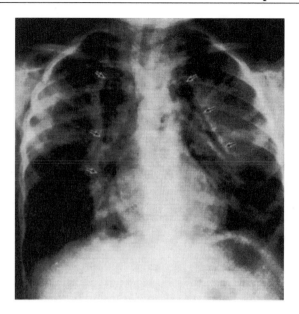

Fig. 1. Massive pneumomediastinum complicating asthma.

as pneumonia and pneumothorax (Fig. 1). Chest x-ray findings in asthma may range from normal to hyperinflation with peribronchial interstitial infiltrate and atelectasis. In a 3-yr study of children hospitalized for asthma (Eggleston 1974), the following abnormalities were seen: 76% had hyperinflation with increased bronchial markings; 20% had infiltrates, atelectasis, pneumonia, or a combination of the three; and 5.4% had pneumomediastinum, often with infiltrates. Pneumothorax occurs rarely and did not occur in this study. Paranasal sinus X-ray studies also should be considered in patients with persistent nocturnal coughing and rhinorrhea.

Allergy Testing

Allergy testing (skin testing or serological testing, such as radioallergosorbent testing [RAST]) is indicated in patients in whom specific allergic factors are believed to be important. Testing is done with extracts of selective allergens based on history and known or potential allergen exposure. Asthma in children is frequently exacerbated by exposure to environmental allergens. In a given patient, the same antigen-specific IgE that can trigger inflammatory events in the airway can be detected in the skin. Antigen applied to the skin reacts with specific mast-cell-bound antibody that induces mediator release. Histamine will create local vasodilation with wheal and flare within 15 min, and a variety of chemotactic factors may create a delayed inflammatory response hours later. Although true positive skin tests indicate that a patient has antigen-specific IgE, it does not prove that exposure will create clinically significant disease. The predictive value of a positive skin test is enhanced if the reactivity is intense and occurs in conjunction with a positive provocative history.

As an alternative to allergen-specific skin tests, serum IgE against a specific antigen can be measured with serological tests such as RAST. In this procedure, antigens are coupled to an inert carrier such as latex or cellulose and mixed with the patient's serum, after which binding of antigen and patient's antibody is measured. In general, RAST is less sensitive and more expensive than skin testing. Its use may be needed in specific situations as when severe skin disease or dermatographism precludes skin testing, or when the subject is taking an agent such as an antihistamine that will suppress skin tests.

THERAPEUTIC CONSIDERATION

Philosophy of Management

A comprehensive approach to treatment of asthma requires an understanding of the disease, the manner in which patients present, and how the disease may affect physical and psychological growth and development. The ultimate goals are to prevent disability and to minimize physical and psychological morbidity. These include facilitating social adjustment of the patient with the family, school, and community, including normal participation in recreational activities and sports. This adjustment is achieved in steps and should begin with early diagnosis and appropriate management of acute episodes. Irritant and allergic factors should be identified and eliminated from the patient's environment. Education of the patient's parents, the patient, or both, to the long-term course of asthma, to the management of exacerbations, and to the importance of ongoing therapy to minimize acute exacerbations is an essential part of asthma treatment. In addition, early intervention with anti-inflammatory therapy may promote remission of disease and prevent chronic changes of airway remodeling.

Achieving these goals requires time, knowledge, and experience. The demands on the physician will vary, depending on the severity of the disease, the age of the patient, and the resources of the patient or family. The family physician or pediatrician who is willing to devote the time can care adequately for the patient with mild or moderate asthma. Allergens and irritants that may be driving this disease should be investigated thoroughly in patients with all forms of asthma. However, the patient with moderate and severe asthma will benefit from referral to an allergist who has the knowledge and experience to modify therapy for special situations, to educate the patient about asthma, to follow the patient's progress, and to act as a co-manager with the primary care physician. Such a referral should help minimize acute attacks and the need for hospitalization or, when hospitalization is necessary, to reduce the length of hospital stay. A team approach that includes regular communication between the primary care physician and the specialist is essential for consistent and comprehensive long-term care.

Compliance by patient, family, or both, is the keystone of any therapy. Compliance is influenced by many factors—the physicians's attitude, the family's and the patient's understanding of the disease, and peer pressure. It is in relation to compliance that psychological factors are of overwhelming importance. The attitude of the patient toward the disease is paramount in his or her willingness to follow the physician's recommendations. The patient's attitude toward asthma and the willingness to comply with recommendations reflect the parents' or peers' attitudes toward the disease. The physician's guidance can prevent overprotection or neglect by helping the family of a younger child to cope with such aspects of asthma as the inconvenience of a

---

Profile of a Child at Risk for Death from Asthma

- Teenager
- Severe asthmatic, requiring daily medication to breathe
- Often from a minority group
- Noncompliant about taking daily, preventive medications
- Significant psychosocial problems in the family

---

medication schedule and environmental control. In older children, the physician should place the responsibility for taking medication on the patient. When medication is needed in school or at play, the patient should be permitted to take it privately without embarrassment. The physician should aid the patient in making decisions on such activities as sports, camping trips, traveling, and other activities when the patient is away from the home environment, while ensuring appropriate control of asthma.

Finally, when a patient fails to comply, the physician should try to learn the reasons and should work out a reasonable solution acceptable to the patient and/or the family. *Noncompliance in the face of severe disease, particularly in an adolescent, places him or her at great risk with regard to both morbidity from the disease and death.*

ENVIRONMENTAL CONTROL

Exposure to allergen and irritants at vulnerable times may significantly increase bronchial reactivity and adversely influence asthma control. The antigens most commonly implicated in chronic asthma are house dust mite, cockroaches, pet-derived antigenic proteins (with cat being the most common) and airborne molds and pollens. While Murray reported on the beneficial influence of bedroom-dust control measures in 1983, subsequent studies add to the information implicating dust mite antigen as a major factor in asthma. Certain environmental efforts are most successful for limiting mite antigen, while others that have been traditionally valued are not particularly helpful.

Dust mites are microscopic creatures that feed on human skin scales, require humidity greater than 50%, and tend to seek darker environments. They are found in carpets, mattresses, and stuffed furniture in homes where the ambient climate is moderate and not too dry. They are not removed by traditional dusting and vacuuming. Encasing mattresses in airtight covers, washing pillows and bedding weekly in hot water (over 130°F), and removing carpeting, particularly if laid on concrete slab floors, will reduce house dust mite levels in the home. The value of acaricides, such as benzyl benzoate, and products that denature mite antigen, such as 3% tannic acid, sprayed on the carpet and stuffed furniture is controversial, and they cannot be recommended with enthusiasm. Measures to reduce humidity to less than 50% will decrease dust mite proliferation. Most physicians concentrate efforts on education that relates to keeping the bedroom and family area as free as possible of house dust mite antigens.

It is unfortunate that pet removal can result in major improvement in asthma symptoms for some highly atopic patients, but that carrying out this removal is so difficult. Families are often unable to deal with the loss of a pet, putting asthma lower on the priority list than other psychosocial issues. If a pet to which a patient is sensitive

Important Environmental Factors in Asthma
Allergens
House dust mite
Cats and dogs
Cockroaches (inner city)
Mold spores
Chemical pollutants
Cigaret smoke
NO_2 (with poor ventilation)
Ozone (outside)

cannot be removed from the home, certain temporizing measures are worthwhile: keeping the pet out of the bedroom and considering an electrostatic or HEPA filter. Studies that have shown that a weekly washing of cats reduces the amount of allergen deposited on carpet and furnishings are now controversial. Many pet antigens are tenacious molecules that travel easily and are difficult to eliminate from the home. The part-time indoor pet may produce the same antigen load as the full-time indoor pet, and it may take months after the pet is removed from the environment for residual allergen to decrease to nonproblematic levels. Also, the chronic inflammatory changes that occur with asthma often prevent patients and families from being able to appreciate improvement in asthma control with a brief period of pet avoidance.

Cockroach antigen is a problem primarily but not exclusively in the eastern and southern United States. Antigen concentration appears to be related in part to lower socioeconomic populations. Cockroach antigen may be more important than dust mite among this population. Attempts at environmental control include removing uncovered food sources and water leaks, exterminating these insects, and repairing squalid and dilapidated conditions that support infestation.

Irritant exposure should also be limited to achieve best asthma control. Exposure to tobacco smoke has been linked to asthma exacerbations, decreased lung growth, and age of onset of asthma. Therefore, smoking in the home should be forbidden. Wood stove heat has been linked to increased emergency room visits for asthma patients and should be avoided in favor of cleaner heating fuels. Atmospheric levels of ozone, SO_2, and NO_2 may be related to asthma exacerbations, though correlations are modest.

The amount of counseling that one offers concerning the environment depends largely on historical issues, level of allergy skin test relativity, and the ability of a family to make changes in their surroundings. The physician should offer firm counseling regarding environmental control if it is pertinent to a specific situation and then show flexibility when there are impasses. This approach is preferable to making an assumption that a family will not deal with avoidance and failing to provide appropriate information.

Home Peak-Flow Monitoring

Another area of management is home peak-flow monitoring, which is important in reviewing overall asthma control. Instruction in peak-flow recording draws the patient or parent in as an active manager of the disease. Home peak-flow monitoring is particularly suited to a subset of patients with asthma: (1) children with fairly severe disease who may not appreciate early deterioration because they do not sense obstruction and hypoxemia; (2) children whose parents are unclear about symptoms and would respond better to objective cues than to vague symptoms; (3) children who are not communicative regarding symptoms; and (4) children who need objective cues to spur compliance with medication regimens. To increase the ease of monitoring, a color-coded system has evolved. A patient's chart contains colored forms in which the green zone means 80–100% of best personal peak-flow rate, yellow is 50–79%, and red is below 50%. The patient is instructed to exercise caution and use supplemental medication when in the yellow zone and to contact the physician for further instructions when in the red zone. Some peak-flow meters are color coded, which aids the subject's assessment.

These nonpharmacological management techniques should be part of an ongoing educational process that involves physician, patient, family, and other health educators such as nurses and respiratory therapists. Education should begin with an explanation of asthma as an inflammatory disease, including an explanation of asthma trigger factors in and outside of the home, and should emphasize environmental control. It should stress the importance of monitoring pulmonary function. Pharmacological intervention should be posed as an important element in the equation of optimal control, but not as the sole desirable intervention.

PHARMACOLOGICAL MANAGEMENT

The goal of pharmacological therapy is to improve pulmonary function and decrease lability to allow patients to have a "normal" life-style and to optimize lung growth. Drugs available in the United States are noted in Table 3. Rarely should patients need to be satisfied with missing school or work time because of asthma limiting physical activity, or sleeping poorly because of nocturnal exacerbations of their disease. This optimal life-style requires compliance with medication as well as avoidance of environmental trigger factors.

The National Heart, Lung, and Blood Institute has supported guidelines for the management of asthma that serve as an excellent foundation for treatment today. These guidelines stress the concept of inflammation in asthma and suggest that patients who require bronchodilator therapy more than twice a week for nonexercise-related asthma should have long-term anti-inflammatory therapy. A schematic view (Tables 4 and 5) of a step-wise approach to asthma care describes the ascent from simple bronchodilator to the use of nonsteroidal or steroidal anti-inflammatory medication, depending on disease severity.

APPROACHES TO CARE

Treatment of Acute Asthma

An acute exacerbation of asthma poses an urgent medical problem as noted in Fig. 2. The best strategy for management is early recognition. Evaluation and treatment decrease worsening and abort further exacerbation and respiratory compromise. Early recognition by the patient and prompt communication between the patient and the health care provider are essential components of the process, allowing the physician to modify the individual patient's medication regimen and control the asthma more effectively.

The intensity of the acute attack and its outcome are influenced by a number of factors: (1) the patient's age; (2) the duration of the episode; (3) a history of previous life-threatening asthma exacerbations requiring hospitalization, intubation, and intensive care, or complications secondary to hypoxia: (4) recent and frequent emergency room visits, and (5) either systemic corticosteroid usage or recent withdrawal from corticosteroids.

Each patient should have available and be familiar with a "plan of action" to follow for acute asthma exacerbations. Peak-flow measurements by the patient are important in this early assessment process and provide a more precise quantitation of airflow obstruction. The basic goal of treatment is to achieve rapid reversal of airflow obstruction. The first line of therapy in this setting is repetitive inhalation of β-2 agonists. Poor or minimal response to β-2 adrenergic agonists is an indication for an emergent evaluation by medical personnel. Parents or patients should be instructed to administer a β-agonist, for example albuterol, either by nebulizer at 0.1 mg/kg/dose (5 mg maximum) or two actuations of a metered-dose inhaler. If the patient's asthma is stable, these regimens can be repeated every 20 min up to three times. If the initial response to treatment is good, based on PEFR $\geq$ 70% of the patient's personal best, then the β-agonist should be continued every 3–4 h along with routine medications. If the patient responds only partially, he or she or the parent should contact the health care provider without further delay, who could initiate oral prednisone therapy at 1–2 mg/kg/dose and arrange for the patient to be seen in an emergent care setting. A β-2 agonist may be given up to every 2 h over the next 6 h.

When a patient with acute asthma is being cared for in the emergency room or clinic, the interaction should begin with a quickly obtained pertinent history and physical examination. It is important to ascertain relevant environmental exposures and infectious triggers such as otitis and sinusitis.

Physical examination often reveals wheezing, accessory muscle use, and tachycardia, These findings are helpful to confirm the diagnosis of acute asthma; unfortunately, they do not reliably indicate the severity of the asthma episode. In the child under 3 yr, one may hear only coughing or signs of croup. Objective measurements include pulmonary functions, such as spirometry or peak expiratory flow rate. In severe asthma with lung function less than 50% of predicted normal and in young children with severe symptoms in whom peak flow cannot be obtained, one should attempt pulse oximetry or arterial blood gas measurements.

Early administration of oral or systemic corticosteroids should allow for more rapid improvement of pulmonary function. During treatment, close monitoring of the patient, with repeated measures of lung function, is essential for optimal management of the exacerbation and directions for changes in therapy. Supplemental oxygen should be administered to keep oxygen saturation above 95%. Nebulized albuterol should be administered at 0.15 mg/kg/dose every 20 min (maximum 5 mg/dose) for up to an hour. Ipratropium aerosol solution 0.25 mg can be added to nebulized albuterol in patients with poor response to albuterol alone. This combination therapy has been shown to decrease hospitalization. Prednisone at a loading dose of 1–2 mg/kg should be administered orally. If the patient responds well, β-agonist therapy should continue every 4 h until symptoms and peak flow measurements show that the patient has reached

(text continues on page 111)

Table 3
Long-Term Controller Medications: Management of Chronic Asthma[a]

Cromolyn sodium/nedocromil sodium

Generic name	Brand name(s)	Dosage form(s)	Dose[b]	Potential adverse effects and therapeutic issues
Cromolyn sodium	Intal®	MDI: 1 mg/puff Nebulizer solution: 20 mg/ampule	1–2 puffs, t.i.d.—q.i.d. 1 ampule, t.i.d.—q.i.d.	Therapeutic response to cromolyn and nedocromil often occurs within 2 wk, but a 4–6-wk trial may be needed to determine maximum benefit. Dose of cromolyn MDI (1 mg/puff) may be inadequate to affect airway hyperresponsiveness. Nebulizer delivery (20 mg/ampule) may be preferred for some children. Safety is the primary advantage of these agents.
Nedocromil sodium	Tilade®	MDI: 1.75 mg/puff	1–2 puffs, b.i.d., q.i.d.	Unpleasant taste for some children

[a]From expert Panel Guidelines for Management of Asthma. NIH, NHLBI, 1997.
[b]These doses are suggested as guides for making clinical decisions. The clinician must use judgment to tailor treatment to the specific needs and circumstances of the child and family.

Long-Term Controller Medications: Inhaled Corticosteroids

Generic name	Brand name(s)	Dosage form(s)	Dose[c] Low	Dose[c] Medium	Dose[c] High	Potential adverse effects and therapeutic issues
Beclomethasone dipropionate	Beclovent™, Vanceril®, Vanceril Double Strength®	MDI: 42 µg/puff MDI: 84 µg/puff	2–8 puffs/d 1–4 puffs/d	8–16 puffs/d 4–8 puffs/d	> 16 puffs/d > 8 puffs/d	*For all inhaled steroids:* Cough, dysphonia, moniliasis; high doses may have systemic effects although studies are not conclusive and clinical significance is not clear. Monitoring growth is recommended.
Budesonide	Pulmicort Turbuhaler®	DPI: 200 µg/puff	1 puff/d	1–2 puffs/d	> 2 puffs/d	The potential risks of inhaled steroids are well balanced by their benefits.
	Pulmicort Respules™d	Nebulizing suspension: 0.125 mg/mL 0.25 mg/mL 0.50 mg/mL per 2 mL respule	0.50 mg/d	1.0 mg/d	2.0 mg/d	
Flunisolide	AeroBid®, AeroBid M®	MDI: 250 µg/puff	2–3 puffs/d	4–5 puffs/d	> 5 puffs/d	To minimize local and systemic adverse events, use a spacer/holding chamber.
Fluticasone propionate	Flovent®	MDI: 44 µg/puff 110 µg/puff 220 µg/puff DPI: 50 µg/puff 100 µg/puff 250 mcg/puff	2–4 puffs/d — — 2–4 puffs/d 1–2 puffs/d —	4–10 puffs/d 2–4 puffs/d 1–2 puffs/d — 2–4 puffs/d 1–2 puffs/d	— > 4 puffs/d > 2 puffs/d — > 4 puffs/d > 2 puffs/d	
Triamcinolone acetonide	Azmacort®	MDI: 100 µg/puff	4–8 puffs/d	8–12 puffs/d	>12 puffs/d	

[c] These doses are suggested as guides for making clinical decisions. The clinician must use judgment to tailor treatment to the specific needs and circumstances of the patient and family.
[d] Not available in the United States at the time of writing.

Table 3 (*Cont.*)

Long-Term Controller Medication: Methylxanthines

Generic name	Brand name(s)	Dosage form(s)	Dose[e]	Potential adverse effects and therapeutic issues
Theophylline	Aerolate® III Aerolate® Jr Aerolate® Sr Choledyl® SA Elixophyllin® Quibron®-T Quibron®-T/SR Slo-bid ® Slo-phyllin® Theo-24® Theochron® Theo-Dur® Theolair® Theolair®-SR T-Phyl® Uni-Dur® Uniphyl®	Capsules, tablets	Starting dose: 10 mg/kg/d. Maximal dose: < 1 yr old: (0.2 × age in wk) + 5 mg/kg/d Maximal dose: ≥ 1 yr old: 16 mg/kg/d, not to exceed the adult maximum (800 mg/d)	Tachycardia, nausea, vomiting, headache, CNS stimulation Monitoring serum levels (5–15 µg/mL) is essential to ensure therapeutic, but not toxic, doses are achieved. Serum levels may be affected by numerous factors (diet, febrile illness, other medications).

[e]These doses are suggested as guides for making clinical decisions. The clinician must use judgment to tailor treatment to the specific needs and circumstances of the child and family.

Long-Term Controller Medications: Long-Acting Bronchodilators

Generic name	Brand name(s)	Dosage form(s)	Dose[f]	Potential adverse effects and therapeutic issues
Salmeterol	Serevent®	MDI: 21 µg/puff DPI: 50 µg/blister	1–2 puffs, bid 1 blister, bid	Tachycardia, tremor. The clinical relevance of potential diminished bronchoprotective effect is uncertain. *DO NOT USE* in place of anti-inflammatory therapy!
Sustained-release albuterol	Volmax® Proventil Repetabs®	Tablet: 4 mg	0.3–0.6 mg/kg/d, not to exceed 8 mg/d, bid	Tachycardia, tremor, irritability
Theophylline[g]	Aerolate® III Aerolate® Jr Aerolate® Sr Choledyl® SA Elixophyllin® Quibron®-T Quibron®-T/SR Slo-bid® Slo-phyllin® Theo-24® Theochron® Theo-Dur® Theolair® Theolair®-SR T-Phyl® Uni-Dur® Uniphyl®	Capsules, tablets	Starting dose: 10 mg/kg/d Maximal dose: < 1 yr old[h]: (0.2 age in wk) + 5 mg/kg/d Maximal dose: ≥1 yr old: 16 mg/kg/d, not to exceed the adult maximum (800 mg/d)	Tachycardia, nausea, vomiting, headache, CNS stimulation Monitoring serum levels (5–15 µg/mL) is essential to ensure therapeutic, but not toxic, doses are achieved. Serum levels may be affected by numerous factors (diet, febrile illness, other medications).

[f] These doses are suggested as guides for making clinical decisions. The clinician must use judgment to tailor treatment to the specific needs and circumstances of the child and family.

[g] Sustained-release theophylline may be considered an alternative, but not preferred, long-term controller medication when issues arise related to cost, adherence, or ability to use inhaled medications.

[h] Sustained release theophylline may have particular risks of adverse effects in infants, who frequently have febrile illnesses that increase theophylline levels. Consider theophylline for infants only if serum levels will be carefully monitored.

Table 3 (*Cont.*)

Quick Relief Medications: Short-Acting Inhaled β₂-Agonists

Generic name	Brand name(s)	Dosage form(s)	Dose [i]	Potential adverse effects and therapeutic issues
Albuterol	Airet® Proventil® Ventolin®	MDI: 90 µg/puff	1–2 puffs, 5–10 min before exercise 2 puffs, tid–qid, prn	*For all short-acting β-agonists:* Tremor, tachycardia, headache
		Nebulizer solution: 5 mg/mL (0.5%); 0.083% (unit dose[j]) containing 2.5 mg	0.05 mg/kg (min: 1.25 mg; max: 2.5 mg)	**NOTE:** Increasing use of short-acting β-agonists, use of >1 canister/mo, or lack of expected effect, indicates inadequate asthma control. See doctor to increase or add long-term controller medication(s).
	Proventil® HFA			
	Ventolin® Rotacaps	MDI: 90 µg/puff	2 puffs, tid–qid, prn	
		DPI: 200 µg/capsule	1 capsule, 5–10 min before exercise 1 capsule tid–qid, prn	
Bitolterol	Tornalate®	MDI[k]: 370 µg/puff	1–2 puffs, 5–10 min before exercise 2 puffs, tid–qid, prn	
Pirbuterol	Maxair®	MDI: 200 µg/puff	1–2 puffs, 5–10 min before exercise 2 puffs, tid–qid, prn	
Terbutaline	Brethaire®	MDI: 200 µg/puff	1–2 puffs, 5–10 min before exercise 2 puffs, tid–qid, prn	

[i] The doses are suggested as guides for making clinical decisions. The clinician must use judgment to tailor treatment to the specific needs and circumstances of the child and family.

[j] Do not use partial unit dose.

[k] Also available as a nebulizer solution (2 mg/mL = 0.2%), but a children's dose has not been established.

Table 3 (Cont.)

Quick-Relief Medications: Short-Acting Inhaled β₂-Agonists

Generic name	Brand name(s)	Dosage form(s)	Dose[1]	Potential adverse effects and therapeutic issues
Levo-albuterol	Xopenex®	Nebulizer solution: Unit dose vials: 0.63 mg/ 3 mL 1.25 mg/ 3 mL	0.63 mg tid for maintenance 1.25 mg tid for acute bronchospasm and for children unresponsive to lower dose	*For all short-acting β-agonists:* Tremor, tachycardia, headache. *Note:* Increasing use of short-acting β-agonists, use of > 1 canister/mo, or lack of effect indicates inadequate asthma control. See doctor to increase or add long-term controller medication(s).

[1]These doses are suggested as guides for making clinical decisions. The clinician must use judgment to tailor treatment to the specific needs and circumstances of the child and family.

Quick Relief Medications: Oral Corticosteroids

Generic name	Brand name(s)	Dosage form(s)	Dose[m]	Potential adverse effects and therapeutic issues
Methylprednisolone	Medrol®	Tablet: 2, 4, 6, 8, 16, 32 mg	Short-course (3- to 10-d) "burst:" 1–2 mg/kg/d (max: 60 mg/d)[n]	*For all oral steroids:* Long-term use is associated with systemic effects. Use at lowest effective dose either daily or on alternate days (which may lessen adrenal suppression). Short courses or "bursts" are effective for establishing control when initiating therapy or during a period of gradual deterioration.
Prednisolone	Prelone® Pediapred®	Tablet: 5 mg Liquid: 15 mg/5 mL; Liquid: 5 mg/5 mL	Short-course course (3- to 10-d) "burst:"; 1–2 mg/kg/d (max: 60 mg/d)[n]	Short-term therapy should continue until child achieves 80% PEF personal best, or until symptoms resolve (usually within 3–10 days, but may take longer). There is no evidence that tapering the dose following improvement prevents relapse.
Prednisone	Prednisone Deltasone® Orasone® Liquid Pred® Prednisone Intensol®	Tablet: 1, 2.5, 5, 10, 20, 25 mg Liquid: 5 mg/5 mL; Liquid: 5 mg/mL	Short-course course (3- to 10-d) "burst:"; 1–2 mg/kg/d (max: 60 mg/d)[n]	

[m] These doses are suggested as guides for making clinical decisions. The clinician must use judgment to tailor treatment to the specific needs and circumstances of the child and family.

[n] A course of 7 d or less is usually sufficient. In some cases, the exacerbation may require up to 10 d of treatment.

Table 3 (Cont.)

Quick-Relief Medications: Anticholinergics

Generic name	Brand name(s)	Dosage form(s)	Dose [o]	Potential adverse effects and therapeutic issues
Ipratropium bromide	Atrovent®	MDI: 18 µg/puff Nebulizer solution: 0.25 mg/mL (0.025%)	1–2 puffs every 6 h 0.25 mg every 6 h	Dry mouth, increased wheezing in some children. May provide additive effect(s) to short-acting β-₂-agonist.

[o] These doses are suggested as guides for making clinical decisions. The clinician must use judgment to tailor treatment to the specific needs and circumstances of the child and family.

New Medications [p]: Long-Term Controller Medications

Generic name	Brand name(s)	Dosage form(s)	Dose [q]	Potential adverse effects and therapeutic issues
Nedocromil sodium	Tilade®	Nebulizer solution	1 ampule, bid–qid	Unpleasant taste for some children

[p] Not available in the U.S. at the time of writing, but pending approval by the FDA.
[q] These doses are suggested as guides for making clinical decisions. The clinician must use judgment to tailor treatment to the specific needs and circumstances of the child and family.

Inhaled corticosteroids

Generic name	Brand name(s)	Dosage form(s)	Dose[r]			Potential adverse effects and therapeutic issues
			Low	Medium	High	
Mometasone furoate	Asmanex®	DPI: 200 µg/puff DPI: 400 µg/puff	2 puffs/d to initiate Tx 1 puff/d for maintenance	2 puffs/d to initiate Tx 1 puff/d for maintenance	2 puffs/d	FOR ALL INHALED STEROIDS: Cough, dysphonia, moniliasis; high doses may have systemic effects although studies are not conclusive and clinical significance is not clear.
Budesonide	Pulmicort Respules™ d	Nebulizing suspension: 0.125 mg/mL 0.25 mg/mL 0.50 mg/mL per 2 mL respule	0.50 mg/d	1.0 mg/d	2.0 mg/d	The potential risks of inhaled steroids are well balanced by their benefits. To minimize local and systemic adverse events, use a spacer/holding chamber.

[r]These doses are suggested as guides for making clinical decisions. The clinician must use judgment to tailor treatment to the specific needs and circumstances of the child and family.

Leukotriene Modifiers

Generic name	Brand name(s)	Dosage form(s)	Dose[s]	Potential adverse effects and therapeutic issues
Montelukast	Singulair®	Tablet: 5 mg, chewable, for ages 6–14 yr; 10 mg for ages >14 yr Tablet: 4 mg chewable, for ages 2–5 yr	1 tablet in evening	Data about adverse effects in children are limited. Increased clinical experience and further study in a wide range of children are needed to determine those children most likely to benefit from leukotriene modifiers and to establish a more specific role for these medications in asthma therapy.
Zafirlukast	Accolate®	Tablet: 20 mg, for ages ≥7 yr	1 tablet, bid	Data about adverse effects in children are limited. Increased clinical experience and further study in a wide range of children are needed to determine those children most likely to benefit from leukotriene modifiers andto establish a more specific role for these medications in asthma therapy. Take 1 h before or 2 h after meals; drug interactions (warfarin); increases prothrombin time.
Zileuton	Zyflo®	Tablet: 600 mg, for ages ≥12 yr	1 tablet, qid	Data about adverse effects in children are limited. Increased clinical experience and further study in a wide range of children are needed to determine those children most likely to benefit from leukotriene modifiers and to establish a more specific role for these medications in asthma therapy. Possible elevation of liver enzymes requires monitoring; drug interactions (terfenadine, warfarin, theophylline).

[s] These doses are suggested as guides for making clinical decisions. The clinician must use judgment to tailor treatment to the specific needs and circumstances of the child and family.

Table 4
Stepwise Asthma Management in Infants and Young Children ($\leq$ 5 Years of age)[a]

	Long-Term Control	Quick Relief
Step 4 Severe Persistent	Daily anti-inflammatory medications: • High-dose inhaled corticosteroid with spacer/holding chamber and face mask AND • If needed, add systemic corticosteroids 2 mg/kg/day and reduce to lowest daily or alternate-day dose that stabilizes symptoms	• Short-acting bronchodilator as needed for symptoms Intensity of treatment depends on severity of exacerbation. • Either: inhaled short-acting β_2-agonist by nebulizer or spacer/holding chamber and face mask. OR oral β_2-agonist **Increasing use indicates need for additional controller therapy.**

Step 3
Moderate
Persistent
	Daily anti-inflammatory medications:
	• Anti-inflammatory
	• Either:
	medium-dose inhaled corticosteroid with spacer/holding chamber and face mask
	   OR once control is established,
	low to medium-dose inhaled corticosteroid and nedocromil
	   OR
	low to medium-dose inhaled corticosteroid and long-acting bronchodilator (theophylline)
		• Short-acting bronchodilator as needed for symptoms
		Intensity of treatment depends on severity of exacerbation.
		• Either:
		inhaled short-acting β_2-agonist by nebulizer or spacer/holding chamber and face mask
		OR
		oral β_2-agonist
		Increasing use indicates need for additional controller therapy.

Step 2 Mild Persistent	Daily anti-inflammatory medications: • Either: Cromolyn (nebulizer preferred, or MDI) or nedocromil (MDI) tid-qid • Infants and young children usually begin with a trial of cromolyn or nedocromil. OR low-dose inhaled corticosteroid with spacer/holding chamber and face mask	• Short-acting bronchodilator as needed for symptoms Intensity of treatment depends on severity of exacerbation. • Either: inhaled short-acting β_2-agonist by nebulizer or spacer/holding chamber and face mask OR oral β_2-agonist **Increasing use indicates need for additional controller therapy.**
Step 1 Intermittent	• No daily medication.	• Short-acting bronchodilator as needed for symptoms <2x/wk. Intensity of treatment depends upon severity of exacerbation. • Either: inhaled short-acting β_2-agonist by nebulizer or spacer/holding chamber and face mask OR oral β_2-agonist **Increasing use indicates need for additional controller therapy.**
	Step Down Review treatment every 1–6 months; a gradual stepwise reduction in treatment may be possible.	**Step Up** If control is not maintained, consider step up. First, review patient medication technique, adherence, and avoidance of allergens and/or other factors that contribute to asthma severity.

[a]From Expert Panel Guidelines for Management of Asthma. NIH, NHLBI, 1997.

Table 5
Stepwise Asthma Management in Children >5 Years[a]

	Long-Term Control	Quick Relief
Step 4 Severe Persistent	Daily medications: High-dose inhaled corticosteroid AND Long-acting bronchodilator: either (e.g., long-acting inhaled β_2-agonist, sustained- release theophylline) AND Corticosteroid tablets or syrup long-term (2mg/kg/day, generally do not exceed 60 mg/d)	Short-acting bronchodilator: inhaled β_2-agonist as needed for symptoms Intensity of treatment depends on severity of exacerbation. **Daily or increasing use of short-acting inhaled β_2-agonist indicates need for additional long-term controller therapy.**

Step 3
Moderate
Persistent
	Daily medication:
	Either
	   Medium dose inhaled corticosteroid
	   OR
	low-medium dose inhaled
	corticosteroid plus a long-acting
	bronchodilator, especially for
	nighttime symptoms (e.g., long-acting
	inhaled β_2-agonist, sustained-release theophylline)
	If needed, medium-high dose
	inhaled corticosteroids and long-acting bronchodilator, especially
	for nighttime symptoms.
		Short-acting bronchodilator: inhaled
		β_2-agonist as needed for symptoms
		Intensity of treatment depends on
		severity of exacerbation.
		Daily or increasing use of short-acting inhaled β_2-agonist indicates need for additional long-term controller therapy.

Step 2
Mild Persistent
	One daily medication:
	Either:
	   Low-dose inhaled corticosteroid
	   OR
	Cromolyn or nedocromil (children
	usually begin with a trial of cromolyn
	or nedocromil)
	Sustained-release theophylline (to
	serum concentration of 5–15
	μg/mL) is an alternative, but not
	preferred, therapy.
	A leukotriene modifier may be
	considered although their position
	in therapy is not fully established.
		Short-acting bronchodilator: inhaled
		β_2-agonist as needed for symptoms
		Intensity of treatment depends on
		severity of exacerbation.
		Daily or increasing use of short-acting inhaled β_2-agonists indicates need for additional long-term controller therapy.

Step 1 Mild Intermittent	No daily medication needed	Short-acting bronchodilator: inhaled β_2-agonist as needed for symptoms Intensity of treatment depends on severity of exacerbation. **Daily or increasing use of short-acting inhaled β_2-agonist indicates need for additional long-term controller therapy.**

Step Down	**Step Up**
Review treatment every 1–6 months; a gradual stepwise reduction in treatment may be possible.	If control is not maintained, consider step up. First, review patient medication technique, adherence, and environmental control (avoidance of allergens and/or other factors that contribute to asthma severity).

[a]From Expert Panel Guidelines for Management of Asthma. NIH, NHLBI, 1997.

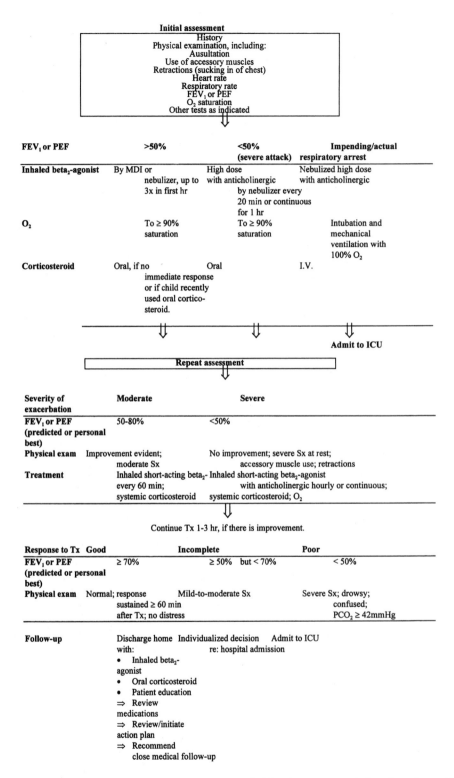

Fig. 2. Management of chronic asthma (from NIH, NHLBI, Management of chronic asthma, 1997).

Triggers of Acute Asthma in Children

- Viral infections
- Weather changes (especially in the fall and spring)
- Exercise
- Allergen exposure
- Irritant exposure (e.g., cigaret smoke)
- Emotional Upset

---

his or her normal baseline, but it can be administered every 1–2 hr if lung function continues to be poor until the response to prednisone is evident. The patient should continue prednisone therapy for at least 4–10 d to ensure adequate anti-inflammatory benefit. While some physicians will give the same total prednisone dose daily for 4 d, others will recommend a tapering dose over 4–10 d. Prednisone can be used as a single morning dose or can be divided during the day. However, the initial loading should be administered as a single dose. Patients with peak flow rates between 40 and 70% of baseline and O_2 saturation between 91 and 95% should be observed for several hours to assess response. The more severe the obstruction, the longer the patient needs to be watched. If the patient continues to demonstrate severe symptoms, if poor peak flow rate continues (<40% of predicted), or if O_2 saturation is diminished (<91%) in room air, hospitalization should be considered. Clinical findings such as the use of accessory muscles, presence of pulsus paradoxus, and increasing dyspnea or cyanosis indicate need for hospitalization.

As an alternative to nebulizer therapy, epinephrine 1 : 1000 can be injected subcutaneously (0.01 mL/kg up to 0.3 mL) and repeated every 15–20 min for up to three treatments, along with supplemental oxygen. This therapy is adequate but involves the pain of injections and cardiovascular side effects of epinephrine that are often unpleasant.

Acute Severe Asthma in Children Requiring Hospitalization

If hospitalized because of poor response, the child should be managed in a facility where vital signs and overall condition can be monitored closely. The PEFR, O_2 saturation, and degree of dyspnea should be assessed frequently. Generally, if the peak flow is above 30% of predicted and the O_2 saturation is above 90% off of oxygen, the child with moderate dyspnea can be observed in an intermediate unit.

Children with more severe airways obstruction should be admitted to an intensive care unit and should have arterialized or arterial blood gases assessed. Supplemental oxygen should be continued, and nebulized albuterol and possibly ipratropium should be administered every 15–60 min as necessary with the administration of intravenous fluids. However, it is important not to overload the patient with fluids because of the danger of causing pulmonary edema. Further doses of systemic corticosteroids should be administered as oral prednisone or iv methylprednisolone or equivalent at 1–2 mg/kg/dose every 6 h. For the patient who is slow to respond, use of iv aminophylline may be considered, though the benefit of this in children is now controversial. A loading dose of 6 mg/kg over 20 min followed by a continuous infusion of 0.9 mg/kg/h may be administered. The loading dose should be eliminated or reduced substantially if the patient has been maintained on therapeutic levels of theophylline pending determination of a stat theophylline serum level. Theophylline serum concentration should be obtained 1½ h after the loading dose, several hours later, and then as indicated by the patient's course, and should be maintained at peak concentrations of less than 15 µg/mL.

If the patient fails to improve, and there are signs of respiratory failure, such as PEFR less than 25% of predicted, pCO_2 greater than 45 mmHg, and a falling pH value, continuous nebulization of a β_2-agonist should be considered. It should be noted that patients with severe asthma usually have CO_2 tensions less than 35 mm Hg. Intravenous terbutaline and mechanical ventilation should be considered in the child with rapidly rising pCO_2 or persistent hypercarbia. Antibiotics should be used only when there are signs of bacterial infection. Sedatives should be avoided, and food and fluid should be given by mouth only when the patient is no longer at risk of requiring mechanical ventilation.

As the child improves, preparation for hospital discharge should include a medication plan with emphasis on long-term medication and a short course of prednisone. Peak-flow monitoring at home should be continued, and a follow-up clinic visit should be planned for shortly after discharge.

COMPLICATIONS OF SEVERE ASTHMA

Complications of asthma may be pulmonary or extrapulmonary. Pulmonary complications include (1) acute respiratory failure, (2) atelectasis, (3) pneumomediastinum and pneumothorax, and (4) superimposed infections (pneumonia, emphysema). Extrapulmonary complications include (1) vasopressin excess, (2) hypokalemia, (3) flaccid paralysis of an arm or leg, (4) sudden alteration in theophylline metabolism with toxicity, (5) cardiac arrhythmia, (6) hypoxic brain damage and hypoxic seizures, and (7) death. Pulmonary and extrapulmonary factors may combine to cause acute respiratory failure, resulting in brain damage or death.

Pulmonary Complications

RESPIRATORY FAILURE

Respiratory failure occurs in a small but significant number of patients admitted to the hospital with status asthmaticus. It often is the result of failure by the physician, patient, or family to recognize the severity of the patient's asthma. Clinical signs of overt respiratory failure include decrease in or absence of pulmonary breath sounds, severe intercostal retractions, pulsus paradoxus, use of accessory muscles of respiration, cyanosis with treatment with a final oxygen concentration (FiO_2) of 40%, reduced response to pain, poor skeletal muscle tone, and profuse diaphoresis. The use of accessory muscles of respiration, as previously noted, is one of the early signs of respiratory failure.

These signs indicate an extreme emergency and mandate immediate treatment for acute respiratory failure.

Arterial blood gas tension and pH must be monitored frequently in a distressed patient. Impending respiratory failure cannot be diagnosed from clinical signs alone. For example, a rise of $PaCO_2$ from 39 to 44 mmHg in 1 h in an exhausted patient who is receiving maximal therapy should be considered progressive respiratory failure and treated as discussed previously.

ATELECTASIS

Up to one third of all hospitalized asthmatic children have had pulmonary complications, such as pneumonia and atelectasis, and 20% have had pulmonary infiltrates involving multiple lobes. Perihilar interstitial infiltrates will vary in severity from increased bronchovascular markings to shaggy, diffuse peribronchial viral pneumonia. Atelectasis of all or part of a lobe, the next most common complication, will occur in 10% of admissions. The right middle lobe is most frequently involved because of anatomical factors, e.g., the right mainstem bronchus tends to twist with hyperinflation, resulting in its partial occlusion. Why right middle-lobe atelectasis develops more frequently in girls than in boys is not clear.

The treatment of atelectasis should be conservative. In most cases it will resolve when the asthma is controlled. Respiratory therapy consisting of postural drainage and clapping as tolerated clinically is helpful. Intermittent positive pressure breathing (IPPB) therapy should be avoided, since it is likely to induce pneumomediastinum or pneumothorax. If atelectasis persists, the presence of a foreign body, an anatomical defect, or an obstructing peribronchial lymph node should be considered. Fiberoptic bronchoscopy may be useful if a foreign body is suspected.

PNEUMOMEDIASTINUM AND PNEUMOTHORAX

In status asthmaticus, 5% of patients may develop extrapulmonary air. Shearing forces, from coughing and bronchospasm, superimposed on hyperinflation also related to atelectasis or pneumonia and possible structural weakness, cause air to rupture alveolar bases and to dissect along blood vessel sheaths (Fig. 3). These effects result in pulmonary interstitial emphysema. It manifests as a worsening clinical course associated with reduced venous return, cardiac output, and blood pressure. Air dissects along the great vessel sheaths to the mediastinum and pericardium and along the aorta to the intestinal wall or along the facial planes into the neck (Fig. 3). While this air remains under high pressure, asthma symptoms worsen and precardiac dullness disappears. Air may escape into the relatively low pressure subcutaneous tissue of the neck and axilla, resulting in crepitant subcutaneous emphysema.

Rarely, pneumothorax complicates childhood asthma. It may be self-limited if small, or tension pneumothorax can occur that may severely compromise breathing. Bilateral pneumothorax can be the cause of sudden death in asthma. Tension pneumothorax that results from rupture of a pleural bleb needs decompression with a chest tube and underwater suction (Fig. 4). A pneumothorax secondary to air rupturing through parietal pleura into the pleural space from a pneumomediastinum is less serious and may be treated conservatively. Often it will clear with treatment of the asthma.

Extrapulmonary Complications

VASOPRESSIN EXCESS (INAPPROPRIATE ADH SECRETION)

The release of ADH is regulated through mechanisms such as (1) pain, fear, and drugs acting on higher central nervous system centers; (2) drops in arterial pressure; (3) increases in plasma concentration (>280 mosM/L) of nondiffusible solute perfusing the hypothalamus, and (4) decreases in stimulation of stretch receptors in the left atrium.

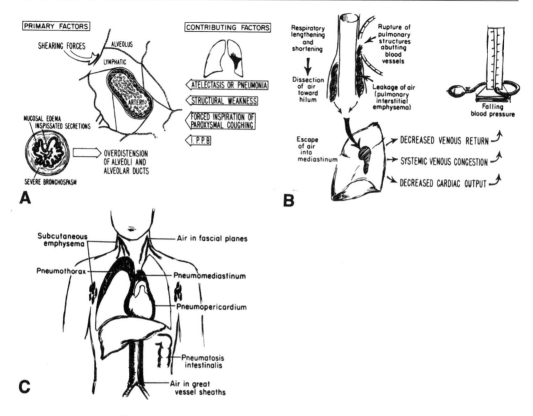

Fig. 3. Mechanism of pneumomediastinum in acute asthma.

When filling of the left atrium is reduced, the vagus nerve stimulates the hypothalamus to secrete vasopressin. In severe asthma, vasopressin levels are elevated regardless of the serum sodium concentrations, apparently because of the effect of severe asthma on the pulmonary circulation. Vasopressin levels fall as the patient improves.

Criteria for the diagnosis of vasopressin excess are as follows:

1. Hyponatremia that is associated with plasma hypo-osmolarity
2. Continuing renal excretion of sodium in presence of hyponatremia
3. Absence of any evidence of dehydration
4. Urinary osmolality value that is greater than plasma osmolality value
5. Normal kidney and adrenal function.

The treatment of excessive vasopressin involves three general principles. (1) Severe asthma must be corrected with appropriate therapy. (2) Water intake and body weight, plasma electrolyte concentration and osmolarity, and urine volume and osmolality must be monitored closely; fluid intake should be restricted to the minimal amount compatible with control of asthma. (3) Complications such as water intoxication with seizures should be treated with hypertonic saline and furosemide. Hypertonic saline and furosemide are rarely needed if the underlying asthma is treated successfully.

HYPOKALEMIA

Both aggressive dosing with β-agonists and corticosteroids have been associated with hypokalemia. This should be considered in the patient who requires prolonged

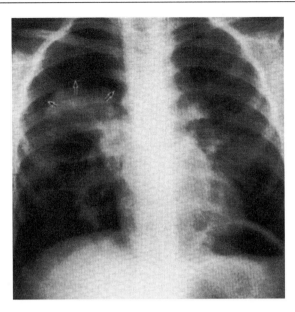

Fig. 4. Pneumothorax secondary to paroxysmal coughing in asthma.

intensive care. The presence of arrhythmia and muscle fatigue should certainly bring this possibility to mind.

NEUROMYOPATHY

In 1974, Hopkins reported 10 children with flaccid paralysis after acute asthma severe enough to require hospitalization. The paralysis developed during the recovery phase from asthma, and all had been immunized for poliomyelitis. In all patients, paralysis was permanent and involved one arm or one leg. To date, over 20 children with this syndrome from Australia, England, Sweden, and the United States have been reported in the medical literature, including one case of areflexic tetraplegia in a 10-yr-old girl. Severe myopathy appears to be an element in some but not all of these pediatric cases as well as in several cases involving adults. Transient phrenic nerve paralysis also has been reported in status asthmaticus, possibly as a complication of assisted ventilation.

CARDIORESPIRATORY ARREST WITH BRAIN DAMAGE

Permanent hypoxic brain damage due to cardiorespiratory arrest can be a complication of severe asthma and is particularly unfortunate because it is preventable with appropriate therapy. In the majority of these patients, it has been the result of the parent's or the physician's failure to recognize the severity of asthma and to institute appropriate therapy.

DEATH

Table 6 lists the causes of death associated with asthma in children. Most are potentially preventable and can be avoided with appropriate education and treatment. Nevertheless, patients with a history of assisted ventilation and severe psychosocial dysfunction are at risk of death even when optimal care appears to be in place.

Table 6
Causes of Death from Asthma[a]

Failure of physician or patient to appreciate severity
    Lack of objective measurements
    Lack of intensified therapy
Inappropriate therapy given:
    Too late because of delay by patient of physician
    Too little (e.g., low steroid dose or recent discontinuation)
    Too much (e.g., β agonists, theophylline, sedative abuse)
Progressive unresponsive asthma
Prolonged attack
Pulmonary complications
    Infection (often undiagnosed)
    Pneumothorax
    Barotrauma
    Aspirations of gastric contents
    Malfunction of ventilator
Cardiac complications
    Arrhythmias
    Hypotension
    Myocardial toxicity
    Sudden cardiac arrest
Underlying cardiopulmonary disease
Hemodynamic
    Hypovolemia, shock
    Pulmonary edema

[a]Mansmann HC Jr, Bierman CW, Pearlman DS. Treatment of acute asthma in children. In: Bierman CW, Pearlman DS, eds. *Allergic Diseases from Infancy to Adulthood*, ed. 2. Philadelphia, WB Saunders, 1988, pp. 571–586.

MANAGEMENT OF CHRONIC ASTHMA

It is important to recognize that chronic asthma may not be obvious in its presentation. Although there may be recurrent episodes of wheezing and shortness of breath, the presentation may be more subtle. Chronic cough may be the sole manifestation of asthma. When cough persists after each upper respiratory infection and when exercise tolerance diminishes markedly with each infection, asthma is a consideration. Patients may complain of exercise intolerance and become noticeably more winded than teammates during sports or may choose a sedentary life-style. The patient with a history of "recurrent bronchitis" or "pneumonia" may also have asthma. Both diagnoses are used as euphemisms to diminish anxiety, which actually prevents families and patients from dealing with the very manageable reality of asthma. Drugs useful in treatment of asthma are noted in Table 3. Asthma medications for daily maintenance use are known as controller medications, while those used intermittently are known as quick-relief medications. While patients who have mild, intermittent disease may need short-acting bronchodilators only occasionally, patients who require these more than a few times each week are candidates for daily therapy with anti-inflammatory medications. An approach to management is summarized in Tables 4 and 5.

For patients with intermittent episodes of mild bronchospasm who appear to be free of wheezing for days or weeks between problem times, intermittent therapy may be appropriate. One may choose an inhaled β-agonist for children over five yr or an oral one for children under five yr of age. An alternative for the young child is a compressor-driven nebulizer that can be used to provide β$_2$-agonists in saline as an aerosol that can be delivered by face mask.

Metered-dose inhalers (MDIs) are effective for children over four yr of age and through adulthood. As the world moves away from Freon-containing propellants, more variations on "classic" MDIs are appearing, including breath-activated aerosol devices, dry-powder devices, and dry-powder capsules for puncture and inhalation.

Holding-chambers devices (e.g., Inspirease®, Aerochamber®, Ace®) used with MDIs should be considered for two reasons: for lowering the age that MDIs are usable to about 4 yr by decreasing the difficulty of synchronizing actuation and inhalation, and also for increasing drug effect by improving lung deposition of drug. Some physicians report success in small children with an inhaled corticosteroid and an aerochamber with face mask. After each actuation, the mask is kept loosely over the child's face, and several inspirations and expirations are allowed before the next actuation. Usually these children continue to use nebulizer therapy with cromolyn and a β-agonist several times daily.

With increasing incidence of symptoms, the patient requires a regular regimen. Obvious clues to this are frequent visits for emergent care, and episodes that affect sleep and school or work attendance. The use of home peak-flow monitoring may well indicate that PEFR is chronically less than 80% of the patient's best baseline, that drops of 20–30% are taking place with some regularity, and/or that there is considerable variability between morning and evening peak flow. At the milder end of this spectrum, patients may do well with bronchodilator alone. However, as asthma becomes more severe, patients should be placed on a regimen of long-term anti-inflammatory therapy. Many younger patients (under 5 yr) do well with cromolyn by nebulizer, while patients over 5 yr can use cromolyn by MDI, and if over 12 yr of age, nedocromil. Therapy usually begins with an ampule of cromolyn or 2 actuations of cromolyn or nedocromil on a regular three or four times/d basis, depending on the patient's particular need and age. Cromolyn and nedocromil can be tapered successfully to twice daily in many cases.

Nonsteroidal anti-inflammatory agents appear to prevent release of mediators from mast cells that induce acute bronchoconstriction and chronic inflammatory airway changes. In addition, these drugs may modulate the activity of neuropeptides and other inflammatory molecules that up-regulate airway hyper-responsiveness. Cromolyn is useful as a maintenance, prophylactic agent for mild to moderate chronic asthma. In addition, cromolyn can be used intermittently to decrease exercise-induced asthma and to prevent antigen-induced episodes. Much of the data concerning cromolyn's anti-inflammatory potential is based on studies using the no-longer available 20-mg capsule delivered by Spinhaler device. Whether the currently available formulation by MDI (1 mg/actuation) provides equivalent action in the recommended dosage of 2 actuations is unclear. Cromolyn is administered by inhalation from the MDI or nebulizer. The nebulizer ampule contains 20 mg/2 ml and probably provides more therapeutic efficacy per dose than the recommended 2 actuations of the MDI.

Nedocromil is a pyranoquinoline that has specific anti-inflammatory effects on the airway. It has been shown to be effective in clinical trials in children and adults with chronic asthma. It appears to have prophylactic properties when used prior to antigen challenge as well as a variety of other challenges including sulfur dioxide, cold air, and exercise. It appears to be similar to cromolyn in anti-asthma potency. Whether its onset of action is faster, whether it is more potent, and whether it has steroid-sparing properties have not yet been determined. Approximately 13% of patients strenuously object to its taste and refuse to use it, while another subset found it unpleasant but tolerable. Nedocromil for asthma is currently available in the United States in MDI form.

Leukotriene antagonists (LTRAs) are newer alternative anti-inflammatory agents for mild persistent asthma. LTRAs are oral agents that block production of receptors for the inflammatory chemicals known as leukotrienes or block the recptors for these compounds. These drugs have been shown to be effective for chronic asthma as well as exercise-induced asthma, when used on a long-term basis. Drugs in this family that are currently approved for use in children include zileuton, zafirlukast, and montelukast. Zileuton blocks formation of leukotrienes. It needs to be taken four times a day and has been associated with liver function abnormalities. These features and FDA approval for ages 12 yr and older limit its use in children. Zafirlukast is a leukotriene receptor antagonist that can be taken on an empty stomach bid and is approved for children over age 7 yr. Montelukast is another receptor antagonist and is taken once at night regardless of food. It has been approved by the FDA for children 4 yr and older and comes in a chewable tablet for youngsters.

LTRAs have not been well studied for potency compared to other agents. While they may be similar to other nonsteroidal agents, they are less potent than inhaled corticosteroids.

If a 1-mo trial of a nonsteroidal anti-inflammatory drug is not beneficial, aerosolized corticosteroid therapy should be initiated. When the patient's condition is stabilized with this, cromolyn, nedocromil, or LTRA can usually be discontinued. β-Agonist bronchodilators should be continued. If they continue to be needed several times a day and if nocturnal asthma continues to be a concern, the long-acting β-agonist salmeterol can be added in hopes of stabilizing the patient's condition without needing a high dose of inhaled corticosteroid. While evidence from controlled trials is not yet available, the use of LTRAs as adjunctive therapy with inhaled steroids for moderate and severe persistent asthma is a growing trend.

Patients with severe asthma are those who have such problems as frequent symptoms affecting sleep and activity as well as emergent visits and occasional hospitalizations. Untreated, their peak-flow rates are markedly depressed and labile. These will require regular use of a β-agonist and an aerosolized steroid, if the child is old enough to use an MDI. Short-acting β-agonist by nebulizer or MDI can be used up to every 4 h. In patients who can use an MDI, salmeterol as a long-acting β-drug administered at night may prevent nocturnal asthma and may simplify the β-agonist regimen using albuterol as needed during the day. Several studies document that salmeterol added to inhaled steroid is as effective as doubling the steroid dose; thus, a long-acting β-agonist is important for minimizing steroid side effects. LTRAs may also be helpful in this regard. Children unable to use an MDI may respond to an inhaled steroid delivered from an MDI into an aerochamber with face mask. Others may require oral steroid

> **Goals of Successful Asthma Management in a Child**
>
> - More "asthma-free" days
> - Less "sleep-less" nights
> - Freedom to run like other children
> - Less "missed" school days
> - Less social, psychological, and financial burden on parents

therapy. If so, a short-acting drug such as prednisone or methylprednisolone used in the morning on alternate days will minimize steroid-induced adverse effects.

Theophylline is another bronchodilator that had great popularity in the United States until the late 1980s. It has lost its popularity for treating asthma because it is relatively difficult to use, safety and efficacy being related to serum levels, which must be monitored regularly for optimal risk benefit ratio. Theophylline may be used as an adjunctive bronchodilator.

Essential points to know concerning theophylline are that: (1) in general, children over 1 yr and under 9 yr of age require a higher dose of theophylline per kilogram than do older children, nonsmoking adolescents, or adults; (2) the ideal therapeutic range for maximizing effectiveness and decreasing adverse effects has been modified to 5–15 µg/mL to lessen risk of adverse effects; and (3) diseases and drugs that affect the P450 cytochrome system in the liver can decrease theophylline clearance as can febrile infections such as influenza markedly elevate the serum theophylline levels.

Oral Corticosteroids

Corticosteroids are potent anti-inflammatory drugs that are available for asthma therapy in oral and inhalable formulations. Steroids are used in a variety of situations: (1) short-term, systemic oral therapy, usually in high doses, is essential for treating acute asthma exacerbations; (2) short-term high-dose iv therapy is useful in status asthmaticus, though high-dose oral therapy can be sometimes used in this situations; (3) inhaled topical corticosteroids are used as long-term maintenance therapy for moderate to severe chronic asthma; 4) low-dose oral daily or alternate-morning therapy is used in severe asthma in which inhaled steroids have not been adequate or in which children are too young to use the aerosolized formulations. For oral use, short-half-life steroids such as prednisone and methylprednisolone are preferable, since they are less likely to affect pituitary–adrenal axis function than the longer-acting drugs.

Inhaled corticosteroids in usually recommended doses are unlikely to cause significant systemic adverse effects, although mild complications such as throat irritation, hoarseness, or pharyngeal candidiasis (often asymptomatic) occur occasionally. As these agents have become more popular for treatment of asthma and as primary care doctors have been encouraged to become comfortable with prescribing them, there has been more discussion of potential risks such as growth retardation, hypothalamic-pituitary-adrenal axis dysfunction and possibly posterior subcapsular cataracts. With dosages that are usual for moderate disease, e.g., 400 µg/day beclomethasone equivalent, clinically significant adverse effects are very uncommon. While higher-dose therapy does increase the possibility of clinically significant evidence of systemic absorption, it is less than one would expect from oral steroid dosage for equivalent disease control.

Aerosolized agents currently available in the United States include beclomethasone diprprionate, triamcinolone acetonide, flunisolide, fluticasone, and budesonide. Their relative potency is summarized in Table 7. It is very important to heed the differences between these agents. The current absence in the United States of a nebulizer aerosol preparation poses a problem in caring for the very young child with severe chronic asthma. Budesonide should soon be available to remedy this deficiency. Some physicians have used an aerochamber spacer with a face mask for very young children who need inhaled steroid and have had varying degrees of success with this delivery system.

Adding to difficulties in winning compliant behavior in the use of corticosteroids, the US Food and Drug Administration (FDA) has added labeling to topical steroid preparations regarding possible increased risk of disseminated varicella in children who use any systemic or topical preparation for asthma or rhinitis. The association between topical steroid use and such increased risk is speculative, while the association between infrequent oral steroid "bursts" for acute asthma and disseminated varicella is statistically real but clinically remote. Now that varicella vaccine is available, children who require these medications who have not had clinical varicella should be immunized. The timing of this should be spaced as distantly as possible from the time of oral steroid therapy to maximize successful immunization, several months being optimal. The adequacy of immunizations can be assessed by measuring serum titers to varicella 1 mo following immunization. Many physicians now institute treatment with oral acyclovir when patients who are taking or have recently been taking oral prednisone and are not immune are exposed to varicella. Such therapy may also be used when patients who are taking inhaled steroid develop varicella lesions.

Considering the potential risk of pituitary-adrenal axis suppression with regular use of oral or inhaled steroids, patients who require these medications and are scheduled for surgery or have experienced severe physical trauma are candidates for oral or parenteral corticosteroid replacement until the high-risk situation has passed.

Allergen Immunotherapy

Immunotherapy may be used as adjunctive therapy in patients who have an IgE-mediated component to asthma. Allergen immunotherapy has been shown to reduce the symptoms of asthma in double-blind studies with a variety of allergens, including house-dust mite, cat dander, grass pollen, and Alternaria. Recent studies have also shown that allergen immunotherapy reduces the late pulmonary reaction to allergen in the lungs. Since immunotherapy modifies the allergic reaction to antigen, it is possible that its use might be most effective if administered early in the course of asthma. Since immunotherapy does carry risk of anaphylaxis, this approach to therapy should be considered in very specific situations and should be carried out by specifically trained physicians. It is very rarely indicated in children under the age of 5 yr.

PSYCHOSOCIAL ISSUES

Psychosocial issues inevitably influence chronic asthma management. For best results in caring for children, physicians must be listeners and educators. The therapeutic

Table 7
Table 7
Estimated Comparative Daily Dosages for Inhaled Corticosteroids

Drug	Low Dose	Medium Dose	High Dose
Adults			
Beclomethasone dipropionate	168–504 µg	504–840 µg	>840 µg
42 µg/puff	(4–12 puff – 42 µg)	(12–20 puffs – 42 µg)	(>20 puffs – 42 µg)
84 µg/puff	(2–6 puffs – 84 µg)	(6–10 puffs – 84 µg)	(>10 puffs – 84 µg)
Budesonide Turbuhaler	200–400 µg	400–600 µg	>600 µg
200 µg/dose	(1–2 inhalations)	(2–3 inhalations)	(>3 inhalations)
Flunisolide	500–1,000 µg	1,000–2,000 µg	>2,000 µg
250 µg/puff	(2–4 puffs)	(4–8 puffs)	(>8 puffs)
Fluticasone	88–264 µg	264–660 µg	>660 µg
MDI: 44, 110, 220 µg/puff	(2–6 puffs – 44 µg) OR	(2–6 puffs – 110 µg)	(>6 puffs – 110 µg)
	(2 puffs – 110 µg)		OR (>3 puffs – 220 µg)
DPI: 50, 100, 250 µg/dose	(2–6 inhalations – 50 µg)	(3–6 inhalations – 100 µg)	(>6 inhalations – 100 µg) OR (>2 inhalations – 250 µg)
Triamcinolone acetonide	400–1,000 µg	1,000–2,000 µg	>2,000 µg
100 µg/puff	(4–10 puffs)	(10–20 puffs)	(>20 puffs)
Children			
Beclomethasone dipropionate	84–336 µg	336–672 µg	>672 µg
42 µg/puff	(2–8 puffs – 42 µg)	(8–16 puffs – 42 µg)	(>16 puffs – 42 µg)
84 µg/puff	(1–4 puffs – 84 µg)	(4–8 puffs – 84 µg)	(>8 puffs – 84 µg)
Budesonide Turbuhaler	100–200 µg	200–400 µg	>400 µg
200 µg/dose		(1–2 inhalations – 200 µg)	(>2 inhalations – 200 µg)
Flunisolide	500–750 µg	1,000–1,250 µg	>1,250 µg
250 µg/puff	(2–3 puffs)	(4–5 puffs)	(>5 puffs)
Fluticasone	88–176 µg	176–440 µg	>440 µg
MDI: 44, 110, 220 µg/puff	(2–4 puffs – 44 µg)	(4–10 puffs – 44 µg) OR (2–4 puffs – 110 µg)	(>4 puffs – 110 µg) OR (>2 puffs – 220 µg)
DPI: 50, 100, 250 µg/dose	(2–4 inhalations – 50 µg)	(2–4 inhalations – 100 µg)	(>4 inhalations – 100 µg) OR (>2 inhalations – 250 µg)
Triamcinolone acetonide	400–800 µg	800–1,200 µg	>1,200 µg
100 µg/puff	(4–8 puffs)	(8–12 puffs)	(>12 puffs)

The most important determinant of appropriate dosing is the clinician's judgment of the patient's response to therapy. The clinician must monitor the patient's response on several clinical parameters and adjust the dose accordingly. The stepwise approach to therapy emphasizes that once control of asthma is achieved, the dose of medication should be carefully titrated to the minimum dose required to maintain control, thus reducing the potential for adverse effect.

The reference point for the range in the dosages for children is data on the safety of inhaled corticosteroids in children, which, in general, suggest that the dose ranges are equivalent to beclomethasone dipropionate 200–400 µg/day (low dose), 400–800 µg/day (medium dose), and >800 µg/day (high dose).

Some dosages may be outside package labeling.

Metered-dose inhaler (MDI) dosages are expressed as the actuater dose (the amount of drug leaving the actuater and delivered to the patient), which is the labeling required in the United States. This is different from the dosage expressed as the valve dose (the amount of drug leaving the valve, all of which is not available to the patient), which is used in many European countries and in some of the scientific literature. Dry powder inhaler (DPI) doses (e.g., Turbuhaler) are expressed as the amount of drug in the inhaler following activation.

regimen should be simplified when possible to encourage compliance. Families should be counseled periodically on giving the child responsibility for his or her disease and its treatment without putting unrealistic expectations on those who are too young to assume it. Educational materials available through groups such as the Asthma and Allergy Foundation of America, Allergy and Asthma Network/Mothers of Asthmatics, and the American Lung Association can be helpful resources to parents and pediatric patients, as can support groups also identifiable through these national organizations.

GOALS

The goal of asthma therapy should be a normal life-style for the patient, as free of restrictions as possible. Usually this can be achieved with appropriate therapy. Patients often benefit from home peak-flow monitoring, objective data being helpful to the patient (and parents) and physician. Most disability from asthma is avoidable with appropriate monitoring and therapy.

SUGGESTED READING

Barnes PJ. Blunted perception and death from asthma. *N Engl J Med* 1994;330:1383–1384.

Barnes PJ, Pedersen S. Efficacy and safety of inhaled corticosteroids in asthma. *Am Rev Respir Dis* 1993;148:S1–S26.

Chilmonczyk B, Salmun LM, Megathlin KN, Neveux LM, Palomaki GE, Knight GJ, et al. Association between exposure to environmental tobacco smoke and exacerbations of asthma in children. *N Engl J Med* 1993;328:1665–1669.

Eggleston PA, Ward BH, Pierson WE, Bierman CW. Radiographic abnormalities in acute asthma in children. *Pediatrics* 1974;54:442–449.

Laitinen LA, Laitinen A, Haahtela T. Airway mucosal inflammation even in patients with newly diagnosed asthma. *Am Rev Respir Dis* 1993;147:697–704.

Management of chronic asthma. From Expert Panel Guidelines for Management of Asthma. NIH, NHLBI, 1997.

Martinez FD, Wright AL, Taussig LM, Holberg CJ, Halonen M, et al. Asthma and wheezing in the first six years of life. *N Engl J Med* 1995;332:133–138.

McFadden Jr ER, Gilbert AA. Asthma. *N Engl J Med* 1992;327:1928–1937.

Peat JK and Li J. Reversing the trend: reducing the prevalence of asthma. *J Clin Allergy Immunol* 1999;103:1–10.

Rachelefsky G. Childhood asthma and allergic rhinitis: the role of leukotrienes. *J Pediatr.* 1997 Sep; 131(3):348–355.

Rachelefsky GS, Katz RM, Siegel SC. Chronic sinus disease with associated reactive airway disease in children. *Pediatrics* 1984;73:526–529.

Rusconi F, Galassi C, Corbo GM, Forastiere F, Biggeri A, Ciccone G, Renzoni E. Risk factors for early, persistent, and late-onset wheezing in young children. SIDRIA Collaborative Group. *Am J Respir Crit Care Med.* 1999 Nov; 160(5 Pt 1):1617–1622.

Sporik R, Holgate ST, Platts-Mills TAE, Cogswell JJ. Exposure to house dust mite allergen and the development of asthma in childhood. *N Engl J Med* 1990;323:502–507.

Strunk RC, Mrazek DA, WolfsooFuhrmann GS, LaBrecque JF. Physiologic and phsychological characteristics associated with deaths due to asthma in childhood. *JAMA* 1985;254:1193–1198.

8 Asthma in Adults
Diagnosis and Management

Michael A. Kaliner, MD

INTRODUCTION

It is estimated that more than 15 million Americans currently have asthma (Table 1) and that the incidence has increased by about 60% in the past decade, not only in the United States but worldwide. Asthma was estimated to cost approximately $9.5 billion in 1997, to be the cause of the most pediatric hospitalizations, to be the sixth most common cause for all hospitalizations, and to cause more than 5000 deaths/yr (an increase of nearly 80% in the past decade).

The word *asthma* was derived from the Greek word for panting, or breathlessness, and thus might be considered a description of the primary symptom of this disease. Asthma can be defined clinically as recurrent airflow obstruction causing intermittent wheezing, breathlessness, chest tightness, and sometimes cough with sputum production. The National Asthma Education Panel, developed in conjunction with the National Heart, Lung and Blood Institute, defined asthma in 1997 as having three components:

1. Airflow obstruction that is reversible (or nearly completely so), either spontaneously or in response to therapy
2. Airway inflammation
3. Increased airway responsiveness to a variety of stimuli

From: *Current Clinical Practice: Allergic Diseases: Diagnosis and Treatment, 2nd Edition*
Edited by: P. Lieberman and J. Anderson © Humana Press Inc., Totowa, NJ

Table 1
Asthma Epidemiology

14–15 million sufferers
5 million children (most common chronic disease)
100 million d with restricted activity
500,000 hospitalizations
1.5 million emergency visits
>5000 deaths (14/d)
$9.5 billion costs (estimated 1997)

CAUSES OF BRONCHIAL ASTHMA (TABLE 2)

Allergic Asthma

About 90% of asthmatics between the ages of 2 and 16 yr are allergic, 70% less than 30 yr of age are allergic, while about 50% older than 30 yr of age are concomitantly allergic. Thus, coincidental allergies are by far the most common underlying condition leading to the development of asthma. One should suspect allergy as a contributing factor when (1) there is a family history of allergic diseases; (2) the clinical presentation includes seasonal exacerbations or exacerbations related to exposures to recognized allergens; (3) there is concomitant allergic rhinitis or other allergic disease; (4) slight-to-moderate eosinophilia is present (300 to 1000/mm^3) or eosinophilia is observed in the sputum; or (5) the patient is less than 40 yr old. Skin testing can be used to confirm IgE directed against incriminated allergens, but does not establish a cause-and-effect relationship. Thus, patients may have a positive skin test but not have clinical symptoms of allergy or asthma when exposed to the incriminated allergen. Consequently, skin testing (or RAST testing) is used only to confirm the history and physical examination that suggest allergy. Levels of total IgE are of limited usefulness; only about 60% of allergic asthmatic subjects have elevated IgE levels.

Because limiting exposure to allergens and allergy immunotherapy are both specifically helpful in treating allergic asthmatic subjects, a careful search for possible allergies is indicated in nearly all asthmatics. Current recommendations are that all asthmatics who wheeze more than 2 d/wk should be observed by an allergist or other physician skilled in identifying allergic disease, to institute prophylactic allergen avoidance measures.

It was once thought that allergic asthma was associated with a milder form of disease, but this contention has not been borne out. Allergic asthma is as severe as asthma of any other cause. If the onset of asthma is between the ages of 2 yr and puberty, generally the prognosis is good, whereas asthma appearing before age 2 may be more severe. Moreover, childhood asthma was once considered a transient disease that might be "outgrown." This philosophy is a serious error in judgment for many reasons, including the availability of excellent effective treatment plans, the impairment of body image an asthmatic child may develop that lasts throughout life, the long-range effects of restricted physical activity on mental and physical health, and the loss of school and recreation time due to a treatable problem. Current recommendations include conditioning of the asthmatic to better prepare him or her for strenuous exercise, selecting swimming or biking in place of running as exercises of choice, and using prophylactic medications in exercise-related airflow obstruction.

Table 2
Conditions That Cause Asthma

Allergic disease
   Allergic asthma
   Allergic bronchopulmonary aspergillosis
Infections
   Bronchiolitis
   Upper respiratory tract infections
   Bronchitis
Industrial-occupational or environmental exposure
   Irritants
   Allergens
Chemical or drug ingestion
   Aspirin or other nonsteroidal anti-inflammatory agents
   Sulfiting agents
   β-Adrenergic antagonists
Vasculitis (Churg and Straus allergic granulomatosis)
Idiopathic (intrinsic)

Conditions That May Worsen Asthma

Sinusitis	Hyperthyroidism
Gastroesophageal reflux	Psychological stress
Pregnancy	

MAST CELLS AND ASTHMA

The essential components of allergic reactions include allergens, IgE antibodies directed at antigenic determinants on the allergen, and activated mast cells that generate and release mediators and cytokines. To initiate allergic responses, exposure to an appropriate antigen and a genetically determined capacity to respond with IgE production are required. Antigen presentation requires access of antigens to the mucous membrane, uptake by antigen-presenting cells, antigen processing, and stimulation of local antibody production. IgE production occurs in the same local environment as antigen presentation, probably in the draining lymph nodes. IgE production is regulated by locally produced helper factors, thought to include cytokines produced by local T helper$_2$ (TH$_2$) cells. The IgE that is produced sensitizes mast cells in the same environment by binding to high-affinity receptors for IgE on the cell surface. Although no one is certain of the precise time involved, the production of sufficient IgE to render a subject allergic is thought to take several years or more. However, children less than 1 yr old with unquestionable allergic diseases are not uncommon.

Once sensitized, mast cells may degranulate upon subsequent allergen exposure. The bridging of IgE receptors by aggregation of IgE molecules bound to multivalent allergens initiates a biochemical reaction that leads to the secretion of a range of chemical mediators from mast cells. These mediators then stimulate the surrounding tissues to elicit the allergic response.

In man, the mast cell is found in the loose connective tissues of all organs, most notably around blood vessels, nerves, and lymphatics. In the lung, mast cells are found

Table 3
Mast Cell-Derived Mediators

Preformed mediators that are rapidly released under physiological conditions	Histamine
	Eosinophil and neutrophil chemotactic factors
	Kininogenase
	Tumor necrosis factor-α
	Endothelin-1
	Arylsulfatase A
	Exoglycosidases
Mediators formed during the degranulation process	Superoxide and other reactive oxygen species
	Leukotrienes C_4, D_4, E_4
	Prostaglandins$_2$, HETEs, HHT
	Prostaglandin-generating factor of anaphylaxis
	Adenosine
	Bradykinin
	Platelet activating factor
Mediators closely associated with the granule matrix	Heparin, chondroitin sulfate E
	Tryptase
	Chymase
	Cathepsin G
	Carboxypeptidase
	Peroxidase
	Arylsulfatase B
	Inflammatory factors
	Superoxide dismutase
Cytokines transcribed after activation	Interleukins-1, 2, 3, 4, 5, 6
	GM-CSF
	Macrophage inflammatory proteins 1 and 1β
	Monocyte chemotactic and activating factor
	TNF-α
	TCA-3
	Endothelin-1

beneath the basement membranes of airways, near blood vessels in the submucosa, adjacent to submucous glands, scattered throughout the muscle bundles, in the intra-alveolar septa, and in the bronchial lumen. Mast cells appear in increased numbers in the epithelium after allergen exposure and are predominant in biopsies obtained during the allergy season. In the airways, there are about 20,000 mast cells/mm^3, and the mast cell represents 1–2% of alveolar cells.

Mediators of Anaphylaxis. There are four sources of mediators generated during the process of mast cell degranulation: preformed soluble molecules stored within the cytoplasmic granules, newly formed molecules quickly generated during the degranulation process, newly synthesized proteins transcribed over a period of hours after the initiation of degranulation, and macromolecular materials that derive from the

Table 4
Pathological Changes in Asthma and Putative Mediators Responsible

Pathological changes	Mast cell mediators responsible
Bronchial smooth-muscle contraction	Histamine
	Leukotrienes C_4, D_4, E_4
	Prostaglandins and thromboxane A_2
	Bradykinin
	Platelet activating factor
Mucosal edema	Histamine
	Leukotrienes C_4, D_4, E_4
	Prostaglandin E_2
	Bradykinin
	Platelet activating factor
	Chymase
	Reactive oxygen species
Mucosal inflammation	Inflammatory factors:
	Cytokines
	Eosinophil and neutrophil
	chemotatic factors
	Leukotriene B_4
	Platelet activating factor
	Interleukins-1,6, tumor necrosis factor
Mucous secretion	Histamine
	Prostaglandins
	HETEs
	Leukotrienes C_4, D_4, E_4
	Chymase
Desquamation	Reactive oxygen species
	Proteolytic enzymes
	Inflammatory factors and cytokines

granule matrix, which may cause actions lasting for a prolonged period (Table 3). The consequences of mediator release occur within minutes (immediate hypersensitivity) or take hours to develop (late-phase allergic reactions). Research has revealed an expanding list of mediators whose actions may contribute to the pathological changes seen in asthma (Table 4).

In addition to the granule-derived mediators, the process of degranulation leads to transcription, synthesis, and secretion of potent cytokines over several hours, which likely contribute to the late-phase allergic response. Thus, mast cells synthesize and release IL-3, IL-4, IL-5, and IL-6 in addition to tumor necrosis factor and other inflammatory cytokines. Mast cells store IL-4 and secrete it as one of the granule mediators, as well. As IL-4 helps regulate IgE production, mast cell activation and release of IL-4 might actually up-regulate IgE production.

Allergens in Asthma. Inhalant allergens are most frequently involved in allergic respiratory diseases such as allergic rhinitis and asthma. These antigens, which directly impact on the respiratory mucosa, are usually derived from natural organic sources such as house dust, pollens, mold spores, and insect and animal emanations. Chemicals and irritants from the workplace have been increasingly recognized as a cause of

> Although allergy is an extremely important cause of asthma, it should be remembered that in about 50% of adults with this disorder no allergy can be found.

rhinitis, asthma, or both. These chemicals can act as allergens or irritants, or they could influence the mucosal environment in such a manner as to predispose the individual toward developing an allergic response. Data suggest that diesel particulates can affect some patients toward becoming allergic. Inhalant allergic diseases may be episodic, seasonal (such as hay fever), or perennial. The most important seasonal allergens are pollens. Despite popular belief, the heavy, sticky pollens of brightly colored flowers seldom cause allergy symptoms, as these pollens are spread by insects and not by wind currents. Exposure to nonseasonal allergens, mainly through inhalation but in some instances by ingestion, accounts for year-round allergies. Among the inhalants, dust mites, mold allergens, cockroaches, and animal emanations are responsible for most perennial allergic asthma.

Diagnosis of Allergy. Despite the development of in vitro methods of detecting IgE antibodies, skin testing (prick or intradermal) with appropriate allergens is the least time consuming, most sensitive, most useful, and also the least expensive method to confirm the presence of allergen-specific IgE. Skin testing can be performed on infants as young as 1–4 mo of age, although age dictates both the choice of allergens used and the clinical conditions for which they can be used. Under the age of 1 yr, food antigens are the likely offenders, causing eczema or asthma. Inhalant allergens are more likely to be involved after 2–4 yr of exposure, although sensitization to indoor allergens can occur much more quickly. In exceptional cases, as in patients with extensive eczema or marked dermatographism that negates use of skin tests, in vitro assays for serum IgE antibodies by radioallergosorbent, fluorescent-allergosorbent, multiple-thread-allergosorbent, or enzyme-linked-immunosorbent test techniques might be substituted for direct testing. With either in vitro testing or skin tests, however, it is essential that the relevance of the results be correlated to the patient's current clinical problems and their detailed history.

Allergic Bronchopulmonary Aspergillosis (ABPA)

ABPA was described in England as a progressive form of asthma leading eventually to pulmonary fibrosis. It was thought that the damp climate in England was responsible for the relatively frequent occurrence there and infrequent occurrence elsewhere. However, recent studies in the United States have revealed the presence of ABPA in the midwestern portion of this country as well.

Compared to other forms of asthma, ABPA is seen infrequently and may be heralded by its specific clinical characteristics. There are five pulmonary disease patterns elicited by exposure to *Aspergillus* species: (1) allergic asthma induced by exposure to mold spores in subjects with IgE antibodies directed at *Aspergillus* antigens; (2) hypersensitivity pneumonitis in response to mold-spore inhalation in nonatopics who develop IgG-class antibodies and cellular immunity to *Aspergillus* antigens; (3) a fungus ball, or aspergilloma, which is a saprophytic colonization of a pre-existing cavity (as in old tuberculosis or sarcoidosis); (4) invasive aspergillosis, which is

Table 5
Diagnostic Criteria for Allergic Bronchopulmonary Aspergillosis

Primary criteria	Asthma
	Eosinophilia ($>1000/mm^3$)
	Positive immediate skin test reactions to *Aspergillus* antigen
	IgG antibodies to *Aspergillus* antigens
	Marked increase in IgE level
	Pulmonary infiltrates, often transitory
	Central, saccular bronchiectasis
	Elevated serum IgE and IgG to *A.* fumigatus compared to control groups
Secondary criteria	*Aspergillus* in sputum
	History of expectorated brown plugs or specks
	Late-phase (or Arthus) skin test results to *Aspergillus* antigen

an overwhelming diffuse pneumonia due to *Aspergillus* in an immunocompromised host; and (5) ABPA, which is a subacute inflammatory reaction elicited by both IgE- and IgG-mediated immune responses directed at *Aspergillus* species growing in the respiratory tree. The precise incidence of ABPA in the United States is not known, but although the disease is not rare, it is seen uncommonly. Diagnostic criteria for ABPA have been established and are summarized in Table 5.

There are five stages of ABPA: Stage 1 is the form of ABPA at which time the diagnostic criteria listed on Table 5 are met. Generally, the patient exhibits moderate to severe asthma, with purulent mucus production, eosinophilia, an abnormal chest X-ray examination; and high IgE levels. Skin testing to *Aspergillus* produces a positive immediate (and oftentimes late) reaction. The possible presence of bronchiectasis is analyzed by computed tomography, and serological testing for IgG antibodies directed at *Aspergillus* is performed. At this point, patients should generally be treated aggressively with corticosteroids, with a resultant remission (Stage 2).

Once the patient has had a remission, corticosteroids are reduced to either every-other-day use or are discontinued entirely. At this stage most experts continue patients on a regimen of moderate doses of inhaled corticosteroids. Stage 3 occurs if an exacerbation eventuates and may lead to the stage at which long-term use of corticosteroids (either daily or every other day) is necessary (Stage 4). Diffuse pulmonary fibrosis (Stage 5) can develop or be the stage at which ABPA is recognized. The importance in making the diagnosis of ABPA rests on the aggressive use of oral and inhaled corticosteroids to try to prevent the development of pulmonary fibrosis.

Infections

All patients with asthma may experience worsening of their symptoms concurrent with upper respiratory tract infections, bronchitis, or influenza-type illnesses. Moreover, children may experience their initial asthma as a consequence of viral bronchiolitis, which commonly develops into chronic asthma. Finally, some patients have no clinical asthma except during concurrent respiratory infections. Some adult asthmatics trace their chronic asthma to a viral respiratory infection that led directly to chronic and often severe, nonallergic asthma.

> The allergy skin test is the method of choice to detect the presence of allergy in the asthmatic.

Bronchiolitis is an acute viral infection of the bronchioles, generally seen only in children less than 2 yr old. It is usually accompanied by upper respiratory tract symptoms, which may precede the lower respiratory tract involvement by 2–3 days. Patients experience cough (sometimes croup), dyspnea, rapid respirations, fever, and sometimes prostration. Physical examination reveals retractions, rapid respiration, occasional rales, and wheezing. Respiratory syncytial virus is the most frequent etiological agent, but adenoviruses, rhinovirus, parainfluenza virus, and others may also cause the disease.

Respiratory-syncytial-virus (RSV)–related bronchiolitis has a mortality risk of 1%. Several studies suggest that atopic children develop IgE antibodies directed at the RSV, which converts the infection into an allergic reaction. About 50% of children with bronchiolitis in whom a family history exists of either allergies or asthma, develop recurring wheezing. In most instances, postbronchiolitis asthma is mild in nature and largely under control or in remission by the age of 8 yr.

Occupational Asthma

The air we breathe may contain allergens of natural origin or generated as a consequence of industrial or environmental processes. In addition, chemicals in the air may irritate the airways and lower the threshold for airway responsiveness. Furthermore, these same irritants may be allergens for susceptible individuals. Besides industrially related exposure, modern life generates pollutants that linger in the air, generally in or around cities, which may damage the lungs. Thus, everyone is at risk of breathing potentially harmful substances, while asthmatics are at much greater risk to react adversely to them. Certain pollutants such as ozone increase airway reactivity even in normal subjects, and asthma may be exacerbated during pollution with either industrial or photochemical smog. Approximately 2–15% of all cases of adult-onset asthma in men are of occupational origin (depending on the level of airway irritants and allergens in any working area).

Suspicion of occupational lung disease should be raised by the history of cough or chest tightness in relationship to the workplace. In asthmatics, worsening of symptoms every week, especially early in the week, may be noted. Such suspicions can be strengthened by evidence of wheezing or abnormal pulmonary function after occupational exposure. Only a few appropriate antigens are available for skin testing, so provocation with the suspected airborne chemical or particulate may be the only confirmatory test available. Some of the more common occupational exposures leading to asthma are listed in Table 6.

The incidence of occupational asthma varies with the exposure and the provocative agent. While only about 5% of workers regularly exposed to toluene diisocyanate (TDI) develop asthma, 10–45% of workers exposed to relatively high concentrations of proteolytic enzymes in laundry detergent in the past were affected. The pattern of response may be immediate, late, or both. The underlying mechanism involves direct irritation and/or the induction of immunological processes, including IgE- or

Table 6
Some Agents Capable of Causing Occupational Asthma

Category	Active substance
Metal salts	Salts of platinum, nickel, chrome
Wood dusts	Oak, western red cedar (plicatic acid), redwood, mahogany
Vegetable dusts	Grain (mite, weevil), flour, castor bean, green coffee, gums, cottonseed, cottondust
Industrial chemicals	Toluene diisocyanate, polyvinyl chloride, phthalic and trimelletic anhydrides, ethylenediamine
Pharmaceutical agents	Penicillins, phenylglycine acid chloride, ethylenediamine
Biological enzymes	*Bacillus subtilis*, pancreatic enzymes
Animal and insect materials	Rodent urine protein, canine or feline saliva or secretions

IgG-type responses. Removal of the worker from the workplace may reduce or reverse the airways disease, although there are many exceptions.

Chemical or Drug Exposure

Aspirin and Nonsteroidal Anti-Inflammatory Drugs (NSAIDs)

It is estimated that 5% of asthmatics will reliably worsen after ingestion of aspirin or other NSAID. Ingestion of aspirin or other NSAID may provoke either of two responses: respiratory responses, including bronchorrhea, rhinorrhea, bronchospasm, conjunctivitis, lacrimation, and flushing; or urticaria and angioedema. Rarely, combinations of the two patterns are seen. Aspirin-sensitive patients may be recognized by the presence of nasal polyps, nonallergic rhinitis, persistent sinusitis, and asthma associated with moderate eosinophilia ($>1000/mm^3$). The frequency of NSAID sensitivity increases with age, although children and families have been described with clear-cut reactivity. There may be a wide range of associated allergies, but many subjects (about 50%) are not allergic.

The mechanism responsible for NSAID sensitivity appears to involve an abnormal modulation of eicosanoid production (increased production of leukotriene(s) (LT) C and D). NSAIDs inhibit the cyclo-oxygenase enzyme system responsible for prostaglandin formation, thereby reducing prostaglandin production and leading to increased production of lipoxygenase products. It has been suggested that NSAIDs cause asthma by reducing the formation of prostaglandins such as PGE that help maintain normal airway function while increasing the formation of asthma-provoking eicosanoids, including hydroxyeicosatetraenoic acids (HETEs) and LTC c and LT d. Recent work in humans has confirmed this suspicion, demonstrating that sensitive subjects exposed to NSAID secrete excessive quantities in LTs in their respiratory tract and develop both rhinitis and asthma.

Aspirin sensitivity should be suspected in any asthmatic with nasal polyposis, chronic sinusitis, and eosinophilia. The polyposis and sinusitis may precede the onset of recognized NSAID sensitivity by years. Under some circumstances, selected patients with this syndrome can be "desensitized" to NSAID by repeated oral challenges with aspirin and may remain unresponsive to subsequent NSAID exposure if oral NSAIDs

> Upper respiratory tract infections, along with allergy, are probably the two most important triggers of asthma episodes.

are given daily. Many asthma investigators believe that LT antagonists are indicated in these patients.

Sulfiting Agents and Asthma

Sulfiting agents include sulfur dioxide and any of its five sulfite salts, which are added to foods to prevent nonenzymatic browning, to inhibit growth of microorganisms, to inhibit enzymatic activity, and to act as antioxidants and reducing agents, as bleaching agents, as processing aids, as pH controls, and for stabilization. In 1986, in response to recognition that sulfites could precipitate asthma, the FDA banned their use on fruits and vegetables served fresh. Other products, like beer and wine, are now labeled as containing sulfites. Sulfites are generally converted under acid conditions to sulfur dioxide (SO_2) and are largely liberated during the processing and cooking of foods. It is thought that ingestion of sulfites leads to the liberation of SO_2 in the mouth and stomach, which is then inspired. In very sensitive asthmatics, inhalation of SO_2, even in small amounts, provokes asthmatic attacks. It may be anticipated that only the most hyper-responsive asthmatics will react to ingested sulfites.

Sulfite sensitivity should be suspected in asthmatics who worsen in relationship to eating processed foods containing sulfites (for example, dried fruit, fruit juices, or processed potatoes) or wine and beer. Sulfite-sensitive asthmatics should be advised to have a Medi-Alert bracelet and to carry a bronchodilator metered-dose inhaler and injectable epinephrine.

β-Adrenergic Antagonists

The β-adrenergic blocking agent propranolol hydrochloride was introduced in 1964, and it was immediately recognized that asthmatics were adversely affected by this drug. β-Adrenergic blocking agents are being used in diverse diseases such as glaucoma, migraine, hypertension, myocardial infarction, and tremor. The underlying mechanism by which β-blockade induces asthma is thought to involve prevention of the normal β-adrenergic inhibitory influences on the parasympathetic ganglia in the airways. The reduction in β-adrenergic inhibitory influences at this level thereby allows relatively unimpaired cholinergic constrictor influences to develop. In the opinion of most specialists, asthmatics should not take β-adrenergic blocking agents. Of note, worsening of the status of a previously stable asthmatic should provoke inquiries as to other medications given by practitioners, in search of possible β-adrenergic blocking agent administration. There is ever widening use of β-blockers and some β-blockers are now "hidden" in combination tablets, along with diuretics.

Vasculitis

In 1951, Churg and Strauss described a vasculitic process that had pathological findings and clinical features warranting the designation of a separate disease entity, allergic angiitis and granulomatosis. The disease is characterized pathologically by necrotizing vasculitis, tissue infiltration by eosinophils, and extravascular granulomas. The disease has three phases: (1) beginning with a prodrome of allergic asthma and allergic rhinitis

> Sinusitis and gastroesophageal reflux are often covert exacerbants of asthma.

that may exist for many years; (2) the second phase includes eosinophilia along with the development of pulmonary eosinophilic infiltrates resembling Löffler's syndrome, eosinophilic pneumonia, or eosinophilic gastroenteritis, and (3) the third phase is the vasculitic phase involving pulmonary vessels (96%), skin (67%), peripheral nerves (63%), the gastrointestinal tract (42%), heart (38%), and kidney (38%).

The syndrome affects males and females equally, the onset of first stage involving allergic rhinitis and asthma occurs around the age of 30 yr, while the vasculitis becomes apparent by the age of 38, and is suggested by the development of eosinophilia >1500/mm^3, infiltrates in chest roentgenogram, hypertension, abdominal pain, purpura, urticaria, subcutaneous nodules, mononeuritis multiplex, general malaise, persistent low-grade fever, and weight loss. Many patients have an increased IgE level and the presence of rheumatoid factor. The prognosis in untreated patients is poor. Treatment generally consists of corticosteroids alone or combined with cytotoxic therapy.

Although this is a rare disease (approximately 1 in 30,000–50,000 asthmatics has Churg and Straus syndrome), the recent introduction of LT antagonists has led to increased recognition. Thus, asthmatics who are weaned off oral corticosteroids and develop a flu-like syndrome with eosinophilia, should be suspect of having Churg and Straus disease. In that circumstance, a chest roentgenogram is indicated to search for pulmonary infiltrates.

Idiopathic or Intrinsic Asthma

Up to 30% of asthmatic patients, particularly those over 30 yr of age, have no apparent cause for their asthma. Often their disease begins with a severe upper or lower respiratory tract infection or sinusitis and progresses to asthma in short order. Such patients often have coexistent sinusitis and nasal polyposis, as well as vasomotor rhinitis. It has been thought that such patients have a worse prognosis than other types of asthmatics, but this is certainly not predictable. In such patients it is necessary to search for factors that might worsen asthma. Many patients with idiopathic asthma regularly produce mucus and have a history of tobacco smoking; such patients may have an asthmatic form of bronchitis.

CONDITIONS ASSOCIATED WITH EXACERBATIONS OF ASTHMA

Several clinical conditions are closely associated with and may worsen asthma by diverse mechanisms.

Sinusitis

An association between asthma and concomitant sinus disease has been recognized since the early part of the century and has been reconfirmed repeatedly both in children and adults. It is estimated that 60–75% of patients with severe asthma have concomitant sinusitis and that 20–30% of sinusitis patients have asthma. Slavin treated 33 adults with asthma and concomitant sinusitis medically or surgically. After therapy, 28 of 33 subjects believed their asthma was improved, and in 15 of 18 their steroid requirement

> Bronchial hyperresponsiveness is a hallmark of asthma and correlates with disease activity.

was reduced by 85%. Anecdotal observations suggest that the difficulty of treating asthmatics with sinusitis is proportional to the degree of sinusitis present. Physicians treating asthmatics should be alert to the possibilities that sinusitis frequently coexists in their patients and that the severity of the sinusitis may influence the course of the bronchial asthma. Although the precise mechanism by which sinusitis worsens asthma is not known with certainty, there is substantial evidence that a nasosinobronchial reflex exists that increases airway irritability and airflow obstruction.

In both children and adults, symptoms from acute sinusitis include purulent nasal discharge, persistent coughing (especially at night), and the presence of purulent mucus in the nasal vault and pharynx. Facial pain, headache, and fever occur less frequently. Most acute episodes of sinusitis follow upper respiratory infections, but some then develop into chronic or recurrent problems. Chronic sinusitis is associated with persistent or recurrent purulent nasal discharge, cough, headache or facial pressure, hyposmia, fetor oris, occasional temperatures, and worsening of asthma.

The physician should consider diagnostic studies for sinusitis whenever symptoms of upper respiratory infection or rhinitis are more protracted than expected, the patient has dull to intense throbbing pain over the involved sinus area, the patient's asthma is not responding appropriately to medications, or the patient has prolonged or persistent bronchitis that has failed to respond to appropriate therapy. On physical examination, edema and discoloration below the eyes may be observed occasionally. The nasal mucosa is inflamed, and a purulent discharge frequently is seen on the floor of the nose, beneath the middle turbinate, or drainging down the throat.

Generally, roentgenograms with the findings of opacification, noticeable membrane thickening, or air-fluid levels within one or more sinuses confirm the suspicion of sinusitis. Computed tomography is much more sensitive than X-ray examination, provides better images, and is the currently recommended diagnostic procedure of choice.

Gastroesophageal Reflux (GERD)

The presence of GERD is suggested by heartburn, especially postprandial, that is increased on bending over, lying down, or straining. Confirmatory tests include roentgenographic demonstration of reflux, the finding of acid in the esophagus after instillation of hydrochloric acid into the stomach, 24-hr monitoring of intraesophageal pH, or Bernstein's test, in which hydrochloric acid is dripped onto the lower esophagus and symptoms are elicited.

It has been reported that as many as 45–65% of adults and children with asthma have GERD. The mechanism by which GERD produces asthma appears to involve triggering intraesophageal reflexes by acid stimulation, resulting in cholinergic reflexes into the airways and resultant bronchial constriction. While GERD may be asymptomatic in asthmatics, the strongest association is with nighttime asthma symptoms—especially night cough and nocturnal wheezing. Gastroesophageal reflux should be highly suspect in patients (especially children) with nocturnal exacerbations (especially cough) and recurrent heartburn. Effective management of GERD may concomitantly reduce asthma in some, but not all, patients.

Pregnancy

Asthma complicates 4% of pregnancies and is the most common chronic disease to do so. About one third of pregnant asthmatics will improve during pregnancy, one third will be unchanged, and one third will worsen. Pregnancy is associated with an increase in tidal volume and a 20–50% increase in minute ventilation. This change has been attributed to a response to increased circulating progesterone, which acts as a respiratory stimulant. Arterial blood gases reflect compensated respiratory alkalosis due to overventilation. Characteristic blood gas findings are pH of 7.40–7.47, partial arterial carbon dioxide pressure of 25–32 mmHg, and partial arterial oxygen pressure of 100–106 mmHg.

Earlier studies suggested the likelihood that prematurity and low-birth-weight infants and both perinatal and maternal death rates were increased in asthmatic women, but current studies do not confirm these problems in properly treated patients. The clinical course of asthma during pregnancy may be predicted by the behavior in the first trimester, and most patients have the same pattern of response with repeated pregnancies. When the condition of a pregnant asthmatic worsens, one should always consider pulmonary emboli as a possible cause.

The management of asthma in pregnancy involves extensive use of inhaled medications and careful avoidance of any medication that might adversely affect the fetus. Because the uterus compromises the thoracic space late in pregnancy, it is very important to keep the pregnant asthmatic under excellent control throughout the pregnancy to avoid exacerbations during the last trimester.

DIFFERENTIAL DIAGNOSIS OF ASTHMA

Not all that wheezes is asthma! Diseases in which wheezing is a component are listed in Table 7. Asthma, chronic bronchitis, and emphysema affect the airways diffusely, cause airway obstruction, and may coexist in the same patient. Generally, chronic bronchitis occurs in cigaret smokers who develop chronic cough that persists for years before airflow becomes symptomatically obstructed. The bronchorrhea may vary in intensity, in relation to infectious or irritant exposure, for example. Chronic bronchitis involves hyperplasia and hypertrophy of the submucosal glands, inflammation of the small airways, and hypersecretion of mucus. Emphysema may also be heralded by long-standing cough and mucous production, but this is a diagnosis confirmed only histologically. Emphysema is suggested by the presence of a reduced diffusing capacity and obstructing airways disease. Most adults have some degree of emphysema at autopsy, but severe emphysema is seen only in about 10%. Emphysema is another disease that usually develops in smokers.

A small number of patients with emphysema and bronchitis have a congenital absence of α_1-antitrypsin, but have bronchitis and wheezing, and may develop emphysema and cirrhosis of the liver.

In children, most conditions likely to be confused with asthma begin in infancy, so it is in the wheezing infant that the differential diagnosis of asthma is important. The most common confusing condition is an aspirated foreign body. A history of

Table 7
Differential Diagnosis of Asthma

Nonasthmatic conditions associated with wheezing
  Pulmonary embolism
  Cardiac failure ("cardiac asthma")
  Foreign bodies[a]
  Tumors in the central airways
  Aspiration (gastroesophageal reflux)[a]
  Carcinoid syndrome
  Laryngotracheobronchomalacia[a]
  Löffler's syndrome
  Bronchiectasis
  Tropical eosinophilia
  Hyperventilation syndrome
  Laryngeal edema
  Vocal cord dysfunction
  Laryngeal or tracheal obstruction[a]
  Factitious wheezing
  α_1-Antitrypsin deficiency
  Immotile cilia syndrome, Kartagener's syndrome[a]
  Bronchopulmonary dysplasia[a]
  Bronchiolitis, croup[a]
Overlapping diseases
  Chronic bronchitis and emphysema
  Cystic fibrosis[a]

[a]Especially important in differential diagnosis in children.

aspiration, findings of unilateral wheezing or hyperinflation on physical examination, or a persistent infiltrate on chest radiology suggests the need for further evaluation. Other illnesses encountered in wheezing infants include bronchopulmonary dysplasia, cystic fibrosis, gastroesophageal reflux, and immunoglobulin deficiency.

PATHOPHYSIOLOGY

Pathologically, the airflow obstruction of asthma is due to combinations of bronchial smooth muscle contraction, mucosal edema and inflammation, and viscid mucous secretion. The disease involves large and small airways but not alveoli. Pathological examination of asthmatic lungs reveals that small bronchi and bronchioles are principally involved, there is extensive airway denudation due to loss or thinning of the epithelium, and the goblet cells are often markedly hyperplastic (Table 8). The basement membrane is thickened because of the deposition of sub-basement membrane collagen, and the lamina propria is infiltrated with CD4+ lymphocytes, mast cells, eosinophils, and neutrophils. The smooth muscle is hyperplastic and contracted. The submucous glands are hyperplastic and are actively secreting mucus. The airway lumen is often filled with secretions containing mucus, edema fluid, eosinophils, inspissated mucous plugs, Charcot-Leyden crystals, and Curschmann's spirals.

The pathophysiological event causing asthma is a reduction in small-airway diameter. This abnormality leads to an increase in airway resistance that makes it difficult for

Table 8
Pathology of Asthma

Denudation of airway epithelium
Sub-basement membrane fibrosis and collagen deposition
Airway wall edema
Mast cell activation
Inflammatory cell infiltration
   Neutrophils
   Eosinophils
   Lymphocytes (TH_2 cells)
Mucous hypersecretion
   Goblet cell hyperplasia
   Mucous gland hyperactivity

inspired air to escape the lungs, leading to a reduction in forced expiratory volumes and flow rates, and hyperinflation of the lung with air trapping. The increase in the work of breathing creates a sense of breathlessness and generates inequities of alveolar ventilation and perfusion, which cause hypoxemia. Initially, blood gases exhibit reduced CO_2 levels, reflecting overventilation in an attempt to maintain O_2 levels. Associated with the dynamics of air trapping are electrocardiographic changes reflecting pneumonia pulmonale, and with hypoxemia, increases in pulmonary arterial pressures. These changes may lead to pulsus paradoxus. The presence of pulsus paradoxus and the need to use the accessory muscles of respiration reflect the severity of the airflow obstruction and may be useful clinical signs.

Bronchial Smooth Muscle Contraction

Because airway obstruction occurs within minutes of an inciting event and can reverse itself within minutes of treatment with β-adrenergic agonists, it is likely that airway smooth muscle constriction contributes significantly to airflow obstruction. Of the recognized factors capable of causing bronchial smooth muscle contraction, mast cell mediators and several neurohormones are probably the most important (Table 4).

Mucosal Edema

Edema of airway mucosa is due to increased capillary permeability with leakage of serum proteins into interstitial areas. In the earliest careful descriptions of asthmatic lungs, the presence of edema was the most striking abnormality. More recently, mucosal edema has been directly observed by bronchoscopy after airway antigen challenge, and plasma protein exudation after antigen challenge has been documented. These observations combine to support the growing appreciation of the importance of airway mucosal edema in asthma.

Vascular permeability occurs within several minutes of allergen challenge and persists for 30–60 min. It is not surprising that edema would occur as a consequence of allergic reactions, as swelling is the primary response to allergen exposure in sensitized individuals in all other parts of the body. The late-phase allergic reaction is thought to be due to a combination of edema of the airways and the presence of increased inflammatory cells.

Airway Inflammation

The mucosa of patients who have died in status asthmaticus contains mixed cellular infiltrates consisting of eosinophils, neutrophils, macrophages, lymphocytes, mast cells, and plasma cells. In the airway lumen, admixed in the abundant secretions are eosinophils and eosinophil-derived Charcot-Leyden crystals, neutrophils, and desquamated clumps of epithelial cells ("Creola bodies"). The same pathological changes are found in the lungs of allergic or nonallergic asthmatics, suggesting that there is a commonality in the pathophysiological events.

Recent biopsy studies of the airways of asthmatics after allergen challenge have shown the following observations: Within minutes of allergen exposure mast cells degranulate (and release mediators detectable in the bronchoalveolar lavage fluid) the superficial vessels swell and become permeable, and edema is formed. Biopsies done several hours later reveal persistent edema, the increased expression of adhesion molecules on blood vessels, and increased cells in the mucosa expressing molecules that can bind to the adhesion molecules. The mucosa becomes infiltrated initially with neutrophils and after 12–24 hr with eosinophils. The eosinophil releases some of its granule contents, as reflected in the presence of major basic protein in airway biopsies or pathological specimens. Eosinophil-derived proteins can cause epithelial denudation, mucous secretion, and irritability of the airway. Of all the infiltrating cells, the eosinophil is the most specific, being seen rather exclusively in asthma and not with other inflammatory diseases of the airway.

Biopsies have also indicated that the lymphocytes in the asthmatic mucosa are primarily CD4+, express genes for the production of IL-4 and IL-5 (suggesting that they are of the TH_2 phenotype associated with increased inflammation, prolonged eosinophil survival, and increased IgE production), and become activated after allergen challenge. The cytokines produced by TH_2 lymphocytes can not only enhance IgE production, but also support many of the pathological events that occur in the airways of asthmatics. It is this population of lymphocytes that appears to be specifically expanded in atopic subjects. Moreover, allergen exposure in allergic individuals is the stimulus for TH_2 expansion during the late-phase allergic reaction and in airways of asthmatics. Thus, there is a growing body of evidence that allergy and asthma are associated with an expanded TH_2 population of lymphocytes that act to support the events occurring in the asthmatic airway.

Mucous Secretion

Pathological examinations of patients who have died in status asthmaticus almost always reveal diffuse collections of mucus, which appear to contribute significantly to obstruction of the airways. The precise mechanisms responsible for increased mucous production have been partly defined (Table 4).

Bronchial Hyperresponsiveness

One of the absolute features of asthma is an exaggerated nonspecific airway reactivity to a variety of irritating stimuli (Table 9). Thus, asthmatics develop airway obstruction in response to natural exposures (cold air, exercise, irritating chemicals, laughing, and coughing) or to provocations in the laboratory (histamine, methacholine, cold-air hyperventilation). Airway hyperresponsiveness is found universally in asthmatics, in a portion of subjects with chronic bronchitis, in some subjects with allergic rhinitis, and in

Table 9
Airway Hyperresponsiveness

Exaggerated bronchoconstriction to a variety of stimuli
Histamine, methacholine, cold air, exercise
Induced by mast cell and lymphocyte mediators, cytokines, and chemokines
Associated with eosinophil and neutrophil infiltration
Improved but not eradicated by anti-inflammatory therapy

3–8% of otherwise normal subjects. There is a close correlation between the degree of increased responsiveness and disease severity: Patients with the most reactive airways often require oral corticosteroids for control, whereas milder degrees of abnormality predict the requirement for fewer medications. Hyperresponsiveness increases after allergen exposure, late-phase allergic reactions, viral infections (especially influenza-type infections), and ozone exposure. Conversely, airway hyperresponsiveness may return toward normal after allergen avoidance, allergy immunotherapy, or treatment with cromolyn or inhaled or oral CCS. In recent years, airway hyperresponsiveness and airway inflammation have become one of the prime targets in asthma therapy, leading to the use of anti-inflammatory agents to reduce airway reactivity.

Other Pathological Events

Denudation of airway epithelial surfaces with the appearance of epithelial clumps in expectorated secretions accompanies severe asthma. The denuded epithelial surfaces may be replaced by goblet cells, resulting in goblet cell hyperplasia and increased mucous secretion. The mechanism for epithelial desquamation has not been systematically examined, although several mediators might participate. Edema of the airway results in movement of edema fluid between epithelial cells and into the airway lumen. This process may also contribute to weakening the epithelial bond. Lymphocyte-derived cytokines may also contribute to these phenomena.

FACTORS PREDISPOSING TO ASTHMA

Genetic Factors

"Asthmatics beget asthmatics." When differentiating asthma from other obstructive airways disease, it is always relevant to ask if family members experience the same symptoms. If the asthmatic is atopic, familial concordance is likely to be present, whereas nonallergic asthmatics have fewer tendencies for genetic transmission. Although the specific gene encoding asthma has not been identified with certainty, several groups are convinced that one or more genes will be identified shortly.

Autonomic Dysfunction

An imbalance of the autonomic nervous system with blunted β-adrenergic responses and hyperresponsiveness of the β- adrenergic and cholinergic systems have been documented in asthmatics, although this defect is not unique for asthma. The exact contributions of the disarray of autonomic imbalances found in asthmatic subjects is not clear. Some of the abnormalities are also found in allergic subjects and in patients suffering from cystic fibrosis. These data suggest that asthmatics have an inherently

Table 10
Asthma Diagnosis: Episodic Symptoms of Airflow Obstruction
(Determine Frequency)

Wheezing
Shortness of breath (with or without exercise)
Chest tightness (below sternum)
Cough (throat versus chest, quantity and quality of sputum)
Nocturnal awakenings
Morning vs evening symptoms
Emergency room visits
Hospitalizations

reduced ability to sustain open airways and a tendency for airflow obstruction based upon an inherent defect in their autonomic balance.

CLINICAL ASTHMA

Symptoms

The classic symptoms of asthma include intermittent, reversible episodes of airflow obstruction (Tables 10 and 11) manifested by cough, wheezing, chest tightness, and dyspnea. When the clinical situation permits, a detailed history should be taken that includes the following: (1) family and personal history of atopic disease; (2) age of onset of asthma, frequency and severity of attacks; (3) times (including seasons) and places of occurrence of asthmatic attacks; (4) known provocative stimuli and any previous correlating skin test reactions; (5) the severity of the disease as reflected in the wheezing episodes per day, the number of missed school or work days per year, whether sleep is interrupted, the necessity for emergency room visits, and the number of hospitalizations for asthma; and (6) previous pharmacological or immunological therapy and its efficacy.

Early symptoms are often a vague, heavy feeling of tightness in the chest, and, in the allergic patient, there may be associated rhinitis and conjunctivitis. The patient may experience coughing, wheezing, and dyspnea. Although the cough (if present) is initially nonproductive, it may progress to expectoration of a viscous, mucoid, or purulent and discolored sputum. There appears to be a subgroup of asthmatics whose asthma is characterized solely by cough without overt wheezing, the "cough variant of asthma." (Just as all that wheezes is not asthma, all that is asthma does not necessarily wheeze.) If this syndrome is suspected, the patient's airways should be examined by spirometry before and after bronchodilator inhalation or after receiving a methacholine inhalation challenge.

Patients who appear to have allergic asthma, as demonstrated by seasonal exacerbations or clearly recognized allergen-related triggering events, may be sensitive to pollens, dust mites, animal danders, feathers, mold spores, occupational dusts, or insects. Less frequently, children may also be allergic to certain foods. If the offending allergen can be identified from the patient's history and avoided, further workup may not be necessary. However, atopic patients may be allergic to many allergens or may react to such small amounts of crude allergens (i.e., dust mite) that the association is not

Table 11
Initial History (Determine Days/Week or Month for Each)

Do you wheeze?
Shortness of breath?
Tightness in the chest?
Exercise? Need pretreatment with bronchodilator?
Cough? Throat vs chest, sputum quality/quantity?
Use of bronchodilator?
Nocturnal awakenings
Peak-flow meter use; average, best, and worst reading?
ER visits, hospitalizations?

Table 12
Peak-flow Meters

Inexpensive
Easy to use
Accurate
Provide "real-life" measurements at worst and best time of day
AM and PM, monitor range between the measurements
Obtain "personal-best" measurement

clear cut. Moreover, allergic asthmatics may respond to many nonallergic conditions (such as cigaret smoke, noxious fumes, upper respiratory tract infections, or weather conditions) by wheezing.

All patients should be asked if they can take aspirin or NSAIDs without ill effects, and this line of inquiry is even more important in patients with sinusitis or nasal polyps. Occupational asthma should be suspected if the patient's condition worsens early each week and then improves during the course of the week, or if asthma is worse during the week as compared to weekends or during travel. It may be necessary to have the patient use a peak-flow meter at work during the course of a week to help determine what exacerbates the disease, or to conduct a bronchial challenge with materials to which the patient is exposed at work.

Chest X-ray studies should be repeated every 3–5 yr, and a yearly complete blood count is a reasonable precaution in most patients. Some subjects worsen reliably with every upper respiratory infection, and it may be necessary to treat them prophylactically with antibiotics and/or corticosteroids to prevent these exacerbations.

Many subjects are unaware of their chest disability and benefit from frequent peak-flow readings. We routinely provide a peak-flow meter to all asthmatics and request that readings be taken twice a day, in the morning and at night. These readings are an invaluable adjunct to the management of most asthmatics (Table 12).

Physical Findings

In the completely asymptomatic patient, results of chest examination will be normal, although head, eye, ear, nose, and throat examination may disclose concomitant serous otitis media, allergic conjunctivitis, rhinitis, nasal polyps, paranasal sinus tenderness, signs of postnasal drip, or pharyngeal mucosal lymphoid hyperplasia. Clubbing of the fingers is extremely rare in uncomplicated asthma, and this finding should direct the physician's attention toward diseases such as bronchiectasis, cystic fibrosis, pulmonary neoplasm, or cardiac disease. With an acute exacerbation, patients may be restless, agitated, orthopneic, tachypneic, breathing through pursed lips with a prolonged expiratory phase, using accessory muscles of respiration, diaphoretic, coughing frequently, or audibly wheezing and cyanotic. Cyanosis occurs only with profound arterial oxygen desaturation and is a grave sign that appears late in the course of severe asthma. Vital signs will confirm the physician's impression that the patient is tachypneic, and evaluation of the blood pressure may show that the patient has a widened pulse pressure and pulsus paradoxus. The latter sign, when present, is a relatively reliable indicator of severe asthma. Although a low-grade fever may be of viral origin, the presence of an elevated temperature should alert the physician to search for a possible bacterial infection requiring antibiotic therapy.

Examination of the chest will often show signs of hyperinflation, such as hyper-resonance on percussion and low, immobile diaphragms. In milder stages of asthma, wheezing may be detected only on forced expiration, but with increasing severity, wheezing may also be heard on inspiration. In some episodes of severe asthma, wheezing may be heard early in the course of disease, but with increasing obstruction of the airways, the wheezing may seem to "improve" as increasing difficulty in ventilating develops. This abatement of wheezing may, unfortunately, be taken as a clinical sign of improvement and result in less than optimal treatment. As the patient does improve, one may notice the reverse situation, namely, that wheezing may increase in intensity. Again, this finding should not be erroneously interpreted as worsening of the asthma. The major point is that in judging the severity of asthma, the physician must rely on many physical findings (such as the use of accessory muscles and the presence of paradoxical pulse) as well as laboratory evaluation. As the patient recovers, the improvement takes place most often in reverse order of the appearance of symptoms, i.e., there is a sequential loss of mental status abnormalities, cyanosis, pulsus paradoxus, use of accessory muscles, dyspnea, tachypnea, and, finally, wheezing. It is important to note, however, that when the attack appears to have ended clinically, abnormal pulmonary function test results are still present and may persist for several days. At this point in the course of the illness, there is usually a residual volume twice that of normal, an FEV_1 60% of that predicted, and a maximum midexpiratory flow rate 30% of that predicted. Such findings support the contention that treatment should be continued well past the symptomatic period and that close outpatient follow-up is indicated.

Classification of Asthma

Asthma may be divided into four clinical phases, based upon symptoms and pulmonary function testing. These stages allow physicians to communicate about asthma severity and provide general guidelines on treatment. The four categories include mild intermittent asthma, mild persistent asthma, moderate persistent asthma, and severe persistent asthma. These categories advance in severity, and a patient may move from one to another depending upon various circumstances. See Table 13 for details of the current classification scheme.

Mild intermittent asthma occurs less than twice weekly and the patient is asymptomatic otherwise. Pulmonary function is normal except during periods of disease and exacerbations are brief and usually easily treated.

Table 13
Classification of Asthma Severity

Category	Symptoms	Nocturnal symptoms	Pulmonary function
Mild intermittent	Less then twice weekly Normal between attacks Attacks brief and usually mild	Less than twice monthly	Both FEV_1 and PEFR >80% predicted
Mild persistent	More than twice a week, less then daily Attacks limit activity	More then twice monthly	Both FEV_1 and PEFR >80% predicted
Moderate persistent	Daily symptoms Daily use of medications Attacks affect activity Attacks usually more than twice a week and may be severe and last days to weeks	More than weekly	FEV_1 and PEFR 60–80% predicted
Severe persistent	Continuous symptoms Limited physical activity Frequent exacerbations	Frequent, up to every night	FEV_1 and PEFR <60% predicted

Mild persistent disease occurs more than two times a week, but less than once a day. Symptoms are severe enough to interfere with daily activities and may interrupt sleep up to twice a month.

Moderate persistent disease occurs on a daily basis and requires regular use of medications. This stage of asthma is moderately inconvenient with patients constantly aware of their disease, requiring medications on a daily basis, having their sleep interrupted at least weekly, and having to accommodate their life-style to the disease.

Severe asthma has continuous symptoms despite medications, which limit activity and are associated with frequent exacerbations and sleep interruptions.

A patient with mild persistent disease can be exposed to allergens or develop a cold and have a severe exacerbation of asthma symptoms that places the disease in the severe persistent classification until the attack is resolved. Conversely, a patient with severe persistent symptoms can be treated effectively and have resolution of symptoms, with reclassification to a mild persistent category while medications are taken.

Table 14
Goals of Asthma Treatment

1. Prevent chronic and troublesome symptoms
2. Maintain (near) normal pulmonary function
3. Maintain normal activity levels
4. Prevent recurrence of the disease and any need for emergency treatment or hospitalization
5. Provide optimal treatment with minimal side effects
6. Meet patient's and family's expectations of asthma control

Exercise-Induced Asthma

Exercise is a well-established nonspecific stimulus to airflow obstruction, and this phenomenon can be demonstrated in most patients with asthma. Thus, exercise-induced asthma might better be thought of as a reflection of increased nonspecific airway hyperresponsiveness than as a distinct form of asthma. It is most common in children and adolescents (probably because they exercise more strenuously than do most adults). The problem is clinically important in at least two thirds of adolescents with asthma because it interferes with school and recreational activities.

The mechanisms by which exercise causes bronchial obstruction is unknown, but a fall in the temperature and humidity of the intrathoracic airways is a critical initiating event. The exact roles of mast-cell-mediator release and reflex responses (perhaps regulating blood flow in response to the temperature change) in this syndrome are unclear. Exercise asthma usually begins after about 6–10 min of exercise or after the exercise is completed. Exercise asthma can be reproduced by having subjects hyperventilate cold, dry air.

Swimming and activities that necessitate only brief intervals of exercise are likely to be best tolerated. Breathing warm and humidified air (as in jogging with a face mask) and the use of prophylactic drug therapy (β-agonists usually) generally afford adequate protection against exercise-induced asthma.

TREATMENT (TABLE 14)

Over the past decade, the treatment of asthma has changed remarkably, largely because of our increased understanding of the pathophysiology of the disease, with recognition of the importance of airway inflammation. Recognizing that the airflow obstruction in asthma is accounted for by a combination of airway-wall edema, increased mucous secretion, increased inflammation, bronchial smooth-muscle contraction, and increased airway irritability, and not just by bronchospasm (as was once thought) has led to a fundamentally altered approach to asthma therapy. One way to summarize this approach is based upon a classification of treatments into specific (long-term controlling) and symptomatic (short-term relieving) agents: Specific treatments are agents that reduce the underlying causes for asthma and thereby reduce the need for symptomatic agents. Symptomatic treatments act only by reducing symptoms of airflow obstruction and have no effect on the underlying causes of asthma. Thus, we can separate the treatments used for asthma into the following:

Specific Treatments (Long-term controlling)	Symptomatic Treatments (Short-term relieving)
Allergy avoidance	β-Agonists
Allergy immunotherapy	Theophylline
Inhaled corticosteroids	Anticholinergics
Cromolyn or nedocromil	
Oral corticosteroids	
Leukotriene modifiers	

All patients should receive one or more specific treatments and may also receive symptomatic treatments, as needed. As a patient's symptoms move him or her into one of the more severe categories of asthma, the patient generally will receive more medications, both specific and symptomatic. Thus, the general approach is to treat initially with combinations of specific and symptomatic therapies to totally control the symptoms and then to reduce the treatments to the least amount required to maintain remission. For example, mild intermittent asthma is treated only with inhaled bronchodilators, on an as-needed basis. At the next level, mild persistent asthma requires more chronic dosing, and the usual approach is to use a low-to-moderate dose of inhaled corticosteroids (CCS) and/or a leukotriene modifier, plus a bronchodilator on an as-needed basis. Moderate asthma is usually treated with a higher dose of inhaled CCS plus a leukotriene antagonist. If symptoms persist, and the patient is using inhaled β-agonists frequently, then a long-acting bronchodilator is added. Alternatively, oral theophylline may be used in addition to or in place of the long-acting β-agonist. The most severe asthmatic patients will be treated with higher doses of inhaled CCS plus more other medications. In all patients, symptomatic therapies are also given, to be used on an as-needed basis. The goal in all of these patients is to tailor the medicines and their doses at the level of the disease, always trying for optimal control with the lowest effective dose of medications. These principles are summarized on Table 15.

To summarize: the basic concepts of asthma management include the following:

1. Daily use of specific treatments (long-term control treatments), often used in combination. Allergy management is superimposed upon other treatment methods.
2. Symptomatic use of bronchodilators (quick-relief medications) used only on an as-needed basis.
3. Step therapy:
   Use whatever dose or combination of therapies that is required to totally control symptoms and achieve a maximum (personal-best) peak flow
   Once the asthma is completely controlled, one should step down the treatment while maintaining symptom control and personal-best peak flow with the lowest effective doses of medication
4. Regular follow-up visits
5. Written management plan (including emergency treatment plan)
6. At-home monitoring with peak-flow meters

Specific Therapies

ALLERGY AVOIDANCE

Allergic diseases are a major cause of asthma, particularly in the pediatric to young-adult populations. Avoidance of allergens, therefore, represents a simple yet important

Table 15
Stepwise Approach to the Treatment of Asthma

Category	Specific, long-term controller medication	Symptomatic medication
Mild intermittent	No daily medication required Allergy treatment as indicated	Inhaled β-agonist prn

Mild persistent	Inhaled corticosteroid (low dose)
	    or leukotriene antagonist
	    or cromolyn or nedocromil
	Allergy treatment as indicated
		Inhaled β-agonist prn

Moderate persistent	Inhaled corticosteroid (moderate
	    dose) plus leukotriene antagonist
	Cromolyn or nedocromil may be
	    tried
	Allergy treatment as indicated
		If inhaled β-agonist
		    is required on a daily
		    basis, long-acting β-
		    agonist (Serevent)
		    should be used
		Theophylline may be added
		    if symptoms persist
		Ipratropium for mucous
		    secretion

Severe persistent	Inhaled corticosteroid (high dose)
	    plus leukotriene antagonist
	Allergy treatment as indicated
		Long-acting β-agonist on a
		    daily basis plus short-
		    acting β-agonist prn
		Theophylline may be
		    added
		Ipratropium may be used
		    if cough and mucous
		    production are a problem

approach to asthma management (Table 16). The status of any patient who wheezes more than 2 d/wk should be evaluated by an allergist (or other physician trained and competent to do allergy assessment) early in the disease process. While almost three fourths of asthmatics are reported to have positive skin test reactions to common inhalant allergens, only significant skin test reactions that closely correlate with clinical symptoms should be targeted for treatment.

There is substantial (although not entirely consistent) evidence supporting the benefits of allergen avoidance as a strategy in asthma care. Avoidance of allergens in dust-mite-allergic asthmatic children leads to improvement in both airflow obstruction and airway reactivity. Similarly, dust-sensitive asthmatic children whose bedrooms are made dust free experience less wheezing, require less medication, and have higher peak-expiratory flow rates than do their counterparts with unmodified bedrooms.

Compliance in preparing allergy-free environments is an issue. Our experience has shown that patients are more likely to comply with written instructions about allergen avoidance than oral instructions, and that these recommendations should be reasonable. For instance, requesting the purchase of allergen encasements for the pillow, mattress, and box springs, along with weekly washing of linens in hot water (>130°F), is reasonable, whereas asking for a carpet to be removed may not be. Thus, we are careful to advise only allergen control measures that the patient can actually carry out.

Table 16
Allergy Advice

1. All patients who wheeze more than 2 d/wk should have an allergy evaluation.
2. Allergy avoidance is fundamental to allergy management.
3. The physician should try allergy avoidance plus pharmacotherapy before considering immunotherapy.
4. The physician should be reasonable in regard to allergen avoidance, advising patients to do what can be done (appropriate dust controls, pets out of the bedroom), not what is impossible.
5. Practical advice should be provided on pollens, molds, dust, dander.

Table 17
Allergy Immunotherapy

1. Indicated if the patient does not respond to avoidance and pharmacotherapy. In some circumstances (dust, dander) avoidance may not be possible.
2. Do not use unless there is a positive history and *significantly positive* confirmatory skin tests
3. Use for 2 yr, and if no improvement, stop!
4. Data supporting its use in asthma in both adults and children are substantial, and it is the only treatment with the long-term chance of remission of asthma.
5. Can be used as an inhaled corticosteroid-sparing agent

IMMUNOTHERAPY (TABLE 17)

In immunotherapy, increasing doses of allergen are subcutaneously injected over time. The use of immunotherapy in asthma has generally been accepted as useful. Data clearly indicate that immunotherapy works well in relatively pure allergic asthmatics, such as those with cat, dog, or pollen-induced asthma. In a large meta-analysis of immunotherapy of asthma, the evidence was considered overwhelming that immunotherapy is helpful. Moreover, current findings are supporting earlier observations that immunotherapy of allergic rhinitis may prevent the development of asthma.

When successful, immunotherapy reduces bronchial reactivity, asthma symptoms, skin test reactivity, and the need for medications. As such, immunotherapy is the only method available in asthma treatment that has the chance of making the patient asymptomatic with less or no medication. Asthmatic patients most likely to benefit from immunotherapy are those who also have concomitant allergic rhinitis, unequivocal immediate sensitivity, a history of asthma with allergen exposure, and an inadequate response to allergen avoidance.

PHARMACOLOGICAL THERAPIES

Inhalers. The use of metered-dose inhalers (MDI) in asthma has revolutionized asthma treatment. The inhaler is a canister containing pressurized fluorohydrocarbons (Freon), in which powdered medications can be suspended. Upon actuation, a metered dose is expelled, containing particles of various sizes. Only those particles less than 5 μm in diameter enter the airstream and reach the lower airways. It is estimated that 5–15% of a metered dose actually reaches the lung; the rest is deposited in the mouth and throat.

Table 18
Proper Use of Metered-dose Inhalers (MDIs)

Shake MDI
Breathe out
Place MDI 2 fingerbreadths in front of open mouth
    (or place in mouth with lips loosely around mouthpiece)
Aim at back of throat
Activate inhaler while breathing in *slowly* (over 3–4 s)
Hold breath 10 s
Wait 30–60 s between activations

Teaching a patient proper inhaler technique is critical to the usefulness of these products. *See* Table 18 for one of the most effective techniques.

The current crop of Freon-propelled MDIs will shortly be replaced with HFA-driven inhalers. These new inhalers will not deplete ozone as does Freon and will have a softer plume that will facilitate deeper penetration of the dose of medication. Some asthma medications are soluble in HFA, allowing for the generation of smaller particle sizes and much greater deposition of the inhaled dose into the lungs (*see* QVAR below).

Until these new medications are available, spacers can be employed to facilitate better inhaler technique. A spacer is a reservoir into which the metered dose is expelled and from which the patient breathes. The major advantage of spacer use is that hand-eye coordination is not necessary, and most large particles impact on the wall of the spacer and do not get inhaled. Thus, the relative fraction of medicine that the patient breathes that actually gets into the lungs is enhanced. Unfortunately, while spacers are an important improvement on inhaler administration, only a small fraction of the total medicine dispelled from the MDI through the spacer actually reaches the lungs.

Another Freon-free choice consists of the dry-powder inhalers that have recently been introduced to the market. These products reduce the eye-hand coordination problem and are very convenient. However, they also suffer from a relatively small respirable fraction.

Antiinflammatory Therapy. CCSs are the most potent of the available pharmacological agents for the specific treatment of asthma and airway hyperresponsiveness. These agents have many actions that make them valuable in the treatment of asthma, including the ability to reduce airway inflammation, mucous secretion, edema, and airway hyperreactivity. Despite their proven value in asthma therapy, CCSs are withheld from many patients who could benefit from their use because of the fear of major side effects. To reduce unwanted systemic effects, the pharmaceutical industry has created highly specific molecules with topical activity but limited systemic effects. It is safe to say that when used properly, inhaled CCS need not cause additional problems for the asthma patient (Table 19).

Inhaled CCSs are the first-line treatment of persistent asthma and are indicated for all patients who wheeze more than twice a week. The dose of CCS is modified for each patient, aiming for the appropriate minimal dose that is effective for the level of severity (Table 20). Thus, patients with mild persistent asthma usually respond to a total dose of 100–600 µg of CCS, with moderate asthma 600–1200 µg/day, and with severe asthma 1000–2000 µg/day.

Table 19
When to Use an Inhaled Corticosteroid

1. For all asthmatics who:
   wheeze more than 2 d/wk
   use a metered-dose inhaler frequently
   have nocturnal awakenings with asthma
   have exercise-induced asthma
   (*All persistent asthmatics!*)
2. Not indicated for the mild intermittent asthmatic who wheezes less than 1–2 d/wk and is asymptomatic otherwise

Table 20
Cautions in Using Inhaled Corticosteroids

1. Rinse mouth after each use (brush teeth)
2. Use to reach personal-best peak flow-rate. Consider using high doses until the peak-flow readings have plateaued. Then back off to lower dose
3. Use spacer or dry-powder inhaler
4. Maximum of bid dosing
5. Try to stay below 1500–2000 µg/d
   Beclomethasone (42 or 84 µg/puff; 35–45 or 17–22 puffs/d)
   Triamcinolone (100 µg/puff; 15–20 puffs/d)
   Flunisolide (250 µg/puff; 6–8 puffs/d)
   Fluticasone (44, 110, and 220 µg/puff; use maximum of 880 µg/day)
   Budesonide (200 µg/inhalation; 8–10 inhalations/d)

CCSs are not equal or interchangeable. Many factors go into the individual choice of CCS. For example, fluticasone is somewhat more potent than several of the other CCSs, but we usually do not prescribe more than a total of 880 µg/d (Flovent 220, 2 puffs bid; maximum dose). On the other hand, many patients respond to fluticasone better then they do to other CCS preparations. For patients with more severe asthma who require higher (1000–2000 µg/d) doses of CCS, the choices are flunisolide (AeroBid, 250 µg/puff), budesonide (Pulmicort, 200 µg/puff; a dry-powder inhaler) and fluticasone (<880 µg/day). In the near future, several more products will be marketed at 250 µg/puff and therefore may be considered for use at high doses.

For lower-dose requirements, there is a wide choice of products, and the choice may be dictated by the availability of a built-in spacer (Azmacort), the desirability of using a dry powder inhaler (Pulmicort), or the wish to avoid using a Freon-propelled MDI (QVAR).

Triamcinolone, flunisolide, and beclomethasone (Beclovent and Vanceril, both at 42 or 84 µg/puff) each have long safety records, while both fluticasone and budesonide have received enormous attention in recent years. In general, daily doses below 1500 µg/day are safe over a long period. Sustained use of higher doses (>1500–2000 µg/day)can be associated with glaucoma, cataracts, increased bone mineral loss, minimal linear growth rate suppression in children, and adrenal suppression, among other unwanted side effects. It is possible to minimize the systemic absorption and side-effect profile of these products by using a spacer (which reduces pharyngal deposition and may enhance the relative fraction actually reaching the lungs in some patients), rinsing the mouth after each use, administering the medications on either qd or bid dosing frequency, and by using the lowest effective dose possible.

Beclomethasone is soon to be marketed in solution in HFA (a substitute for Freon that is ozone friendly) in a novel MDI that generates an aerosol consisting of smaller particle sizes than are generated by currently available CCS preparations. This new product, QVAR (50 and 100 µg/puff), will be capable of achieving extraordinary deposition rates into the lungs, far into the small airways (Fig. 1). It is therefore likely that this new preparation will be more effective than current preparations of beclomethasone.

One objective way to decide if the dose of inhaled CCS is adequate is to monitor the morning peak flow rates. Thus, a patient is started on a chosen dose of inhaled CCS and the peak flow is followed until it peaks and plateaus. The initial dose of CCS is either maintained or increased until the peak flow increases and plateaus, arriving at the patient's personal-best peak flow. Thereafter, the dose of CCS can be reduced while the peak flow is monitored. The aim is to achieve the lowest dose of CCS that maintains the personal-best peak flow.

Peak flows are also useful for helping in the management of emergency situations by helping the physician estimate the degree of severity of an asthma attack. Finally, peak flows allow patient self-management. Each patient is shown his or her "personal-best" peak flow (the plateau number), and alerted as to what to do if the peak flow falls 10–20%, 20–50%, and >50% (*see* Table 21). Thus, proper use of peak flows substantially enhances the management of asthma, and many asthma specialists routinely provide peak flow meters to each of their patients.

Oral CCS therapy is used to achieve control during exacerbations, when the peak flow falls to 50% or more from the patient's personal best. Oral CCSs are also useful at the first sign of a cold or sinusitis in patients known to have exacerbations under these conditions. Oral CCSs are usually considered as a treatment of a last resort for those asthmatics who have failed to respond to other drugs, largely because of concern over the risk of serious adverse effects. Despite these concerns, if oral steroids are to be used, clinicians must be sure to give adequate doses—often 20–30 mg/d or more—for a sufficient time to achieve a meaningful effect. The initial daily dose can be given in a single dose or divided doses, recognizing that divided doses are both more effective and more dangerous. Patients should be given a written schedule of their individualized treatment plan. As soon as possible after a remission is achieved, the dosing schedule should either be reduced to an alternate-day regimen or tapered-off entirely.

If a patient requires frequent bursts of daily CCS, it might be more efficient to treat with alternate-day CCS—a dose one day and then none for 48 h. This alternate-day schedule reduces most of the untoward side effects of oral CCS.

Nonsteroidal Drugs: Cromolyn and Nedocromil. The nonsteroidal agents cromolyn sodium (Intal) and nedocromil sodium (Tilade) can be used to reduce the inflammatory response and mast cell reactivity in patients with asthma (Table 22). They are more useful in younger, allergic asthmatics and best used for prophylaxis. In addition, prophylactic use of these agents can prevent allergen-induced early asthmatic responses, late asthmatic responses, and the increased airway reactivity associated with these reactions.

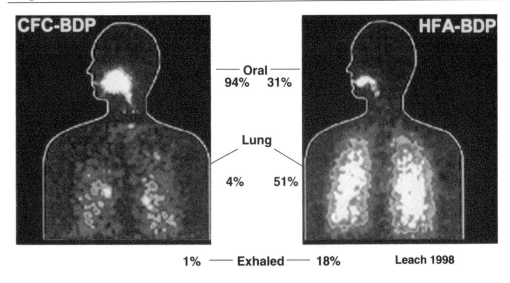

Fig. 1. Comparison between the inhalation of beclomethasone in HFA vs Freon. Six healthy males inhaled BDP from canisters in which the propellant was HFA (*right panel*) or Freon (*left panel*). The average deposition into the lungs was 55–60% for the HFA preparation (QVAR) and 4–7% for Freon. Asthmatics (n=16 also demonstrated 56Å 6% deposition from the HFA preparation. The solution of beclomethasone into HFA markedly facilitated the deposition of inhaled CCS for asthma treatment. (From: Leach CL, Davidson PJ, Boudreau PJ. Improved airway targeting with the CFC-free HFA-beclomethasone metered dose-inhaler compared with CFC-beclomethasone. *Eur Respir J* 12:1346–53,1998.)

Cromolyn is used to maintain control in cases of mild to moderate asthma. Although the exact mechanism of action is not fully understood, cromolyn appears to stabilize the mast cell, preventing the release of mast cell mediators, and to protect against bronchospasm. Cromolyn is particularly beneficial in the younger allergic asthmatic, but can also be used in adults and children with nonallergic asthma. Cromolyn causes only minimal side effects. A 4–6-wk trial may be required to determine efficacy in individual patients.

Nedocromil is similar in action to cromolyn and may be somewhat more effective. Evidence suggests that nedocromil is safe and effective in decreasing asthma symptoms and bronchial reactivity in allergic and nonallergic adult asthma patients. Both agents are categorized as pregnancy category B. Both agents can be used as first-line treatment of mild persistent asthma, especially in children, and both agents could be added to inhaled CCS in more moderately affected patients.

Cromolyn is often given to small children through nebulization and has been useful in preventing exercise-induced asthma.

Nonsteroidal Drugs: Leukotriene Modifiers. Currently, there are two classes of leukotriene (LT) modifiers on the market (Table 23): zafirlukast (Accolate, 20 mg bid on empty stomach) and montelukast (Singulair, 10 mg qhs) are leukotriene receptor antagonists and zileuton (Zyflo, 600 mg qid) is a LT synthesis inhibitor. These products have been on the market for a few years, and experience suggests that Accolate and Singulair can be tried as monotherapy in mild disease, with about 30–50% of patients

Table 21
Patient "Self-Management"

(Based upon personal best peak-flow measurements)
Peak flow falls 10–20%: double use of inhaled CCS
Peak flow falls >20%: use short–acting bronchodilator Q 4–6 h; call office (determine if infection is present)
Peak flow falls 40–50%: add oral CCS; call office
Peak flow falls greater than 50%: emergency visit
Provide written emergency management plan

Table 22
When to Use Cromolyn or Nedocromil

1. Most useful in younger, allergic asthmatics.
2. Best if used for prophylaxis. Might add after patient is well controlled with CCS, as a means to reduce CCS dose.
3. Try for coughing patient.
4. Try prophylactically for exercise-induced asthma.
5. Try larger doses if standard dose fails (more than 2 puffs at a time).
6. Try nedocromil in the office. If taste is a problem, do not prescribe.
7. Use nebulized form for younger asthmatics.

responding. As these are oral medications, and patients tend to prefer pills to inhalers, they may be worth a try in mild cases. These agents exhibit some anti-inflammatory actions and bronchodilator capacity, and they are generally quite safe. In moderate and severe asthma, both Accolate and Singulair can be added to inhaled CCS to allow reduction in the dose of CCS. Zyflo is the most powerful of the group and provides potential beneficial actions in both moderate and severe asthma. However, the side effects of Zyflo limit its usefulness; 3% of patients will experience an increase in liver enzymes, up to threefold to fivefold baseline. Therefore, liver enzymes must be measured whenever Zyflo is used. Moreover, a qid product is hard to administer, even though the frequency of dosing can be reduced to bid once improvement has occurred.

These products should be tried in all patients with aspirin sensitivity, and they are useful in some patients with sinusitis, polyposis, or urticaria. Because of drug-drug interactions, theophylline, coumadin, propranolol (Zyflo) and coumadin (Accolate) doses may need adjustment.

Symptomatic Agents

β-Adrenergic Agonists (Table 24)

β-agonists have been available for three decades and are now the most commonly prescribed medications for asthma. This class of agents is selective for the β_2-receptor of the airway, resulting in relaxation of the airway smooth muscle and, possibly, modulation of mediator release from mast cells and basophils.

The role of β-agonists in the treatment of asthma has undergone a significant change in recent years. While formerly considered the first choice in asthma treatment, experts now agree that these agents should be used only on an as-needed basis. This change

Table 23
When to Use Leukotriene Modifiers

1. Currently, two classes: Zafirlukast (Accolate, 20 mg bid on empty stomach) and Montelukast (Singulair, 10 mg qhs) are leukotriene receptor antagonists, and Zileuton (Zyflo, 600
   mg qid) is a leukotriene synthesis inhibitor.
2. Try Accolate or Singulair in mild to moderate disease and Zyflo with moderate to severe
   disease.
3. Try in aspirin-sensitive patients and patients with sinusitis, polyposis, urticaria.
4. Must adjust theophylline and warfarin doses (Zyflo) and warfarin (Accolate).
5. Experience indicates that about 30–50% of patients will improve with each product, some
   dramatically. Zyflo is probably the most potent but also has the most serious potential
   side effects.
6. Need to follow liver function tests with Zyflo, q mo × 3, q 3–6 mo thereafter.
7. Zyflo can be tapered to tid and bid after 1–2 mo.
8. All of these agents have the capacity to allow reduction in CCS dosing.

came about in part because of concern that regular and heavy use of β-agonists might
lead to increased mortality, a contention that has not been confirmed by carefully
conducted prospective studies. Nonetheless, it is now recommended that β-agonists
be used only when symptoms require prompt bronchodilation and that the dose and
frequency of administration be as low as possible. Generally, one canister per month
(which is about 200 puffs or 7 puffs/d) should be adequate for any patient. (Table 25).
In patients using two or more canisters per month, asthma should be considered to
be inadequately controlled and should be aggressively treated with anti-inflammatory
agents. β-Agonists are excellent preventive treatment for exercise-induced asthma and
should be administered 10–20 min before exercise. Some patients respond better to
bronchodilation through the Ventolin Rotacap system (a dry-powder inhaler system)
or Maxair (a breath-activated MDI) because of easier coordination between breathing
and activation of the product.

There are a variety of inhaled β-agonists on the market, although albuterol is the
most popular. While albuterol is relatively fast acting, it still takes up to 15 min for its
maximal effect. Oral β-agonists are also available, with actions that may last from 4
to 8 h. In general, inhaled β-agonists are preferred as they have fewer side effects and
work more quickly than oral preparations. Albuterol is also available in a dry-powder
form (Rotacaps), that has proven very useful for pretreatment of exercise-induced
asthma. An alternative is the breath-activated MDI, Maxair, which removes part of the
hand-eye coordination problems seen with ordinary MDI. Proventil is the first albuterol
product available in the ozone-friendly propellent, HFA. A novel form of albuterol
recently became available as a nebulized treatment of emergency asthma, Xepenex
(levalbuterol solution). This product is the isolated r-enantiomer of albuterol, removing
the l-form, which is purported to have some toxicity. The r-enantiomer will become
available as a possibly safer inhaled bronchodilator in the near future.

LONG-ACTING β-AGONISTS

The long-acting inhaled β-agonist, salmeterol xinafoate (Serevent), offers 12-h
duration of bronchodilation and has been shown to be effective in the treatment of

Table 24
When to Use a β-Agonist (Short-Acting)

1. With symptomatic disease, *as needed*
2. With exacerbations, at a peak flow 20% below personal best
3. Prior to exercise
4. *Do not use on a regular basis*
   Do not prescribe qid
   instead, use *"as often as qid"*

Table 25
Cautions with Short-Acting β-agonists

1. Be aware of canister use. Aim for <1 canister per month (1 canister per month is 200 puffs of albuterol = patient is using inhaler multiple times, every day)
2. Always ask how many times per day the β-agonist is being used, before refilling prescription.
3. Consider Ventolin Rotacap or Maxair for patients with difficulty using a MDI.
4. Consider Proventil HFA, which is albuterol in HFA, an ozone-friendly propellent.

mild, moderate, and severe asthma. This drug is indicated for patients who require multiple doses of a short-acting β-agonist despite concomitant use of inhaled CCS at appropriate doses (Table 26), for nocturnal wheezing despite appropriate treatment, and, in some cases, for prevention of exercise-induced asthma. Salmeterol may also have a role in some cases of occupational asthma, as prophylaxis for patients who are intermittently exposed to irritants in the workplace. Addition of Serevent to the treatment plan in moderate or severe asthma may allow reduction in the required dose of inhaled CCS.

Serevent has a delayed and progressive onset of action, achieving maximal brochodilation hours after its use. Thus it is not useful in emergency treatment or when a patient's asthma isworsening. However, as a prophylactic bonchodilator, it is very helpful in selected patients (Table 27). Serevent is available both as a MDI and as a dry-powder inhaler. We usually use Serevent through a spacer to reduce swallowing of the product. Generally, Serevent is added to the treatment plan that includes inhaled CCS and other specific therapies. Preferred use is in the moderate or severe asthmatic both to provide symptomatic bronchodilation and reduce the need for inhaled CCS.

THEOPHYLLINE

Although declining in popularity, theophylline has been used for many years as both emergency and routine therapy and is still an extremely useful symptomatic agent to treat chronic asthma (Table 28). Theophylline is often recommended for patients whose disease is not adequately controlled by other medications, those who have nocturnal diseases, and those in whom a long-acting oral bronchodilator is needed (such as the rare patient with chlorofluorocarbon sensitivity). The recommended dose for most patients aims to achieve a blood level of 5–15 μg/mL.

Table 26
When to Add Serevent

1. When patient requires multiple inhalations of short-acting
   β-agonist per day despite appropriate therapy.
2. When patient is experiencing nocturnal wheezing despite
   appropriate therapy.
3. Consider use for prevention of exercise-induced asthma when use
   of short-acting β-agonist is inconvenient.
4. Consider for patient who is intermittently exposed to irritants in the
   environment (work exposures, fumes) as prophylaxis.
5. Consider as an inhaled CCS-sparing agent.

Table 27
Cautions in Use of Serevent

1. Never start during exacerbations or when patient's condition is
   worsening, add when condition is stable.
2. Start cautiously in older patients (1 puff bid if patient >60–65 yr).
3. Use spacer or dry-powder inhaler to reduce swallowing and
   systemic exposure.
4. Advise patients not to carry this product; it is for prophylaxis only.
   Recommend that it be used in the bathroom, not when needed.

Although a staple for the treatment of asthma for many years, theophylline is associated with several drawbacks. Dose-related side effects include gastrointestinal discomfort, headache, insomnia, and seizures. In addition, use of theophylline is thought to affect behavior, mood, and learning in both adults and children; however, these possible actions are controversial. Drug-drug interactions are also of concern, with some agents increasing theophylline levels and others reducing it (Table 29). Some of the agents implicated include allopurinol, cimetidine, ciprofloxacin, erythromycin, and birth control pills. Despite these drawbacks, theophylline should be considered an important third-line agent in the treatment of moderate to severe asthma, to be used in conjunction with specific treatments and β-agonists.

Theophylline is a category B product in pregnancy and can prove very useful in asthmatics who worsen significantly during pregnancy. Appropriate serum levels of theophylline in pregnancy are 5–12 µg/mL. Studies have shown that compliance is higher with oral theophylline than with inhaled agents, especially with teenagers. Theophylline is available as once or twice-daily sustained-release tablets.

ANTICHOLINERGICS (TABLE 30)

Ipratropium bromide (Atrovent) and atropine sulfate are the only anticholinergic drugs available in the United States for treatment of asthma. An inhaled formulation of ipratropium may be beneficial in the treatment of asthmatics with excessive mucous secretion (the asthmatic-bronchitis patient). The availability of nebulized ipratropium has led to its increased use in emergency treatment of asthma and in patients (many of whom are children) who use nebulizers. Ipratropium is also available in combination

Table 28
When to Use Theophylline

1. When patient's condition is not adequately controlled symptomatically with short- or long-acting β-agonists
2. With persistent nocturnal awakenings
3. When a long-acting, oral bronchodilator is preferred
4. Consider as an inhaled CCS-sparing agent
5. In pregnancy, when a safe long-acting bronchodilator is necessary

Table 29
Cautions with Theophylline

1. Yearly blood levels (5–15, μg/ml; <12 ug/ml if pregnant)
2. Agents that affect theophylline metabolism:
    Decreased metabolism *(elevated blood levels):*
    liver failure, >55 yr old, heart failure, high temperature, <1 yr old, allopurinol, cimetidine, ciprofloxacin, erythromycin, TAO, BCP, propranolol, ketoconazole, chlorethromycin, and others
    Increased metabolism *(reduced blood levels):*
    cigaret or marijuana smokers, phenytoin, rifampin, charcoal foods, and others

with albuterol (Combivent), and the combination has more bronchodilating properties than either agent alone.

Treatment of Concomitant Diseases and Conditions

Many asthmatics will respond only when their concomitant sinusitis, GERD, thyroiditis, emotional stress, or pregnancy is under control. Moreover, the treatment of asthma requires close attention to concomitant colds, flu, bronchitis, irritant or pollutant inhalation, recreational drug use, and emotional changes. Compliance is a significant problem, both with medication use and allergen avoidance and inhaler techniques. Thus, the physician who treats asthma needs to keep the whole patient in focus, as well as the patient's work and family environment. On the other hand, proper treatment is nearly always effective and can be extraordinarily gratifying. It is common to convert "pulmonary cripples" into totally functioning humans in a matter of weeks.

The proper treatment of asthma involves a close partnership between primary care physicians (PCP) and specialists. Referral to specialists should result in significant insight in the cause and treatment of this disease, and the patient should receive important education in allergen avoidance and medication use, as well as written emergency treatment plans. Evidence for an important role of immunotherapy in allergic asthmatics as an important long-term controlling (specific treatment) influence is gaining popularity again. In today's market. most immunotherapy is started by the allergist and provided in the PCP's office. Thus, immunotherapy and allergen avoidance techniques, much like other approaches to asthma, can be started and explained by the specialist and supported and provided by the PCP.

Table 30
Anticholinergics

1. Most useful in the asthmatic with bronchitis to help reduce mucous production.
2. Atrovent solution adds to β-agonist inhalation in emergency settings.
3. Combivent (an MDI-combining albuterol with ipratropium) may be useful for asthma and bronchitis.

SUGGESTED READING

Expert panel report 1: *Guidelines for the diagnosis and management of asthma*. National Asthma Education Program. US Department of Health and Human Services. NIH Publication 91–3642. Bethesda, MD. 1991.

Expert panel report 2: *Guidelines for the diagnosis and management of asthma*. National Asthma Education and Prevention Program. US Department of Health and Human Services. NIH Publication 97–4051. Bethesda, MD. 1997.

Global initiative for asthma. National Institute for Heart, Lung and Blood. NIH Publication 95–3659. Bethesda, MD. 1995.

International asthma management panel. *International Consensus Report on Diagnosis and Management of Asthma*. US Department of Health and Human Services. NIH Publication 92–3091, Bethesda, MD. 1992

Kaliner MA. Current Review of Allergic Disease. Philadelphia, Current Medicine, 1999.

Lemanske RF, Busse WW. Asthma. *JAMA* 1997;278:1855–1873.

9 Rhinitis

Dennis K. Ledford, MD

CONTENTS

INTRODUCTION

The nasal airway, which includes the nasal cavity and the nasopharynx, begins at the nasal vestibule and extends through the nasopharynx (Fig. 1). The epithelium is a ciliated, pseudostratified, columnar mucosa except for the squamous epithelium lining the vestibule and anterior third of the nasal airway. The mucosa of the nasal airway is contiguous with that of the paranasal sinuses and eustachian tubes. The blood flow to the nasal mucosa is one of the highest for any tissue of the body, with the flow controlled by a combination of resistance and capicitance vessels. The latter permit pooling of blood in the submucosa, resulting in swelling or congestion. The microcirculation is fenestrated to facilitate the transfer of water from the vascular space to the mucosa. The high blood flow and fenestrated vessels facilitate heating and humidification of the airstream.

Rhinitis is a term loosely used to refer to symptomatic disorders of the nasal airway. Some authors prefer the general term rhinopathy, as opposed to rhinitis, for symptomatic nasal airway disease because of the absence of inflammation in some of these disorders. The term *rhinitis* will be used in this review when referring to symptomatic disorders of the nasal airway. The differential diagnosis of nasal airway symptoms can be subdivided arbitrarily into eight groups based upon probable etiology or association: allergy, idiopathic perennial nonallergic rhinitis, infection, medication or hormone effects, nasal mucosal atrophy, neoplasm, systemic disease, and structural abnormalities (Table 1).

From: *Current Clinical Practice: Allergic Diseases: Diagnosis and Treatment, 2nd Edition*
Edited by: P. Lieberman and J. Anderson © Humana Press Inc., Totowa, NJ

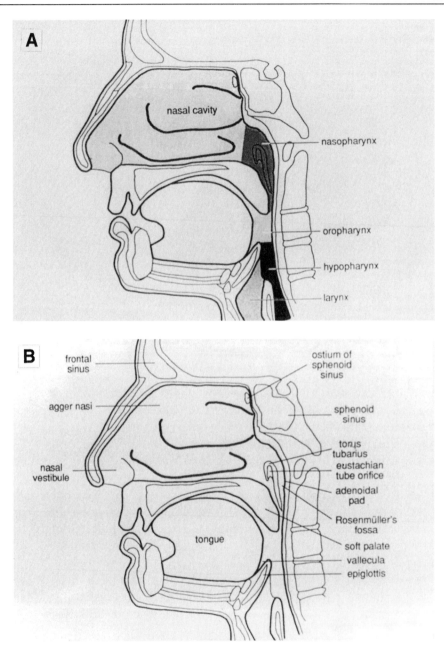

Fig. 1. Schematic of the upper airway with designation of anatomical structures.

ALLERGIC RHINITIS

Allergic rhinitis results from inhaled allergen cross linking specific IgE on the surface of mucosal and submucosal mast cells. The result is the release of a series of stored mediators and the synthesis of other mediators and cytokines. These mast cell products are responsible, directly or indirectly, for the symptoms of allergic rhinitis. Allergic rhinitis affects more than 20% of the population, with one study showing an

Table 1
Differential Diagnosis of Rhinitis

Disease	Major Classification	Cause
Allergic Rhinitis	Seasonal Perennial	
Infectious Rhinitis	Viral	Adenovirus Influenza virus Parainfluenza virus Respiratory syncytial virus Rhinovirus
	Bacterial	Streptococcus Hemophilus
Structural Nasal Disorders	Nasal septal deviation Nasal polyps Adenoid hyperplasia or cyst Choanal atresia	

	Neoplasm	Squamous cell carcinoma (more
		  common in cigaret smokers)
		Angiofibroma (more common
		  in adolescent boys)
		Esthesioneuroblastoma
		  (resembles a benign
		  nasal polyp)
		Lymphoma
		Sarcoma
		Inverted papilloma

	Foreign body Encephalocele	

Other Forms of Rhinitis	Atrophic rhinitis
	Perennial nonallergic rhinitis
	  (vasomotor rhinitis)
	Nonallergic rhinitis with
	  eosinophilia (NARES)	

	Rhinitis medicamentosa	Topical decongestants
		  Oxymetazoline
		  Cocaine
		  Neosynephrine
		Systemic therapies
		  β blockers
		  α antagonists
		  Estrogen supplements or
		    oral contraceptives
		  Nonsteroidal anti-inflammatory
		    drugs

	Systemic diseases	Endocrine/hormonal
		  Hypothyroidism
		  Pregnancy or breast feeding
		  Diabetes mellitus
		Inflammatory
		  Sarcoidosis
		  Wegener's granulomatosis
		  Relapsing polychondritis
		  Reticular histiocytosis
		    (lethal midline granuloma)
		Infiltrative
		  Amyloidosis

incidence of 42% in children older than 6 yr. The severity is variable, dependent upon the degree of allergic sensitivity, allergen exposure and aggravating factors such as septal deviation, adenoid hyperplasia, coexisting sinusitis or nasal polyps. Rhinitis is not life threatening but is a significant epidemiological factor in the health of a population. This significance is due to the following:

- Quality of life of subjects with moderate allergic rhinitis is lower than of subjects with moderate asthma, thus influencing the perceived health of affected subjects.
- Allergic rhinitis increases the incidence and prevalence of sinusitis and otitis media.
- 60–80% of subjects with allergic rhinitis have bronchial hyperreactivity.
- Subjects with seasonal allergic rhinitis develop asthma 3–5 times more often than subjects without rhinitis.
- The incidence of allergic rhinitis is increasing, with one study showing a doubling from 1971–1981.

The reasons for the increasing prevalence of allergic rhinitis are unknown but indoor environmental issues, cigaret smoking, increasing populations in urban environments and the effects of air pollution are likely possibilities. Thus, allergic rhinitis adversely affects the lives of many people, and identifies individuals at risk of expensive medical complications with significant morbidity.

The cost of allergic rhinitis care is difficult to estimate because of the overlap with upper and lower airway complications and the various rhinitis syndromes. It was estimated that in 1990 the annual direct medical expense for the care of seasonal allergic rhinitis was $1.8 billion. This is a very conservative figure, since care of perennial allergic rhinitis is not included. The indirect costs include absenteeism and decreased productivity, with estimates of 3.4 million work-loss days for 12.8 million individuals employed outside of the home. Approximately 30 million cases of sinusitis occur per annum in the United States, and allergic rhinitis is a predisposing factor in 25–70%. Upper respiratory symptoms are one of the most common reasons people seek outpatient medical care, and allergic rhinitis is frequently either the cause or a cofactor for these symptoms. Thus, the significance of allergic rhinitis extends from a cause of common nuisance symptoms to a major contributor to population health issues.

Pathophysiology

Allergic rhinitis is the result of production of specific IgE coupled with exposure to allergen. Seasonal allergic rhinitis is usually due to pollen, with typical patterns of spring symptoms due to tree pollen, summer symptoms due to grass pollen and autumn symptoms due to weed pollen. These idealized patterns are subject to local climate and botanical influences. For example, the "spring" tree season in Florida occurs in January–March, and weed pollen is not prevalent in the mountains and the western US. Mold seasons occur in certain areas, such as the late fall in the Gulf Coast of the United States. Perennial allergic rhinitis is generally due to the indoor allergens from dust mites, animal proteins and possibly mold. Cockroach allergen, an important cause of perennial allergic asthma, may be a contributor to allergic rhinitis. The vulnerability of the nasal mucosa to allergic disease is in large part a result of the efficient filtering of the inhaled, nasal airstream. Approximately 100% of particles greater than or equal to 10-μm in diameter are captured in the nasal mucosa, 80% of 5-μm particles and

Table 2
Mast Cell Mediators of Allergy

Cell type	Mediator	Action
Preformed	Histamine	Increases vascular permeability, increases mucous production, anti-inflammatory effects via H_2 receptors
	Neutral proteases Tryptase(s) Chymotryptases(s) Carboxypeptidase(s)	Protein degradation and activation of protein precursors
Synthesized During Cellular Activation	Leukotriene C_4 (LTC_4)	Increases vascular permeability, increases mucous production
	Leukotriene B_4 (LTB_4)	Increases neutrophil chemotaxis
	Prostaglandin D_2 (PGD_2)	Smooth muscle contraction
	Thromboxane A_2	Platelet aggregation, vasoconstriction
	Platelet activating factor (PAF)	Platelet aggregation. Increases neutrophil and eosinophil chemotaxis and activation. Increases vascular permeability, smooth muscle contraction
Cytokines	Interleukin-4 (IL-4)	Increases endothelial expression of VCAM-1, increases IgE production, stimulation of TH_2, and inhibition of TH_1 lymphocytes
	Tumor necrosis factor (TNF-α)	Increases endothelial ICAM-1 expression
	Interleukin-5 (IL-5)	Activates eosinophils and basophils
	Interleukin-3 (IL-3)	Activates esoinophils and basophils, growth factor for mast cells
	Granulocyte-monocyte-colony-stimulating factor (GM-CSF)	Activates eosinophils and basophils, growth factor for mast cells
	Select chemokines	Neutrophil, eosinophil and basophil chemotaxis, enhances mast cell and basophil mediator release

almost none of the 1- to 2-μm particles. Pollen grains vary in size from 10–100 μm, an ideal size for nasal deposition.

The allergic response in respiratory disease is a two-phase process. An initial sensitization phase is required to produce specific IgE. The second phase is the interaction of allergen with specific IgE bound to high-affinity IgE Fc receptors on mast cells and possibly basophils. The crosslinking of IgE on the cell surface triggers a series of biochemical events resulting in the release of preformed mediators and the synthesis of other mediators (Table 2). The result is an acute-phase or immediate allergic reaction in the nose characterized by sneezing, pruritus and rhinorrhea. The sneezing decreases within minutes of exposure, but the rhinorrhea requres more than 20 min to abate (Fig. 2). The sneezing and pruritus are primarily due to the release of the mediator histamine. Congestion is slower in onset and persists for more than

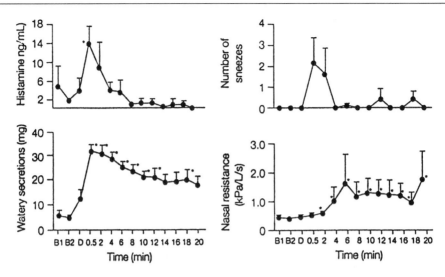

Fig. 2. Sneezing, watery secretions and swelling (increased nasal resistance) are among the first indications of allergic rhinitis. They occur within minutes after a single-dose antigen challenge and are mediated primarily by histamine. The graphs illustrate the time course of histamine production (by mast cells), which correlates with these early phase physiological events. Notice, however, that even after histamine levels have diminished and sneezing has subsided, the production of watery secretions and swelling persists (p<0.05 vs diluent; B1 and B2, baseline measurements; D, diluent.) (From Naclerio RM. Allergy 1997.)

20 min following a single, experimental allergen exposure. This initial, acute-phase response is followed by a late-phase allergic response 4–6 h after allergen exposure. The late phase is characterized by more persistent symptoms, primarily congestion. The nasal mucosa is infiltrated with eosinophils, neutrophils, basophils, moncytes and T-lymphoctyes, resulting in an inflammatory reaction. Cytokines are the major modulators of this inflammation. These cytokines include interleukin-4 (IL-4) primarily from mast cells, IL-3, IL-4, IL-5 and granulocyte-monocyte-colony-stimulating factor (GM-CSF) from helper T-lymphocytes and mast cells, and IL-6, IL-8, GM-CSF and RANTES (a chemokine or chemoattractant for eosinophils) from the epithelial cells. The late-phase response occurs in more than 50% of experimental challenges, depending on the sensitivity of the individual and amount of allergen administered. Understanding the early- and late-phase responses requires an awareness of the various cell types involved.

ANTIGEN PRESENTING CELLS

Specific IgE production requires sufficient exposure to the allergen and a predisposed host. Allergen exposure to the immune system necessitates antigen processing by antigen-presenting cells, such as Langerhans' cells (CD1+ dendritic cells) and macrophages. These cells are present in the nasal epithelium and lamina propria, and their number increases in symptomatic subjects. This increase is not specific for allergic rhinitis, as nasal macrophage number increases following nonspecific, nonimmunological stimulation of the mucosa, e.g., daily saline lavage or brushing of the mucosa. Thus, nonimmunological irritation may increase the likelihood of allergen presentation to immunocytes.

T-Lymphocytes

The T-lymphocyte must recognize antigen presented by antigen-presenting cells, initiate a specific immune response and regulate this response before specific immunity such as IgE production occurs. Populations of T-lymphocytes or individual T-lymphocytes with a phenotype designated TH_2 are of primary importance in the IgE response. TH_2 cells produce cytokines that augment IgE production and decrease IgG and IgA production. These cytokines include IL-4 and IL-13. These TH_2 cells also release IL-3, IL-5 and GM-CSF, which activate and enhance survival of eosinophils. Local production of these regulatory cytokines has been verified by analysis of nasal lavage or nasal biopsies. These analyses have shown either the cytokines or the messenger RNA for the cytokines in these nasal samples.

Eosinophils

The distinguishing inflammatory cells in allergic inflammation are eosinophils. These leukocytes are recruited locally and activated primarily during the late phase allergic response. Their movement to inflammatory sites and subsequent activation appear to be directed by specific cytokines, such as IL-3, IL-5, GM-CSF and factors regulated on activation of normal T-cells expressed and secreted (RANTES; a cytokine or chemoattractanct for various cells, particularly eosinophils). Adhesion to the nasal vascular endothelium via E-selelctin is important for the eosinophil's initial emergence from the circulation.

The first contact of the eosinophil with the nasal vascular endothelium is termed the rolling phase because the eosinophil loosely and reversibly adheres to the endothelium via E-selectin. Subsequently, the eosinophil adheres more tightly to the endothelium because specific ligands (or integrins) on the surface of the eosinophil interact with adhesion molecules (up-regulated by cytokines) on the vascular endothelial cell surfaces. Thus:

- Very late antigen 4 (VLA-4) binds to the vascular cell adhesion molecule 1 (VCAM-1).
- Leukocyte functional antigen 1 (LFA-1) binds to the intercellular adhesion molecule 1 (ICAM-1).
- An unknown eosinophil ligand binds to the endothelial cell leukocyte adhesion molecule 1 (ELAM-1).

Only the VLA-4 / VCAM interaction is specific for the eosinophil. Following antigen challenge, expression of E-selectin and VCAM-1 up-regulates on the surfaces of nasal endothelial cells of subjects with allergic rhinitis. Expression of ICAM-1 does not increase (Fig. 3).

The most potent chemoattractant for eosinophils is probably RANTES. Other chemoattractants and activators of eosinophils include membrane cofactor protein (MCP-3), LTB_4, histamine, eosinophil chemoattractant of anaphylaxis (ECF-A) from mast cells, platelet activating factor (PAF), IL-3, IL-5, GM-CSF, and the complement protein fragment C5a.

Eosinophils are pro-inflammatory, with the capacity to release preformed cytotoxic proteins such as major basic protein and eosinophil cationic protein, various proteinases and toxic superoxide radicals. Other inflammatory substances produced by eosinophils include LTC_4, GM-CSF, IL-1, IL-3, and transforming growth factor α.

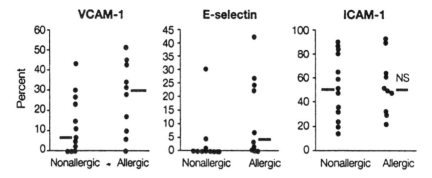

Fig. 3. Expression of adhesion molecules, such as E-selectin and the vascular adhesion molecule 1 (VCAM-1), on the surfaces of vascular endothelial cells in the nasal submocusa is up-regulated in patients with allergic rhinitis ($n = 10$), but not in nonallergic rhinitis ($n = 13$; $p < 0.05$), 24 h after allergen challenge. The expression of the intercellular adhesion molecule 1 (ICAM-1; NS, not significant) does not increase. Regulation of these factors is mediated primarily by cytokines released from helper T-lymphocytes and mast cells. The adhesion molecules bind with integrins (VCAM-1 binds with very late antigen 4) on the surfaces of eosinophils that are recruited during the late-phase response. This mechanism facilitates movement of a vast array of immune cells from the circulatory spaces to the nasal submucosa and mucosa, where they release mediators that further the inflammatory process. (From Lee BJ, et al. J Allergy Clin Immunol 1994.)

MAST CELLS/BASOPHILS

Mast cells and basophils are the only cells that express high-affinity IgE Fc receptors and are the most important cells in IgE-dependent allergic reactions. Nasal biopsies from symptomatic subjects with allergic rhinitis have an increased number of subepithelial and intraepithelial mast cells, many of which are degranulated. Mediators released from mast cells following crosslinking of high-affinity IgE Fc receptors include histamine, tryptase, chymotryptase, leukotrienes (primarily LTC$_4$) and prostaglandins (primarily PGD$_2$). Mast cells also produce the cytokines tumor necrosis factor α (TNF-α), IL-4, IL-5, and IL-6 (Table 2). Basophils provide a similar constellation of mediators and cytokines except that PGD$_2$ is not produced. The absence of PGD$_2$ and presence of histamine in nasal lavage of late-phase allergic reactions support the importance of basophils in this delayed, inflammatory allergic response. Basophils can be identified in nasal secretions, in contrast to the absence of mast cells in secretions, and the number increases following allergen challenge.

NEUTROPHILS

Neutrophils are a major infiltrating cell type in the airway epithelium during the late-phase allergic reaction. These cells release inflammatory mediators, including LTB$_4$ and platelet activating factor (PAF). Neutrophils contribute significantly to the inflammation following allergen challenge.

EPITHELIAL CELLS

Airway epithelial cells not only act as a barrier but are also effector cells that secrete inflammatory mediators and cytokines. These include chemotactic factors, colony-stimulating factors, prostaglandins and leukotrienes. Cellular adhesion factors, such as ICAM-1, are also expressed on epithelial surfaces and serve as viral receptors as well

> The most useful tool in the differential diagnosis of rhinitis is the history. Two most common forms of chronic rhinitis are allergic and chronic nonallergic. These can usually be distinguished by features of the history.
>
> Features that suggest allergy are:
> • Seasonal variation with exacerbations in spring and fall
> • Exacerbation on exposure to aeroallergens (e.g., animals and freshly cut grass)
> • Association with other allergic conditions, especially conjunctivitis

as binding to inflammatory cells. The regulation of these receptors may be important in the interaction of viral infection and allergic respiratory disease.

ENDOTHELIAL CELLS

Endothelial cells help regulate vascular tone and permeability, thus influencing nasal edema and congestion. Endothelial cells also influence cellular traffic following allergen exposure. The inflammatory cells involved in the late-phase allergic response are attracted by a selective recruitment process. Endothelial receptors stimulate increased adherence and the tissue immigration of circulating eosinophils, basophils and T-lymphocytes. The initial selective cellular recruitment occurs in response to cytokine-induced up-regulation of leukocyte adhesion molecules and cell-surface ligands, particularly VCAM-1 and E-selectin (Fig. 3). ICAM-1 is the predominant endothelial cell adhesion molecule but does not increase following antigen challenge and is not selective for cells involved in allergic inflammation.

ADDITIONAL PATHOPHYSIOLOGICAL FACTORS

In addition to the factors described above, the signs and symptoms of allergic rhinitis are modified by other factors not directly dependent on allergic inflammation. These include:

- *Neural reflexes*: The role of the autonomic nervous system in allergic rhinitis has been demonstrated by the development of congestion in the contralateral nasal airway following nasal challenge with allergen. The effect is antagonized by atropine suggesting parasympathetic mediation. Neurogenic influence on the late-phase response is suggested by a slight increase in histamine and basophils in the contralateral nasal airway following allergen challenge. The mechanism for this neurogenic inflammation is unknown.
- *The "priming effect"*: The phenomenon of heightened sensitivity to allergen challenge following a prior challenge is probably a result of inflammation following the initial exposure. This theory is supported by the mitigation of the priming effect by pretreatment with topical or systemic corticosteroid therapy. Even if the acute phase allergic response is unaffected, the priming effect diminishes.
- *Nasal hyperreactivity*: Patients with symptomatic allergic rhinitis are hyperresponsive to nonantigenic stimuli such as methacholine, histamine and cold, dry air. Heightened sensitivity is not a specific result of allergic inflammation, since subjects with nonallergic rhinitis are also hyperreactive to cold, dry air. Symptoms resulting from hyperreactivity to nonantigenic, environmental factors may modify or augment the symptoms of allergic rhinitis.

Table 3
Allergy Symptoms and Responsible Mediators

Symptom	Mediator
Itching/Sneezing	Histamine
	Prostaglandins
Nasal blockage/	Histamine
Microvascular Leakage	Prostaglandins
	Leukotrienes
	Platelet Activating Factor (PAF)
	Kinins
	Chymase
	Substance P
Mucous Secretion	Histamine
	Eicosanoids
	Platelet Activating Factor (PAF)
	Kinins

Clinical Presentation and Diagnosis

The primary symptoms of allergic rhinitis are itching, rhinorrhea and sneezing (Table 3). Increased mucous secretion, nasal congestion, postnasal drip and facial pressure are common but nonspecific. Seasonal or intermittent perennial allergen exposure is more likely to result in the typical symptoms of allergic rhinitis, whereas perennial allergen exposure may result primarily in congestion. Sneezing paroxysms of four or more in succession and itching, especially intense itching or itching of tissues other than the nose, are relatively specific for allergic disease. The family history, age of onset and environmental association with symptoms are supportive of the diagnosis. A primary family member with atopy increases the probability of allergic disease to over 40%; two family members increase probability to over 60%. Most subjects with allergic rhinitis develop symptoms during childhood and adolescence, but up to 30% of affected subjects develop symptoms after the age of 20 yr.

Physical findings of allergic rhinitis are limited. The typical allergic facies is one with open mouth breathing and puffiness around the eyes (Dennie's sign, Morgan line of the lower eyelid secondary to conjunctival edema) (Fig. 4). A narrow face, high-arched palate and recessed mandible are associated with chronic rhinitis. A transverse nasal crease of the nasal tip may result following incessant rubbing of the nose. The nasal mucosa is classically pale, but this is detected in a minority of affected subjects (Fig. 5). The secretions are usually clear and watery but may be mucoid or even cloudy yellow. Nasal smears of secretions or turbinate biopsies demonstrating eosinophils are a potentially useful clinical test to support the diagnosis. Nasal smears are positive in approximately 60% of adults with allergic rhinitis; less in children under the age of 5 yr. Elevations of total serum IgE and/or peripheral eosinophil counts also support the diagnosis but are generally not cost-effective, since more than 20% of subjects with allergic rhinitis will be normal. Testing for specific IgE by skin test or radioallergosorbent test (RAST) or other in vitro testing is necessary to confirm the diagnosis. Knowledge of the local environment and correlation with symptoms is essential in the interpretation of test information. Skin testing generally is more

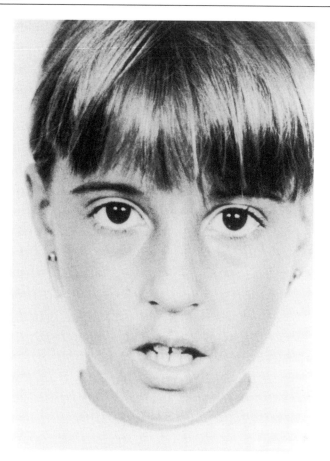

Fig. 4. Typical allergic facies in a child. The open-mouth breathing, dark color beneath the eyes ("allergic shiners") and narrow, elongated face (adenoid facies) are characteristic but not specific or sensitive for allergic rhinitis.

sensitive. Various concerns about skin tests can be addressed with adequate attention to technique and to the quality of reagents. These concerns include false-positive and false-negative results, variation with skin test site, variable reproducibility, inconsistent potency of allergen extracts and medical therapy that minimizes skin test reactivity. Standardized allergen extracts coupled with efforts to standardize techniques have helped overcome many of these objections, and skin testing remains the most cost-effective means of diagnosing allergic rhinitis.

The differential diagnosis of allergic rhinitis includes perennial nonallergic rhinitis (vasomotor rhinitis), rhinitis medicamentosa, anatomical nasal obstruction (including nasal polyps, septal deviation, malignant disease, choanal atresia, adenoid hyperplasia), nonallergic rhinitis with eosinophilia (NARES) and chronic sinusitis (Table 1). These other conditions should be considered or evaluated in the diagnosis of allergic rhinitis (*see* below).

Treatment

The therapy of allergic rhinitis is a three-pronged approach—avoidance or reduction of exposure to allergens, pharmacological treatment and immunotherapy. In addition,

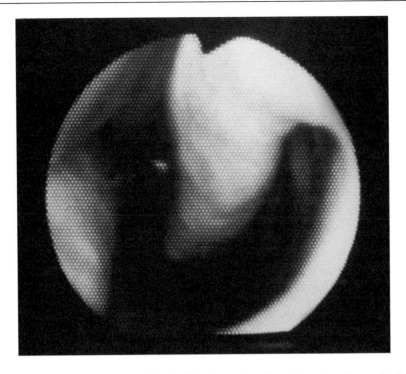

Fig. 5. Nasal mucosa in a patient with allergic rhinitis, as visualized through a fiberoptic rhinolaryngoscope. The pale, mucosal surface with clear, watery secretions is typical.

nonimmunological factors and complications of allergic rhinitis should be identified and treated if possible. These include bacterial sinusitis, rhinitis medicamentosa and structural abnormalities such as a significant septal deviation, nasal polyps or adenoidal hyperplasia (Fig. 6). A stepwise approach to the treatment of allergic rhinitis is provided in Table 4.

ALLERGEN AVOIDANCE AND CONTROL

Allergen avoidance is the most direct means for controlling, or even curing, allergic rhinitis (Table 5). Although avoidance is an important component of overall care, the pervasive presence of most antigens and nonadherence are major limitations. The conflict of separation from the indoor family pet and the restriction of staying indoors when pollen or mold counts are elevated are but two examples of the difficulties encountered. Despite the limitations, this effective and generally efficient means of limiting allergic rhinitis should be reviewed with every affected subject. The association of allergic rhinitis with medical complications, including but not limited to sinusitis, otitis media, and asthma, should not be emphasized to instill in the subject a commitment to environmental control. The limitations of medications, need for long-term use, cost and potential side effects of medical therapy should be reviewed also.

PHARMACOLOGICAL THERAPY

Antihistamine therapy is efficacious for the symptoms of itching, rhinorrhea and sneezing. Fifty years of experience substantiate the beneficial effects and general tolerance to this treatment. The mechanism of action is a competitive blockade of

Table 4

Stepwise Approach to the Treatment of Seasonal Allergic Rhinitis

Allergen avoidance, pharmacological therapy	
Mild disease or with occasional symptoms	Oral nonsedating H_1-antihistamine when symptomatic (fexofenadine, loratidine, or possibly cetirizine)[a]
	OR
	Topical nasal azelastine when symptomatic or sodium cromoglycate to eyes, nose or both/ alternative for intermittent eye symptoms is topical ocular antihistamine or topical nonsteroidal anti-inflammatory (ketorolac tromethamine)[b]
Moderate disease with prominent nasal symptoms	Intranasal corticosteroid daily (start early in season)
	PLUS
	Antihistamine or topical eye therapy with sodium cromoglycate or lodoxamide tromethamine or olopatadine hydrochloride[b]
Moderate disease with prominent eye symptoms	Oral nonsedating H_1-antihistamine\daily[a]
	OR
	Intranasal corticosteroid and topical eye therapy with sodium cromoglycate or lodoxamide tromethamine or olopatadine hydrochloride/topical nonsteroidal antiinflammatory (ketorolac tromethamine) additional therapy for exacerbations[b]
If above ineffective	Review possibility of coexisting disease or complications (e.g., sinusitis)
	Consider immunotherapy
	Systemic corticosteroid therapy for a few days for severe symptoms
	Topical ipratropium bromide if rhinorrhea a major problem
Perennial allergic rhinitis in adults	
Intermittent disease	Allergen avoidance
	Intranasal corticosteroids if long-term exposure
	Oral nonsedating H_1-antihistamine therapy
	Oral decongestants

[a]Sedating, traditional (first-generation) antihistamine therapy is a consideration because of cost of second-generation antihistamines. However, functional impairment occurs with first-generation antihistamine therapy even if treated subjects do not perceive impairment. Therefore, it is difficult to evaluate the risk/benefit ratio, and a treating physician may be at legal risk if any accident occurs while a patient is being treated with a sedating antihistamine without first trying nonsedating antihistamine therapy. Fexofenadine and loratidine are safe, effective, nonsedating antihistamine therapies that have almost no side effects. There is no concern with combining these treatments with other therapies, including macrolide antibiotics and azole antifungals. Cetirizine is mildly sedating with clinical trial results variable as to the importance of this sedation. Azelastine (a topical antihistamine therapy for rhinitis) is also mildly sedating, but some authorities debate the clinical significance of this effect. Azelastine improves eye symptoms, suggesting that absorption is clinically significant or that aspiration of the agent into the lacrimal duct provides topical eye therapy.

[b]Topical ocular therapy is not recommended with contact lens use.

171

Table 5
Allergen Avoidance Measures

For mite allergen	For cat allergen
Bedrooms	Remove cat from the house (allergen
Cover mattresses and pillows with	reduction sufficient to affect symptoms may
impermeable covers	take > 12–16 wk or longer)
Wash bedding regularly at 130° F	Measures to reduce cat allergen if cat remains
Remove carpets, stuffed animals, and	in home
clutter from bedrooms	Minimize cat contact with carpets,
Eliminate wall-to-wall carpet	upholstered furniture and bedding
Vacuum clean weekly (wearing a mask	Use vacuum cleaners with an effective
or using a HEPA-filtered vacuum	filtration system
cleaner)	Increase ventilation
Rest of house	Consider a high-efficiency air filtration
Minimize carpets and upholstered	system (HEPA) to remove small airborne
furniture (particularly in basements	particles
or overlying concrete)	Consider washing of cat every 2 wk
Reduce humidity below 45% relative	
humidity, or 6 g/kg (may not be feasible	
in many climates)	
Consider treatment of carpets with benzyl	
benzoate powder or tannic acid spray	
(questionable efficacy)	

Adapted from Platts-Mills TAE, Solomon WR. Aerobiology and inhalant allergens. In: Middleton E Jr, Reed CE, Ellis EF, Adkinson NF, Yunginger JW, Busse WW eds. *Allergy:Principles and Practice*, ed. 5 St. Louis, Mosby, 1998; p399.

the H_1 receptor. Antihistamine therapy may also affect expression of cell recruitment ligands and eosinophil chemotaxis, potential anti-inflammatory effects.

The originally synthesized antihistamines are termed first generation. Examples of first-generation antihistamines include diphenhydramine, chlorpheniramine, triprolidine and hydroxyzine. First-generation antihistamines are highly lipophilic and readily penetrate the blood-brain barrier, resulting in sedation or somnolence in 10 to 25% of treated subjects. First-generation antihistamines bind to muscarinic receptors causing anticholinergic side effects such as dry mouth, urinary hesitancy, tachycardia, blurred vision, constipation and reduced seizure threshold. A first-generation antihistamine, triprolidine, has the same effect on a driving test as a blood alcohol level of 0.05 mg/dL, according to one study. Many affected subjects are unaware of the functional impairment associated with first-generation antihistamine therapy. Second-generation antihistamines are lipophobic molecules with charged side chains These structural features result in minimal penetration of the blood-brain barrier. Second-generation antihistamines also do not bind to the muscarininc receptors. Thus, significant sedation or anticholinergic side effects do not occur with their use. Examples of second-generation antihistamines include cetirizine, fexofenadine, and loratidine. Astemizole and terfenadine are second-generation antihistamines no longer on the market owing to adverse effects on heart rhythm in a small percentage of subjects.

Drugs Useful in the Therapy of Rhinitis

- Antihistamines—especially good for sneezing and rhinorrhea
- Decongestants—useful only for nasal stuffiness and congestion
- Anticholinergic agents—useful for anterior rhinorrhea
- Mast cell stabilizers—especially useful for pretreatment prior to aeroallergen exposure, such as before mowing the lawn
- Corticosteroids—the most potent of all agents and useful for all symptoms

---

All of the first-generation and most of the second-generation antihistamines are metabolized by the cytochrome P-450 hepatic enzyme system. Half-life values range from <24 h for cetirizine, fexofenadine, loratidine and terfenadine, to approximately 24 h for chlorpheniramine and azelastine, and up to 9.5 d for astemizole and its active metabolites. Therapeutic agents that inhibit or compete for the cytochrome P-450 enzyme system will result in an increase in the half-life of most antihistamines. Examples of drugs interacting with cytochrome P-450 include macrolide antibiotics and azole antifungal agents.

Most, but not all, antihstamines increase the QT interval of the electrocardiogram because of inhibition of a slow-potassium, rectifier current required for membrane repolarization of the cardiac myocyte. Significant prolongation of the QT interval may result in a potentially fatal ventricular arrhythmia, torsades de pointes. Astemizole, terfenadine or most first-generation antihistamines should not be combined with therapies that affect the cytochrome P-450 metabolic pathway. Cetirizine, fexofenadine or loratidine has no effect on QT interval and therefore may be combined with macrolide antibiotics, azole antifungals or other agents that affect cytochrome P-450 (Table 6).

Decongestants stimulate α-adrenergic receptors, resulting in blood vessel constriction and reduced blood flow to the mucosa. The net result is less blood volume in the nasopharyngeal and sinus mucosa with attenuated swelling and edema. Decongestants can be administered topically or orally. The former is more rapid in onset but is not recommended for long-term use. Oral decongestants are often combined with antihistamines. The most common side effects are insomnia, irritability and impairment of bladder emptying.

Corticosteroids reduce mucosal inflammation by reducing fluid movement from the vascular space into tissues; by reducing adhesion molecule expression, thereby decreasing inflammatory cell recruitment; by reducing mediator and cytokine synthesis; by reducing arachidonic acid metabolism; by minimizing nasal irritant receptor sensitivity and by reducing inflammatory cell activation (Table 7). Topical corticosteroids applied to the nasal mucosa reduce the inflammatory changes and symptoms of the early- and late-phase response following allergen challenge. Pretreatment, for as short a time as 48 h, inhibits the acute-phase response. Reduction in the number of mucosal and submucosal mast cells following topical corticosteroid therapy is an important mechanism for minimizing the acute-phase response.

The onset, duration and magnitude of the effect of topical corticosteroid therapy are related receptor-binding activity, tissue concentration, sensitivity of the naspopha-

Table 6
Antihistamine and Antihistamine/Decongestant Options for Allergic Rhinitis

Drug type	Drug	Dosage
Oral (nonsedating) antihistamine[a]	Astemizole[b]	10 mg once a day
	Cetirizine	5 or 10 mg once a day
	Fexofenadine	60 mg twice a day or 180 mg once a day
	Loratadine	10 mg once a day
Oral (nonsedating) antihistamine/ decongestant combinations	Fexofenadine/ pseudoephedrine	1 tablet (60 mg of fexofenadine, 120 mg of pseudoephedrine) twice a day
	Loratadine/ pseudoephedrine	1 tablet (5 mg of loratadine, 120 mg of pseudoephedrine) twice a day, or extended-release tablet (10 mg of loratadine, 240 mg of pseudoephedrine) once a day
Topical antihistamine	Azelastine	2 sprays per nostril twice a day

[a]A number of oral sedating antihistamines are also available, such as chlorpheniramine, diphenhydramine and promethazine.

[b]May cause potentially fatal ventricular arrhythmia; do not administer with macrolide antibiotics, azole antifungal agents or other agents that increase the effective dose by inhibiting or competing for cytochrome P-450. No longer sold in the U.S.

ryngeal mucosa and the tissue half-life of the corticosteroid. Quantifying the topical potencies of the various corticosteroids to facilitate comparisons is difficult. All currently available topical corticosteroids (beclomethasone diproprionate, budesonide, flunisolide, fluticasone propionate, mometasone and triamcinolone acetonide) are effective in reducing the nasal symptoms of allergic rhinitis (Table 8). Available data suggest comparable efficacy on a microgram to microgram basis. Topical corticosteroids provide a favorable risk/benefit ratio in the treatment of allergic rhinitis. However, there is a potential, though unlikely, of systemic side effects from inhaled corticosteroids. Local side effects of nasal bleeding and mucosal irritation are common but rarely significant.

Other therapies of allergic rhinitis include sodium cromolyn and ipratropium bromide. Sodium cromolyn is effective for prevention of symptoms but is not useful to relieve current symptoms. The major limiting factor for sodium cromolyn therapy is the frequency of administration required for optimal efficacy, four times a day or more. The large body of data attesting to the safety of sodium cromolyn is an important factor in its favor. Ipratropium bromide is effective for both perennial and seasonal allergic rhinitis, but primarily only relieves rhinorrhea.

IMMUNOTHERAPY

The goal of immunotherapy is to reduce the specific immunological reactivity of an individual to the allergens responsible for symptoms. Immunotherapy is not desensitization, since clinical improvement occurs despite the persistence, and occasional increase, of specific IgE antibody. The mechanism by which immunotherapy is effective in allergic disorders remains incompletely defined with various theories offered (Table 9).

Table 7
Effects of Corticosteroids on Inflammatory Cells

Cells affected	Corticosteroid effect

T-lymphocytes	Reduction of circulating cell number
	Increase in apoptosis
	Inhibition of:
	  Lymphocyte activation
	  Interleukin-2 (IL-2) production
	  IL-2 receptor expression
	  IL-4 production
	  Proliferation following antigen exposure

Eosinophils	Reduction of circulating cell number Increase in apoptosis Reduction of immigration into epithelial and mucosal tissues Reduction of cell activation during late-phase allergic response Reduction of cell recruitment during late-phase allergic response Inhibition of IL-4 and IL-5 enhanced cell survival
Mast cells/basophils	Reduction of circulating cell number Reduction of cell recruitment during late-phase allergic response Reduction of mast cell mediators following allergen challenge Reduction of histamine content and release Reduction of epithelial and mucosal numbers following topical application
Neutrophils	Reduction of cell recruitment after antigen challenge

Macrophages/ monocytes	Reduction of circulating cell number
	Inhibition of release of:
	  IL-1
	  Interferon gamma
	  Tumor necrosis factor alpha
	  Granulocyte-monocyte colony-stimulating factor

Adapted from Meltzer EO. *Allergy* 1997;52(suppl 36):33–40; and Kamada AK, Szefler SJ. In: *Asthma and Rhinitis*. Boston, Blackwell Scientific, 1995: pp. 1255–1266.

A variety of clinical trials, with variable blinding and control groups, have been carried out for seasonal and perennial allergic rhinitis since 1954. Thirty of the thirty-four best designed, double-blind trials demonstrate efficacy. Twenty-five of the thirty studies with clinical benefits demonstrate an increase in specific IgG or a decrease in specific IgE or both in two studies. Four of the remaining five did not measure humoral responses, and the one study showing clinical benefit without confirmatory humoral changes was of 3 mo duration and measured only specific-IgE. Skin tests with allergens before and after immunotherapy are documented in 13 of the 30 beneficial studies; 4 show no change, and 9 demonstrate decreased skin test reactivity. Nasal or conjunctival allergen challenges were performed before and after immunotherapy in 13 of the studies showing efficacy; 12 of the 13 demonstrate decreased nasal or conjunctival reactivity to the allergen used for immunotherapy. Basophil histamine

Table 8
Anti-Inflammatory Options for Allergic Rhinitis

Drug type[a]	Drug	Dosage
Nasal corticosteroids	Beclomethasone	2 sprays in each nostril twice a day; for double-strength formulation, 2 sprays in each nostril once a day
	Budesonide	2 sprays in each nostril twice a day or 4 sprays in each nostril once a day
	Flunisolide	2 sprays in each nostril twice a day
	Fluticasone[b]	2 sprays in each nostril once a day
	Mometasone	2 sprays in each nostril once a day
	Triamcinolone	2 sprays in each nostril once a day
Nasal nonsteroidal anti-inflammatory	Cromolyn	1 spray in each nostril 3–6 times daily at regular intervals
Oral corticosteroid	Prednisone[c]	15–30 mg/day for 3–7 d; discontinue without taper

[a] To relieve rhinorrhea, consider ipratropium nasal solution, 2 sprays in each nostril 2 or 3 times a day.
[b] Approved for use in children 4 yr of age and older. All others approved for 6 yr of age and older.
[c] Use minimally because of potential side effects.

release decreased in 1 study following immunotherapy but was unchanged in 3 others in which it was measured.

The four double-blind studies that do not demonstrate clinical improvement were similar in design to the positive trials. Immunological changes observed in three of these studies include increased specific IgG and decreased IgE in one. Skin test reactivity decreased in one of the two negative studies in which it was measured; in vitro basophil histamine release was unchanged in one study; and nasal provocation with antigen was decreased in the one negative study in which it was measured. Thus, there is no obvious explanation for the negative results in these four trials.

In summary, the majority of the controlled trials with immunotherapy demonstrate beneficial clinical effects in both seasonal and perennial allergic rhinitis. Laboratory tests and challenge studies, in general, correlate with the clinical findings. The most consistent humoral change is an increase in specific IgG, with some studies showing a switch from specific IgG1 to IgG4. However, the many exceptions indicate that there is not a specific confirmatory test to demonstrate clinical benefit. Symptomatic improvement remains the standard response variable. Treatment of rhinitis with immunotherapy may reduce the likelihood of the development of asthma.

The indications for immunotherapy include severe symptoms, poor response to medications, intolerance to or side effects from medications or reluctance to take medications. Beneficial effects include the reduction of symptoms of allergic rhinitis and possibly limitation of the development of complications, including asthma. Relative contraindications include uncontrolled asthma, β-blocker therapy, autoimmune disease and malignant disease. Immunotherapy should be initiated and supervised by a trained specialist but can be administered by any physician who is prepared to treat anaphylaxis, the most serious adverse effect of the treatment.

Table 9
Mechanisms of Action of Immunotherapy

Increase in T-suppressor activity
Decrease in histamine-releasing factors
Increase in specific IgG
Decrease in specific IgE
Decrease in mediator release from basophils

PERENNIAL NONALLERGIC RHINITIS (PNAR)

Perennial nonallergic rhinitis (PNAR) is a term used to designate a heterogeneous group of disorders that share clinical features. The pathophysiology is unknown, and nasal histology does not correlate with symptoms. PNAR is common, representing 28–60% of subjects referred to an allergy/immunology or otolaryngology clinic for evaluation. No vasomotor dysfunction has been identified in PNAR; therefore, the term *vasomotor rhinitis* is not descriptive and should be avoided. No mucosal inflammation typically occurs, so the term *rhinitis* is a misnomer as well, but *PNAR* is the term used in this review.

The typical presentation is one of nasal obstruction with or without rhinorrhea, exacerbated by physical stimuli such as odor, air temperature changes, moving air, body position, airborne irritants such as cigaret smoke, food or beverage. Sneezing and itching are less common. Neurogenic mechanisms may play a pathophysiological role, but this has not been confirmed by electrophysiological studies. Some affected subjects hyperrespond with nasal congestion following challenge with cholinergic agents, suggesting a type of nasal hyperreactivity similar to that occurring in the bronchial airway with asthma. Spicy foods or alcohol ingestion may also trigger symptoms. A variant of PNAR with copious rhinorrhea associated with eating or prepartion for eating is termed gustatory rhinitis. Exercise may improve the symptoms of PNAR, contrasting with allergic rhinitis. The degranulation of nasal mast cells, by undefined allergens or by physical stimuli such as cold, dry air and hyperosmolar mucosal fluid, is not likely a critical part of the pathophysiology, since the symptoms of itching and sneezing paroxysms are typically absent. However, mast cell mediators are measurable in PNAR nasal lavage following cold air challenge.

The diagnosis of PNAR is suggested by the history of symptoms, the nature of provoking stimuli and absence of a family history of allergy. The nasal mucosa is variable in appearance but generally is congested with normal to erythematous color (Fig. 6). The secretions are usually clear and do not contain a significant number of eosinophils or neutrophils. Other causes of nasal symptoms should be excluded because of the lack of a confirmatory diagnostic test for PNAR. The exclusion of perennial allergic rhinitis is particularly important since the symptoms of the two are similar, and some subjects have both conditions. Sinusitis should also be considered since many symptoms are common to both.

The treatment of PNAR is symptomatic since the pathophysiology is unknown. The physician should focus the therapy on the primary symptom. Decongestants, nasal saline to lavage irritants from the mucosa and topical ipratropium bromide for rhinorrhea are often helpful. Antihistamine therapy offers limited benefits, although the

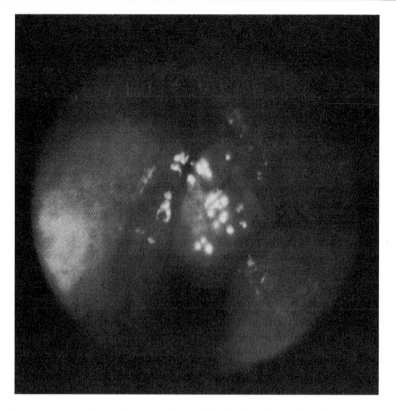

Fig. 6. Nasal mucosa in a patient with perennial nonallergic rhinitis, as visualized through a fiberoptic rhinolaryngoscope.

anticholinergic effects of first-generation antihistamines may be helpful for rhinorrhea. Topical corticosteroid therapy relieves symptoms probably by reducing glandular secretion and blood flow to the nose, since mucosal inflammation is not usually present. The response to topical nasal corticosteroids is variable and not as consistent as with allergic rhinitis. Regular aerobic exercise, 20–30 min two to three times a week, may help reduce symptoms. Nasal congestion and sinus pressure are often the most bothersome symptoms, so emphasis on avoidance of regular topical decongestants is important. Oral lozenges containing menthol may relieve symptoms of nasal congestion, but menthol does not decongest the nose. Finally, affected subjects need reassurance and sensitive care to reduce "doctor shopping," unnecessary surgery, overuse of antibiotics and overinterpretation of allergy tests.

Nonallergic Rhinitis with Eosinophilia (NARES)

NARES is a syndrome that may or may not be a separate diagnostic entity but is classified with PNAR because of common clinical features. Affected subjects are described as suffering from perennial nasal congestion, rhinorrhea, sneezing and pruritus but do not have specific IgE for allergens, an increase in total IgE or a personal or family history of atopy. The nasal secretions contain eosinophils, which distinguishes this condition from other forms of PNAR. The lack of an atopic personal and family history in NARES makes an undefined allergy unlikely as the cause. The condition

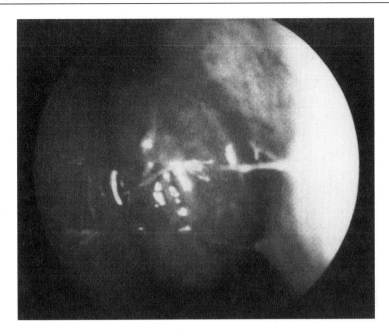

Fig. 7. Intranasal polyp, as visualized through a fiberoptic rhinolaryngoscope.

may be part of the spectrum of eosinophilic rhinitis and nasal polyposis, but there are no epidemiological studies demonstrating progression of NARES to nasal polyposis. However, subjects with the aspirin triad (nasal polyps with eosinophils, asthma, aspirin sensitivity) experience rhinorrhea and nasal congestion prior to development of nasal polyps, suggesting a spectrum of disease (Fig. 7).

Allergic rhinitis and nasal polyposis are the principal diagnoses to be excluded when one is assessing NARES. Treatment is symptomatic with a topical nasal corticosteroid generally the most effective pharmacological agent. Symptom relief often requires a higher dosage of corticosteroid than that generally required for allergic rhinitis.

RHINITIS INDUCED BY DRUGS OR HORMONES (RHINITIS MEDICAMENTOSA)

Topical use of α-adrenergic decongestant sprays for more than 5–7 d in succession may result in rebound nasal congestion upon discontinuation of treatment. Continued use of the decongestant to control withdrawal congestion can lead to an erythematous, congested nasal mucosa termed rhinitis medicamentosa. Regular use of intranasal cocaine will have the same effect and should be considered in the differential diagnosis. Other systemic changes associated with medications and hormones may also be associated with nasal symptoms, although the nasal mucosa may not always appear the same.

The mechanisms responsible for nasal symptoms associated with medications and hormones are variable. Antihypertensive therapies with β-blockers and α-adrenergic antagonists probably affect regulation of nasal blood flow. α-Adrenergic antagonists are also commonly utilized for symptom relief of prostate enlargement. Topical ophthalmic β-blocker therapy may also result in nasal congestion by the same mechanism. Nasal congestion and/or rhinorrhea also may result from changes in estrogen and

> It is important to note that a significant number of patients with chronic rhinitis (especially adults) do not have allergies.

possibly progesterone, either from exogenous administration, pregnancy or menstrual cycle variations. Hypothyroidism is associated with nasal congestion, rhinorrhea and pale, allergic-like nasal mucosa. Aspirin and other nonsteroidal antiinflammatory drugs (NSAIDs) may result in congestion and rhinorrhea. Subjects with intermittent symptoms associated with aspirin or NSAIDs may be part of the evolving spectrum of chronic, eosinophilic rhinosinusitis with nasal polyps. Reassurance that the nasal symptoms are the result of the medications or hormonal changes may be sufficient to discourage other unnecessary investigations.

The primary treatment of rhinitis medicamentosa is discontinuation of the offending agent or correction of the hormonal imbalance, if possible. Symptomatic treatment may be helpful. Treatment of rebound nasal congestion associated with topical decongestant use may require 20–30 mg/d of oral prednisone or equivalent, for 5–7 d followed by topical intranasal corticosteroid therapy.

ATROPHIC RHINITIS

Atrophic rhinitis usually occurs in elderly patients. Affected subjects report nasal congestion, crusting of the nasal airway and a bad smell (ozena). The examination reveals a patent nasal airway with atrophic turbinates despite the symptoms of congestion (Fig. 8). The prevalence of this condition is variable, with a greater occurrence in select geographic areas, such as southeastern Europe, China, Egypt or India, than in northern Europe or the United States. The cause of atrophic rhinitis is unknown with the leading theory being age-related mucosal atrophy complicated by secondary bacterial infection. Primary atrophic rhinitis resembles the rhinitis associated with Sjögren's syndrome, previous nasal surgery including extensive turbinectomy, chronic granulomatous disease such as Wegener's granulomatosis or previous local irradiation. Symptomatic treatment with low-dose decongestants and nasal saline lavage is minimally effective. Topical antibiotic therapy, such as gentamicin or tobramycin 15 mg/mL or ciprofloxacin 0.15 mg/mL in saline, may offer some benefit. The addition of proplylene glycol, 3–15%, to nasal saline may prolong the benefits of topical moisture by reducing the water's surface tension.

OTHER NASAL DISORDERS

The differential diagnosis of chronic rhinitis includes the systemic diseases and structural disorders listed in Table 1. Select laboratory tests listed in Table 10 may facilitate diagnosing or excluding some of the systemic conditions, although biopsy is usually necessary to confirm the diagnosis. Unilateral or asymmetric symptoms or progressive symptoms of nasal obstruction increase the suspicion for malignancy or foreign body. These possibilities are best evaluated by radiographs and/or fiberoptic rhinolaryngoscopy followed by referral to a surgical specialist if an abnormality is identified.

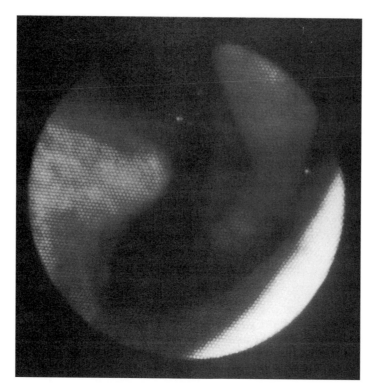

Fig. 8. Nasal mucosa in a patient with atrophic rhinitis, as visualized through a fiberoptic rhinonlaryngoscope.

Table 10
Laboratory Tests for Systemic Diseases Associated with Nasal Symptoms

Test	Diagnosis
Erythrocyte Sedimentation Rate	Wegener's granulomatosis
	Relapsing polychondritis
	Sarcoidosis
Delayed-Type Hypersensitivity	Tuberculosis
Testing	Sarcoidosis
VDRL	Syphilis
Sweat Chloride	Cystic fibrosis
Antineutrophil Cytoplasmic Antibody	Wegener's granulomatosis
Angiotension Converting Enzyme Level	Sarcoidosis
Quantitative Immunoglobulins	Common variable immunodeficiency
	IgA deficiency
Thyroid-Stimulating Hormone	Hypothyroidism
Saccharin Taste Test[a]	Immotile cilia syndrome

[a]Saccharin is placed with a cotton swab on the inferior turbinate, at the junction of the anterior and middle thirds of the turbinate. The time required for tasting is recorded, with normal usually less than 20 min. Greater than 30 min before tasting is considered indicative of dysfunction of ciliary motility. The patient must be instructed not to sniff, blow the nose or use any topical nasal therapies during the test. (Stanley P, MacWilliam L, Greenstone M, et al. Efficacy of a saccharine test for screening to detect abnormal mucociliary clearance. *Br J Dis Chest* 1984;78:62. Corbo GM, Foresi A, Bonfitto P, et al. Measurement of nasal mucociliary clearance. *Arch Dis Child* 1989;64:546.).

181

CONCLUSIONS

Rhinitis or nasal/sinus complaints are probably the most common reason people seek care from a physician. Rhinitis is not associated with significant mortality, but decreases the quality of life of affected subjects. Allergic rhinitis, the most common form of rhinitis, is associated with or increases the probability of several medical conditions with additional morbidity and expense of treatment. These include bacterial sinusitis, otitis media and asthma. Additional complications of chronic rhinits include maxillofacial maldevelopment with poor occlusion of teeth and nocturnal sleep disturbance with fatigue and sleep apnea. The physician who recognizes and treats rhinitis in a cost-effective manner will provide a valuable service to a large portion of his or her practice.

SUGGESTED READING

Beckman DB, Grammer LC. Pharmacotherapy to prevent the complications of allergic rhinitis. *Allergy Ashtma Proc* 1999;20:215–223.

Dykewicz MS, Fineman S, Skoner D, et al. Diagnosis and management of rhinitis: complete guidelines of the joint task force on practice parameters in allergy, asthma and immunology. *Ann Allergy Asthma Immunol* 1998;81:478–518.

Howarth P. The cellular basis for allergic rhinitis. *Clin Exp Allergy* 1995;50(Suppl 23):6–10.

Ledford DK. Efficacy of immunotherapy. In: Bukantz S, Lockey RF, eds. *Allergens and allergen immunotherapy*, ed. 2nd. New York, Marcel Dekker Inc., 1998, pp. 359–381.

Lee BJ, Naclerio RM, Bochner BS, et al. Nasal challenge with allergen upregulates the local expression of vascular endothelial cell adhesion molecules. *J Allergy Clin Immunol* 1994;94:1006–16.

Meltzer EO. The pharmacological basis for the treatment of perennial allergic rhinitis and non-allergic rhinitis with topical corticosteroids. *Allergy* 1997;52(Suppl 36):33–40.

Mygind N, Naclerio RM. Definition, classification, terminology. In: Mygind N, Naclerio RM, Eds. *Allergic and non-allergic rhinitis*. Copenhagen, Bunksgaard, 1993, pp. 11–14.

Naclerio RM. Pathophysiology of perennial allergic rhinitis. *Allergy* 1997;52(Suppl 36):7–13.

Philip G, Togias AC. Nonallergic rhinitis: pathophysiology and models of study. *Eur Arch Otorhinolaryngol* 1995;1:27–32.

Settipane R, Hagy G, Settipane G. Long-term risk factors for developing asthma and allergic rhinitis:a 23-year follow-up study of college students. *Allergy Proc* 1994;15:21–25.

Sims TC, Reece LM, Hilsmeier KA. et al. Secretions of chemokines and other cytokines in allergen-induced nasal responses: inhibition by topical steroid treatment. *Am J Respir Crit Care Med* 1995;152:922–933.

10 Sinusitis and Otitis Media

Jonathan Corren, MD
and Gary Rachelefsky, MD

CONTENTS

SINUSITIS
OTITIS MEDIA
SUGGESTED READING

SINUSITIS

Definitions and Epidemiology

Sinusitis is a clinical condition characterized by mucosal inflammation of the paranasal sinuses. Acute sinusitis is a rapid-onset bacterial infection that has been present for less than 1 mo and most commonly affects the maxillary sinuses. Subacute sinusitis, with symptoms present between 1 and 3 mo, usually develops when an acute episode of bacterial sinusitis has not been adequately treated. Chronic sinusitis has been present for at least 3 mo and is often associated with persistent mucosal changes.

Sinus disease is frequently encountered in general practice. It has been estimated that 0.5% of viral upper respiratory infections result in acute sinusitis. Chronic sinusitis is also a very common condition and afflicts at least 31 million people in the United States.

Pathogenesis

Four host factors determine the susceptibility to sinusitis, including patency of the ostia, ciliary function, quality of secretions, and local host immunity. Obstruction of the sinus ostium leads to reduced oxygen content and the development of mucosal edema and serum transudation within the sinus cavity. These alterations foster bacterial growth, reduce ciliary movement and alter leukocyte function. If an acute episode of sinusitis occurs, the sinus will usually return to normal following effective antibiotic treatment. However, if therapy is incomplete or underlying etiological factors are not treated, persistent changes may occur in sinus anatomy and physiology. Factors that have been associated with sinusitis are listed in Table 1.

From: *Current Clinical Practice: Allergic Diseases: Diagnosis and Treatment, 2nd Edition*
Edited by: P. Lieberman and J. Anderson © Humana Press Inc., Totowa, NJ

Table 1
Conditions Associated with Sinusitis

Obstruction of the sinus ostia
    Acute viral rhinitis
    Chronic rhinitis (allergic and nonallergic)
    Nasal polyps
    Adenoidal inflammation and enlargement
    Septal deviation
    Aerated middle turbinate
    Foreign body (nasogastric tube)
Dental infection
Physical phenomena
    Barotrauma (flying, diving, swimming)
    Air pollution
Systemic diseases
    Antibody deficiency syndrome
    Down's syndrome
    Cystic fibrosis
    Wegener's granulomatosis
    Ciliary dyskinesia syndrome

Clinical Presentation

ACUTE SINUSITIS

The most consistent feature distinguishing acute bacterial sinusitis from a viral respiratory infection is persistence of symptoms beyond 7 to 10 d. Cough and nasal discharge are the two most common complaints in children, while headache and facial pain are unusual in children younger than age 10. Adult patients with acute sinusitis most often complain of discolored nasal discharge, unilateral facial pain, headache and cough. Although reported in only a minority of patients, upper tooth pain is a complaint very specific for sinusitis.

On examination, high temperature and signs of toxicity are unusual and should prompt a search for complications such as meningitis or periorbital abscess. Anterior rhinoscopy frequently reveals erythematous, swollen turbinates and purulent secretions on the floor of the nose. However, the absence of pus does not rule out active infection, since sinus drainage may be intermittent. Facial tenderness elicited by palpation is an unreliable sign in differentiating sinusitis from acute rhinitis. Transillumination may be useful in evaluating acute maxillary and frontal sinusitis in adults if interpretation is confined to extremes of light transmission (i.e., clear vs opacified sinus cavity).

CHRONIC SINUSITIS

Patients with chronic sinusitis usually have indolent symptoms of nasal congestion, thick postnasal drip, and cough. Adult patients may also complain of facial fullness and headache. Secondary eustachian tube obstruction or middle ear fluid may result in popping of the ears and muffled hearing. In addition to these chronic complaints, patients may also experience recurrent exacerbations of symptoms resembling acute sinusitis.

Symptoms Suggestive of Sinusitis

- Acute disease
  - Persistence of URI symptoms, usually without fever, beyond 7–10 d
  - Children: cough, nasal discharge; adults: discolored nasal discharge, unilateral facial pain, headache, cough
- Chronic disease: long-standing nasal congestion, thick postnasal drip, cough, facial fullness, sore throat, and hearing problems

---

Physical examination often demonstrates swelling and erythema of the inferior and middle turbinates and occasionally mucopurulent secretions on the floor of the nose and middle meatus. Nasal polyps may be present and usually originate from the middle meatus. In children, middle ear effusions are present in half of all cases and serve as excellent clues to the presence of sinusitis. Transillumination is not useful in evaluating chronic sinus disease since mucosal thickening usually yields equivocal results.

Flexible fiberoptic rhinoscopy is a useful and easily learned procedure that can help identify important anatomical lesions not visible by anterior rhinoscopy, including posterior deviation of the nasal septum, nasal polyps, enlargement or inflammation of the adenoid and tumor.

Diagnostic Tests

In many patients with acute and chronic sinusitis, diagnosis and subsequent therapy can be based upon the history and physical findings. However, in a significant number of patients, signs and symptoms may be equivocal, and additonal testing is required to make a diagnosis.

LABORATORY TESTS

Cytological examination of freshly stained nasal secretions (using Hansel's or modified Wright-Giemsa medium) is a convenient and inexpensive technique for evaluating nasal complaints. Significant neutrophilia (>5 neutrophils/high power field) is a sensitive but nonspecific predictor of sinusitis, while nasal eosinophilia is highly predictive of allergic rhinitis and normal sinus X-rays. Nasal cytology is most helpful in excluding the possibility of sinusitis when eosinophils are present and/or neutrophils are absent.

The peripheral white blood count/differential and nasal swab cultures have no utility in determining the presence of infection or in accurately identifying pathogenic bacteria in sinusitis.

IMAGING STUDIES

Although plain radiography has recently fallen out of favor in evaluating sinusitis, we feel that this technique continues to play a helpful role in selected patients. While plain X-rays accurately visualize the maxillary and frontal sinuses (particularly the Water's occipitomental view), the ethmoid and sphenoid sinuses are difficult to assess. Water's view findings that are diagnostic of sinusitis include a sinus air–fluid level,

---

Treatment of Chronic Sinusitis

- Medical therapy
  - Nasal corticosteroid
  - Nasal irrigation with saline
  - Antibiotic for 3–6 wk
  - Allergen avoidance

- Surgery
  - Only used for medically refractory cases
  - Success variable

---

sinus opacification or severe mucosal thickening (>50% of antral diameter in children and >8 mm in adults). In patients with possible acute sinusitis in whom initial medical therapy has failed, a plain film is useful in documenting infection before additional, more expensive antibiotics are prescribed. A Waters' view is also helpful in evaluating possible chronic sinusitis in children, since the maxillary sinuses are usually the principal sinuses involved. In adults with chronic sinusitis, however, plain films may yield false-negative results, since infection is limited to the ethmoid sinuses in up to 40% of cases.

Computed tomography (CT) provides a detailed view of the ethmoid and sphenoid sinuses and the ostiomeatal complex regions. Recently, "screening" sinus CT (4 to 10 cuts) has become widely available. In conjunction with an otolaryngologist or allergist, CT should be performed in patients who have persistent or recurrent symptoms suggestive of sinusitis despite adequate medical therapy. CT should be delayed if a viral upper respiratory infection has recently occurred, since 85% of patients have transient abnormalities on CT following a cold. CT of the sinuses should always be used judiciously, since even the screening scan remains a relatively expensive test and does require sedation for most children younger than 8 yr of age.

Magnetic resonance imaging (MRI) is extremely sensitive in detecting subtle soft tissue abnormalities of the paranasal sinuses. For this reason, it is the technique of choice in imaging suspected sinus neoplasms, fungal infections and complicated infections that extend intracranially. MRI should not be used for routine diagnosis of sinusitis, since it is very costly and does not adequately visualize the bony landmarks required for surgical planning.

Sinus ultrasound is rarely used as a diagnostic test owing to its poor sensitivity and specificity in patients with both acute and chronic sinusitis.

MAXILLARY ASPIRATION AND CULTURE

Referral should be made to an otolaryngologist for maxillary aspiration when acute sinusitis is associated with signs of severe toxicity (particularly in hospitalized or immunosuppressed patients) or is unresponsive to an adequate trial of appropriate antibiotics.

```
┌─────────────────────────────────────────────────────────────┐
│                    Diagnosis of Sinusitis                     │
│  • Acute                                                      │
│     • Clinical symptoms usually suffice                       │
│     • Plain films may be helpful                              │
│  • Chronic                                                    │
│     • CT is gold standard                                     │
│     • Plain films of limited utility                          │
└─────────────────────────────────────────────────────────────┘
```

Microbiology

ACUTE SINUSITIS

The most commonly identified organisms in children with acute sinusitis are *Streptococcus pneumoniae* in 30–40%, Haemophilus influenzae in 20–25%, and Moraxella catarrhalis in 20%. In adults, S. pnemoniae and H. influenzae are the two leading causes of sinusitis while Moraxella is unusual. Anaerobic organisms are primarily identified in cases of acute sinusitis originating from dental root infections, but are otherwise uncommon. Hospital-acquired sinusitis is most often seen as a complication of nastogastric tube placement and is typically caused by Gram-negative enteric organisms such as *Pseudomonas* and *Klebsiella*.

CHRONIC SINUSITIS

Bacterial isolates in children with chronic sinusitis are usually the same as those seen in acute disease. In children with more severe and protracted symptoms, anaerobic species (such as bacteroides) and staphylococci are cultured more frequently. Anaerobic organisms and increasingly Staphylococcus epidermidis predominate in adults with chronic sinusitis. Among the anaerobes, species of *Bacteroides* and anaerobic cocci account for nearly 90% of the isolates.

Fungi are a common cause of sinus disease in immunocompromised hosts, including diabetics and patients with defective cell-mediated immunity. *Aspergillus*, *Nocardia*, and *Bipolaris* species have also been recently identified as causes of sinusitis in patients who are otherwise healthy; they should be considered in all cases of sinusitis that have proven resistant to agressive medical and/or surgical therapy. Allergic fungal sinusitis is a syndrome that often occurs in adults with asthma and has been attributed to *Aspergillus*, *Bipolaris*, and *Curvularia* species. It is characterized by severe, hyperplastic sinusitis and nasal polyposis and is associated with significant eosinophilia of sinus tissue and blood.

Medical Therapy

ACUTE SINUSITIS

Antibiotics are the primary form of treatment for acute sinusitis. Amoxicillin remains the initial drug of choice for most patients with mild to moderate symptoms of sinusits. Patients allergic to penicillin should be treated initially with trimethoprim-sulfamethoxazole or a new-generation macrolide (e.g., clarithromycin or azithromycin). A good rule of thumb for duration of antibiotic therapy is to treat for 7 d beyond the point of symptom improvement; in most cases this requires 10–14 d.

Patients with more severe symptoms or who do not improve within approximately 5 d should be given an alternative, β-lactamase resistant agent for at least 10 additional days. While many antibiotics have proven effective in treating acute sinusitis, amoxicillin-clavulenate, cefuroxime, and cefpodoxime have consistently demonstrated excellent coverage of S. pneumoniae, H. influenzae and M. catarrhalis and are good choices for second-line antimicrobial therapy. Failure of the patient to respond to this treatment may indicate the presence of resistant S. pneumoniae or may reflect the possibility of severe nasal/sinus edema preventing adequate drainage of infected secretions. If symptoms are typical of acute sinusitis (e.g., purulent nasal drainage), a third-line antibiotic can be started in conjunction with aggressive ancillary therapies (see below). Newer quinolones (e.g., levofloxacin, grepafloxacin) provide excellent coverage against a wide range of bacteria, including resistant species of S. pneumoniae. In view of the rising incidence of antimicrobial resistance, we reserve these powerful drugs for patients in whom other antibiotics have failed. If patients do not respond to this empiric approach, sinus aspiration and culture should be undertaken to guide the need for additional treatment.

Symptoms recurring soon after a course of antibiotics are usually due to the original organism and should be treated with an alternative β-lactamase–resistant agent for 21 d.

Topical and oral decongestants reduce nasal congestion associated with acute sinusitis and may reduce ostial edema, allowing for improved sinus drainage. Mucolytic agents such as guaifenesin are commonly employed in sinusitis to reduce mucous viscosity and may be helpful in selected patients. Older antihistamines with strong anticholinergic effects such as diphenhydramine and hydroxyzine may cause mucous inspissation and impede sinus drainage. However, the newer, second- and third-generation antihistamines such as loratadine, cetirizine, and fexofenadine have virtually no anticholinergic effects and can be continued in patients who require these agents for concomitant allergic rhinitis.

CHRONIC SINUSITIS

While there are few published data regarding antimicrobial therapy for chronic sinusitis, anecdotal evidence suggests that patients should be treated for a minimum of 21 d. In patients who have not been previously treated with antibiotics, amoxicillin is a cost-effective choice for first-line therapy. In patients who are allergic to penicillin, clarithromycin provides good coverage against most relevant pathogens. If the patient has demonstrated no response to these drugs within 10 d, an alternative β-lactamase–resistant antibiotic (per acute sinusitis) should be given for 21 d. For adult patients who do not improve with this treatment, agents with increased anaerobic coverage such as clindamycin or metronidazole may be effective.

In addition to antibiotics, topical nasal corticosteroids should be prescribed for 3–6 wk to reduce chronic mucosal edema and inflammation. If severe turbinate swelling or nasal polyps are present, a 5–7-day course of prednisone (0.5 mg/kg/day given in 2–3 divided doses) is often very effective. Both topical and oral corticosteroids appear to be safe in chronic sinusitis, and there is no evidence that they increase the risk of intracranial extension or fulminant infection when given to patients with normal immune function. In allergic patients and patients with nasal polyposis, long-term use of nasal corticosteroids may be helpful in preventing recurrences of sinusitis.

Nasal irrigations, performed 2–3 times daily with a bulb syringe and saline, can be very helpful in removing dried secretions. Other methods to increase nasal humidification (hot showers, room humidifiers, and steam inhalers) are easy to use and may provide symptomatic relief for short periods.

Surgical Therapy

Patients with chronic sinusitis refractory to medical therapy should be referred to an otolaryngologist for consideration of surgery. In children with persistent maxillary sinus disease, antral lavage (with or without adenoidectomy) effectively removes purulent material and often provides long-lasting symptom relief. In adults, however, functional endoscopic surgery has largely supplanted other surgical procedures and is effective in 50–80% of patients. Patients with aspirin-sensitive asthma, nasal polyposis and pansinusitis are more likely to have recurrent disease and should be discouraged from undergoing multiple repeat surgical procedures.

Patients suspected of having intracranial complications (e.g., periorbital abscess, brain abscess or meningitis) of acute sinusitis should be referred for immediate surgical consultation. Cardinal signs and symptoms include high fever, severe headache, proptosis and changes in mental status.

Evaluaton of Patients with Recurrent or Persistent Sinusitis

Fifty percent of children and 30–40% of adults with recurrent or chronic sinusitis are sensitized to common aeroallergens such as plant pollens, house dust mite and animal danders. Allergy skin testing should be performed in these patients, since they often benefit from a comprehensive program of allergen avoidance, antiallergic drug therapy and, in selected cases, immunotherapy. Patients with severe, recurrent episodes of sinusitis associated with other infections (e.g., otitis, bronchitis, and pneumonia) may suffer from one of the antibody deficiency syndromes and should undergo a screening assessment of their immunoglobulin levels. If a deficiency is noted, or still suspected after the initial testing, these patients should be referred to an allergist/immunologist for further evaluation.

OTITIS MEDIA

Definitions and Epidemiology

Acute otitis media (AOM) refers to an acute suppurative infection of the middle ear space that usually lasts for 3 wk or less. Otitis media with effusion (OME; previously referred to as secretory or serous otitis media) represents persistent middle ear fluid that most often follows an episode of AOM and may last for many months. Recurrent acute otitis media is defined as three or more episodes of acute otitis media during the preceding 6 mo.

AOM is the most frequently diagnosed disease of children and is unusual in adult patients. It occurs in roughly 60% of children by the age of 1 yr and in 80% by age 3. Half of all children have had three or more episodes of AOM by age 3. Otitis media with effusion is similarly common, noted in approximately 50% of patients during the first year of life.

Pathogenesis

The two factors that contribute most significantly to otitis media are eustachian tube dysfunction and bacterial proliferation in the nasopharynx. The functions of

Table 2
Conditions Associated with Otitis Media

Anatomical causes of eustachian tube dysfunction	Systemic diseases
Viral upper respiratory infection	Down's syndrome
Allergic rhinitis	Ciliary dyskinesia syndrome
Chronic sinusitis	Immunodeficiency
Tonsillar hypertrophy (including adenoids)	
Cleft palate disease	
Variants of eustachian tube anatomy	

the eustachian tube include pressure equalization, protection of the middle ear from nasopharyngeal secretions and mucociliary clearance of the middle ear. Eustachian tube obstruction results in the development of negative pressure that is followed by serum transudation into the middle ear. This sterile effusion may become infected by bacteria refluxing from the nasopharynx into the middle ear. Incomplete eradication of an initial infection or prolonged underventilation of the middle ear may ultimately result in a chronic, mucoid effusion. Table 2 lists conditions commonly associated with otitis media.

Clinical Presentation

AOM

Children with AOM typically complain of acute unilateral ear pain that occurs several days after a viral upper respiratory infection. The symptoms frequently start early in the morning and are associated with irritability and fever, although nausea, vomiting and diarrhea are not uncommon. Otoscopy usually reveals a red, thickened and bulging tympanic membrane. Insufflation (pneumatic otoscopy) generally demonstrates poor mobility of the drum. Importantly, the drum may also appear red in a crying child (because of increased vascularity of the tympanic membrane) and may lead to an incorrect diagnosis of AOM.

OME

Children with this chronic condition are usually asymptomatic, but may have subtle loss of hearing. There is usually no recent history of fever, irritability or other systemic symptoms. The eardrum may appear yellow, orange or blue and is often retracted. Air-fluid levels or bubbles may be present, and the drum moves poorly with insufflation. Unfortunately, if midldle ear fluid is very thin, mobility may appear normal even to highly trained observers. Physical findings suggestive of allergic rhinitis, sinusitis or tonsillar hypertrophy should be sought, since these condtions may play important pathogenic roles in OME.

Diagnostic Tests

ELECTROACOUSTIC IMPEDANCE (TYMPANOMETRY)

Tympanometry is easy to perform and is far more sensitive than pneumatic otoscopy in detecting middle ear fluid. If findings are normal, OME can be confidently ruled out.

AUDIOMETRY

In children older than 18 mo, audiometry is an important test in determining whether OME has resulted in hearing loss. Fluid may cause up to a 40 dB hearing loss. This test should be employed when middle ear fluid has been present for at least 3 mo before deciding whether ventilation of the middle ear is necessary.

DIAGNOSTIC TYMPANOCENTESIS

Tympanocentesis with culture of middle ear fluid is indicated in children who are are extremely ill with AOM, children who have not responded to an adequate trial of appropriate medical therapy and children in intensive care nurseries.

Microbiology

The three principal organsims identified in middle ear effusions from both AOM and OME are the same as those isolated from patients with acute sinusitis. Streptococcus pneumoniae, nontypeable Haemophilus influenzae and Moraxella catarrhalis are isolated in 35, 23 and 14% of effusions, respectively. Other organisms that are occasionally cultured include Staphylococcus aureus, alpha streptococus, and group A streptococcus. Special exceptions include very young infants and children in intensive care nurseries, in whom group B streptococci and gram-negative organisms are very common causes of AOM.

Medical Therapy

AOM

While placebo-controlled studies have demonstrated that most children will recover from AOM without treatment, antibiotics do reduce the duration and severity of signs and symptoms. More importantly, antibiotics have reduced the incidence of and death rate from suppurative complications of AOM. For initial episodes, amoxicillin remains the drug of choice and should be given for 10 d. Trimethoprim-sulfamethoxazole is a good alternative in penicillin-allergic patients. In most cases, symptoms should improve significantly within 2–3 d. If symptoms persist, a second-line antibiotic with β-lactamase resistance (see Acute Sinusitis) should be given for an additional 10 d.

Adjunctive measures, including antihistamine-decongestant combinations and topical nasal corticosteroids have not been proven to be effective in randomly chosen children with AOM. However, these agents may have a beneficial effect in children with concomitant allergic rhinitis.

RECURRENT AOM

Prophylactic antibiotics have been shown to be effective in reducing the number of episodes of AOM in children who are prone to recurrence. Amoxicillin (20 mg/kg/d) and sulfisoxazole (50 mg/kg/d) are used most commonly, and treatment should be continued through the high-risk URI seasons (late fall to early spring). Pneumococcal vaccine should also be encouraged in all children over age 2 who suffer from recurrent otitis.

OME

While at least 80% of effusions resolve spontaneously within 2 mo, effusions that persist for longer than 3 mo will not usually improve without therapy. The most effective medical therapy for OME is probably a 14-d trial of amoxicillin. More potent antimicrobial agents or longer courses of antibiotics have not been shown to be helpful. Adjunctive measures (antihistamine-decongestants, topical corticosteroids) have also not been shown to be effective. Antibiotic therapy for OME should be considered in children who have associated sinusitis, documented conductive hearing loss, vertigo or tinnitus, or structural changes in the tympanic membrane or middle ear or in infants who are unable to describe symptoms. Following antibiotic therapy, the effusion must be followed carefully to ensure resolution.

Surgical Therapy

If medical therapy for recurrent AOM or OME is ineffective or poorly tolerated, a patient should be referred to an otolaryngologist for evaluation of the condition. Myringotomy with tube placement is effective in reducing the frequency of acute infections and in decreasing the duration of chronic effusions and their associated hearing loss. If tube placements are not effective, or a child has persistent adenoidal infection or enlargement, adenoidectomy with repeat tube placements has been shown to be beneficial in children older than age 4. Tonsillectomy has not been shown to provide any additional benefit over adenoidectomy alone.

Evaluation of Patients with Recurrent AOM or OME

Thirty to forty percent of children with recurrent AOM and OME have associated nasal allergy. These patients should undergo allergy testing and, if indicated, a complete program of allergen avoidance and antiallergic drug therapy prior to surgical intervention. Children with very severe, recurrent episodes of AOM associated with intracranial complications or bronchial infections should undergo an evaluation of their humoral immunity.

SUGGESTED READING

Sinusitis

Corren J. Sinusitis in primary care: making the clinical diagnosis. *Patient Care* (suppl.) p.11, December 15, 1993

Evans FO, Sydnor JB, Moore WEC, et al. Sinusitis of the maxillary antrum. *N Engl J Med* 293:735, 1975.

Gwaltney JM, Scheld WM, Sande MA, Syndor AS. The microbial etiology and antimicrobial therapy of adults with acute community-acquired sinusitis: a fifteen-year experience at the University of Virginia and reivew of other selected studies. *J Allergy Clin Immunol* 90 (suppl):457, 1992.

Wald ER, Milmore GJ, Bowen A, et al. Acute maxillary sinusitis in childhood. *New Engl J Med* 304, 1981.

Williams JW, Simel DI, Robers L, Samsa GP. Clinical evaluation for sinusitis: making the diagnosis by history and physical examination. *Ann Intern Med* 117:705, 1992.

Otitis Media

Bluestone CD, et al. Workshop on epidemiology of otitis media. *Ann Otol Rhinol Laryngol Suppl* 1; 1990.

Cantekin EI, Mandell EM, Bluestone CD, et al. Lack of efficacy of a decongestant–antihistamine combination for otitis media with effusion (secretory otitis media) in children. *N Engl J Med* 308:297, 1983.

Sade J, Luntz M. Adenoidectomy and otitis media: A review. *Ann Otol Rhinol Laryngol* 100:226, 1991.

11 Diagnosis and Treatment of Ocular Allergy

Leonard Bielory, MD

CONTENTS

INTRODUCTION
THE OCULAR SURFACE
ALLERGIC DISEASES OF THE EYE
OCULAR EXAMINATION
OPHTHALMIC PROCEDURES AND TESTING
OCULAR DRUG FORMULATIONS
DRUGS USED IN THE TREATMENT OF OCULAR ALLERGIC DISORDERS
SUGGESTED READING

INTRODUCTION

The eye is probably the most common site for the development of allergic inflammatory disorders, since it has no mechanical barrier to prevent impact of allergens such as pollen on its surface. Primary care providers frequently encounter various forms of allergic diseases of the eye that present as "red eyes" in their general practice. However, the eye is rarely the only target for an immediate allergic-type response. Typically, many patients have other combinations of allergic disorder such as rhinoconjunctivitis, rhinosinusitis, asthma, urticaria and/or eczema; there also exists a systemic allergic component. Even so, ocular signs and symptoms can frequently be the most prominent features of the entire allergic response for which these patients come to see their physician.

The primary care physician also needs to be aware of the various other ocular conditions that present as a red eye, some of which can produce profound visual loss if not treated appropriately. The signs and symptoms associated with these various conditions often overlap and can be difficult to differentiate. Therefore, an understanding of ophthalmological examination techniques and diagnostic procedures can further assist the primary care provider to make an accurate diagnosis of ocular allergy. (See Table 1.)

From: *Current Clinical Practice: Allergic Diseases: Diagnosis and Treatment, 2nd Edition*
Edited by: P. Lieberman and J. Anderson © Humana Press Inc., Totowa, NJ

Table 1
Differential Diagnosis of the Red Eye

Allergic	Infectious	Autoimmune	Nonspecific
Acute	Viral	Episcleritis	Dry Eye Syndromes
Seasonal	Bacterial	Pemphigoid	Foreign Body
Perennial	Inclusion	Uveitis	Acne Rosacea
Chronic	Fungal	Vsculitis	Chemical Induced
Vernal	Parasitic		
Atopic			
Giant Papillary			

This chapter provides a review of the various forms of allergic inflammation and focuses on the clinical characteristics that help to differentiate one allergic disorder from another as well as from other ocular conditions.

THE OCULAR SURFACE

Allergens and other ocular irritants are easily deposited directly onto the surface of the eye. Many agents that are systemically absorbed can be also concentrated and secreted in tears, causing allergic conjunctivitis or an irritant form of conjunctivitis. Other causes of the red eye may also include intraocular conditions associated with systemic autoimmune disorders such as uveitis or scleritis. In addition, allergic inflammatory disorders such as those that may affect surrounding skin, mucosa or even sinuses and release various mediators of inflammation, including histamine, leukotrienes, and neuropeptides, can have effects on the local ocular tissue.

ALLERGIC DISEASES OF THE EYE

Conjunctivitis, in its entirety, is a broad term that describes conjunctival inflammation. There are many causes of conjunctivitis. The clinical presentation of ocular surface allergic disorders is quite varied and depends, in part, on the immunological mechanism involved and the specific ocular tissues that are affected. Based on these differences, the most common forms of allergic ocular disease can be divided into seasonal allergic conjunctivitis, perennial allergic conjunctivitis, vernal conjunctivitis, atopic keratoconjunctivitis, and giant papillary conjunctivitis. Of all the possible ocular manifestations of allergic disease, allergic conjunctivitis is the most common (Table 2).

Clinical Examination

The clinical examination of the eyes for signs of ocular allergy begins with the external components that surround the eye and the eye itself. First, one examines the eyelids and eyelashes, focusing on the presence of erythema on the lid margin, as well as telangiectasias, scaling, thickening, swelling (blepharitis, dermatitis) and collarettes of debris at the base of the eyelashes, and evidence of periorbital discoloration, blepharospasm, or ptosis. Next the conjunctivae are directly examined for chemosis (clear swelling), hyperemia (injection), palpebral and bulbar papillae, and cicatrization

Table 2
Differential Diagnosis of Conjunctival Inflammatory Disorders

SIGNS

	AC	VC	AKC	GPC	CONTACT	BACTERIAL	VIRAL	CHLAMYDIAL	KCS
Predominant Cell type	Mast cell EOS	Lymph EOS	Lymph EOS	Lymph EOS	Lymph	PMN	PMN Mono Lymph	Mono Lymph	Lymph Mono
Chemosis	+	+/-	+/-	+/-	-	+/-	+/-	+/-	-
Lymph node	-	-	-	-	-	+	++	+/-	-
Cobblestoning	-	++	++	++	-	- ++	+/-	+ ++	-
Discharge	clear, mucoid	stringy, mucoid	stringy, mucoid	clear, white	+/-	mucopurulent	clear, mucoid	mucopurulent	+/- mucoid
LID Involvement	-	+	+	-	++	-	-	-	-

SYMPTOMS

	AC	VC	AKC	GPC	CONTACT	BACTERIAL	VIRAL	CHLAMYDIAL	KCS
Pruritus	+	++	++	++	+	-	-	-	-
Gritty sensation	+/-	+/-	+/-	+	-	+	+	+	+++
Seasonal variation	+	+	+/-	+/-	-	+/-	+/-	+	-

AC = allergic conjunctivitis; VC = vernal conjunctivitis; AKC = atopic keratoconjunctivitis; GPC = grant papillary conjunctivitis; KCS = keratoconjunctivitis sicca; BC = blepharoconjunctivitis; PMN = polymorphonuclear cells; Lymph = lymphocyte; Mono = monocyte; EOS = eosinophil

Table 3.
Common Clinical Signs and Symptoms of Ocular Inflammation

Trichiasis: inturned eyelashes
Epiphora: excessive tearing
Blepharospasm: spasm of the orbicularis oculi muscles
Subconjunctival hemorrhages: benign lesions occurring spontaneously, but may follow vigorous
    rubbing of the eye, vomiting, coughing or Valsalva's maneuvers
Blepharitis: inflammation of the eyelids
Madarosis: loss of eyelashes
Chalazion: inflammation of the meibomian gland
Hordeolum: a sty
Cicatrization: shrinkage and scarring of the conjunctival surface
Episcleritis: benign self-limiting sometimes bilateral inflammatory process of the tunic that
    surrounds the ocular globe
Scleritis: inflammatory process of the outer tunic surrounding the globe associated with
    autoimmune disorders, e.g., systemic lupus erythematosus, rheumatoid arthritis

(scarring). The discharge from the eye is also noted for increase or discoloration. It is important to differentiate between the injection associated with inflammation of the sclera (scleritis) that tends to develop over the course of several days. Scleritis is also commonly associated with autoimmune disorders such as systemic lupus erythematosus, rheumatoid arthritis and Wegener's granulomatosis. Another major clinical differential point is that scleritis and/or episcleritis commonly is associated with moderate and severe ocular pain on motion whereas conjunctivitis is commonly painless. The primary care provider should also be aware of a form of ocular infection that is described as a ring of erythema around the limbal junction of the cornea (ciliary flush) which is a clinical sign for uveitis, a serious form of intraocular pathology (Table 3).

The presence of follicles or papillae involving the bulbar and tarsal conjunctivae should be noted. Follicles can be distinguished as grayish, clear or yellow bumps varying in size from pinpoint to 2 mm in diameter with conjunctival vessels on their surface, while papillae contain a centrally located tuft of blood vessels.

Corneal involvement is more commonly seen in the chronic forms of ocular allergy, e.g., vernal keratoconjunctivitis and atopic keratoconjunctivitis. The slit-lamp biomiocroscope is the optimum device for examination of the cornea, although many important clinical features can be seen with the naked eye or with the use of a hand-held direct ophthalmoscope. The direct ophthalmoscope can provide the desired magnification by "plus" (convex) and "minus" (concave) lenses. The cobalt blue filter on the new hand-held ophthalmoscopic heads assists in highlighting anatomical anomalies affecting the cornea or the conjunctiva that has been stained with fluorescein.

The cornea should be perfectly smooth and transparent. Mucus adhering to the corneal or conjunctival surfaces is considered pathological. Dusting of the cornea may indicate punctate epithelial keratitis. A localized corneal defect may develop into erosion or a larger ulcer. A corneal plaque may be present if the surface appears dry and white or yellow.

The limbus is the zone immediately surrounding the cornea and is normally invisible to the naked eye, but when inflamed this area becomes visible as a pale or pink swelling.

**Key Features of the Diagnosis
of IgE-Mediated Allergic Eye Disease**

There are three key features of IgE-mediated allergic eye disease:
• Pruritus, which is usually intense
• Bilateral involvement
• Associated with atopic respiratory tract disease
    The absence of any of these is strong evidence against allergy as a cause of the condition.

Discrete swellings with small white dots (Trantas-Horner's dots) are indicative of degenerating cellular debris that is commonly seen in chronic forms of conjunctivitis.

In addition, since the eye has thin layers of tissue surrounding it, there is an increased tendency to develop secondary infections that can further complicate the clinical presentation.

Acute Allergic Conjunctivitis

Ocular disorders mediated by mast cells are the most common hypersensitivity responses of the eye. Allergic conjunctivitis (AC) is due to the direct exposure of the ocular mucosal surfaces to environmental allergens such as pollens from trees, grasses and weeds interacting with the pollen-specific IgE found on the mast cells of the eye. Of all the various pollens, ragweed has been identified as the cause in the United States in approximately 75% of cases of allergic rhinoconjunctivits. Common conjunctival symptoms are itching, tearing and perhaps burning. Involvement of the cornea is rare, with blurring of vision being the most common corneal symptom. Clinical signs include a milky or pale pink conjunctiva with vascular congestion that may progress to conjunctival swelling (chemosis). A white exudate may form during the acute state, which becomes stringy in the chronic form. While ocular signs are typically mild, the conjunctiva frequently takes on a pale, boggy appearance that often evolves into diffuse areas of papillae (small vascularized nodules). These papillae tend to be most prominent on the superior palpebral conjunctiva. Occasionally, dark circles beneath the eyes (allergic shiners) are present as a result of localized venous congestion. *Perennial allergic conjunctivitis* (PAC), like seasonal allergic conjunctivitis, also exhibits the classic IgE/mast cell–mediated hypersensitivity to airborne allergens. But, instead of being sensitive to grass or weed pollens, patients with perennial allergic conjunctivitis are more commonly sensitive to common household allergens such as dust mites, animal dander and, possibly, cockroach. The ocular reaction seen in both seasonal allergic conjunctivitis and perennial allergic conjunctivitis often resolves quickly once the offending allergen is removed. Obtaining a detailed history from the patient can make the diagnosis of these disorders. Both eyes are typically affected simultaneously, and quite often, a family history of hay fever or atopy may be elicited.

Vernal Keratoconjunctivitis

Vernal conjunctivitis is a chronic mast cell/lymphocyte–mediated allergic disorder of the conjunctiva appearing more in males prior to pubescence, after which it is equally distributed among the sexes and "burns out" by the third decade of life (about 4–10 yr after onset). This condition is seasonally recurrent and chronic in nature, occasionally lasting up to 10 yr. Vernal conjunctivitis usually begins in the spring with symptoms that include intense pruritus exacerbated by time, exposure to wind, dust, bright light, hot weather or physical exertion associated with sweating. Associated symptoms involving the cornea include photophobia, foreign body sensation and lacrimation. The most remarkable finding of vernal conjunctivitis is intense itching and giant papillae on the tarsal conjunctiva (Fig. 1). The "giant" papillae reaching 7–8 mm in diameter of the upper tarsal plate can result in large masses of them leading to the cobblestone effect seen on examination. In addition, patients may develop a thin copious milk-white fibrinous secretion; limbal or conjunctival "yellowish-white points" (Horner's points and Trantas' dots); an extra lower eyelid crease (Dennie's line); corneal ulcers or pseudomembrane formation of the upper lid when everted and exposed to heat (Maxwell-Lyons' sign). The effects of vernal conjunctivitis can be so severe that blindness may result, affecting one eye more than the other. Diffuse areas of punctate corneal epithelial defects can occur in some cases. These defects are best appreciated with a cobalt blue light after the instillation of topical fluorescein dye. In severe cases, these superficial punctate defects may progress to epithelial "shield ulcers." Conjunctival biopsies reveal increased numbers of eosinophils, basophils and mast cells, as well as plasma cells and lymphocytes.

Atopic Keratoconjunctivitis (AKC)

AKC is a chronic inflammatory process of the eye associated with a familial history for atopy such as eczema and asthma; primary care physicians should expect to see 25% of their elderly patients with eczema to also have some form of AKC. AKC can be seen in individuals as early as their late teens; it commonly persists until the fourth and fifth decades of life. AKC is an eye disorder with disabling symptoms; when it involves the cornea, it can lead to blindness. Ocular symptoms of AKC are similar to the cutaneous symptoms of eczema and include intense pruritus and edematous, coarse and thickened eyelids. Severe AKC is associated with complications such as blepharoconjunctivitis, cataract, corneal disease and ocular herpes simplex; it is primarily associated in 40% of the older patients, with the peak incidence occurring in the 30–50 year-old age group. The symptoms of AKC commonly include itching, burning and tearing, which are much more severe than in AC or PAC and tend to be present throughout the year. Seasonal exacerbations are reported in many patients, especially in the winter or summer months, as well as exposure to animal dander, dust and certain foods. Ocular disease activity has been shown to correlate with exacerbations and remissions of the dermatitis. Cataracts associated with AKC occur in 8–12% of patients with the severe forms of atopic dermatitis, but especially in young adults, approximately 10 yr after the onset of the atopic dermatitis. A unique feature of AKC cataracts is that they predominantly involve the anterior portion of the lens and may evolve rapidly into complete opacification within 6 mo while AKC patients may develop posterior polar type cataracts; these are more commonly associated with prolonged use of topical corticosteroid therapy. Keratoconus occurs in a small percentage of patients with atopic dermatitis. Retinal detachment appears to be increased in patients with AKC, although it is also increased in patients with atopic dermatitis in general.

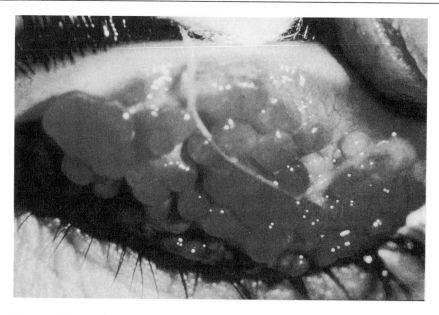

Fig. 1. Giant papillae on the tarsal conjunctiva of a patient with vernal conjunctivitis. Photograph courtesy of Barbara Jennings.

Blepharoconjunctivitis

Blepharitis is inflammation of the eyelid margins that is most often misdiagnosed as an ocular allergy, since it commonly causes conjunctivitis as well. Infection or seborrhea commonly causes it. As in patients with atopic dermatitis, the most important organism isolated from the lid margin is *Staphylococcus aureus*. Antigenic products and not the colonization itself are thought to play the primary role in the induction of chronic eczema of the eyelid margins. The symptoms include persistent burning, itching, tearing and "a feeling of dryness." Patients commonly complain of more symptoms in the morning than in the evening. This is in contradistinction to patients with dry eye syndromes who complain of more symptoms in the evening than in the morning because of drying out of the tear film during the day. The crusted exudate that develops in these patients may cause the eye to be "glued shut" when the patient awakens in the morning. The signs of staphylococcal blepharitis include dilated blood vessels, erythema, scales, collarettes of exudative material around the eyelash bases and foamy exudates in the tear film. Blepharitis can be controlled with improved eyelid hygiene with detergents (e.g., nonstinging baby shampoos) and with steroid ointments applied to the lid margin with a cotton tip applicator that loosens the exudate and scales.

Contact Dermatitis of the Eyelids

In contradistinction to ocular allergy, which is predominantly associated with the activation of mast cells, contact dermatitis is predominantly a lymphocytic delayed type of hypersensitivity reaction involving the eyelids. Because the eyelid skin is soft, pliable and thin, contact dermatitis of the eyelids frequently causes the patient to seek medical attention for a cutaneous reaction that elsewhere on the skin normally would be less of concern. The eyelid skin is capable of developing significant swelling

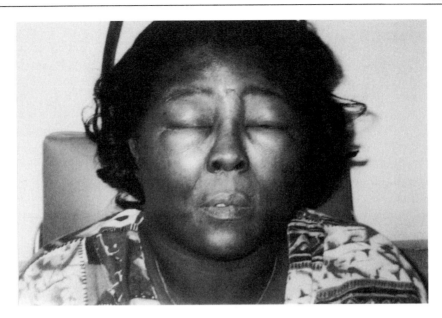

Fig. 2. Angioedema around the eyes 24 h after exposure to hair dye. Patient had a similar reaction to hair dye 2 mo previously.

and redness with minor degrees of inflammation. Contact dermatitis of the lids and periorbital area more often is caused by cosmetics applied to the hair, face or fingernails than by cosmetics applied to the eye area. It is important to bear in mind that the sites to which some of these cosmetics are applied may not be affected. This is particularly true for hair dye (Fig. 2) and nail polish. Preservatives such as thimerosal found in contact lens cleaning solutions have been shown by patch tests to be major culprits. Stinging and burning of the eyes and lids are the most common complaints. These subjective symptoms are usually transitory and unaccompanied by objective signs of irritation. Two principal forms of contact dermatitis attributable to eye area cosmetics are recognized: allergic contact dermatitis and irritant (toxic) contact dermatitis. The patch test can assist in pinpointing the causative antigen, but interpretation of patch-test results may consequently be difficult, and the likelihood of irritant false-positive reactions must be borne in mind.

Giant Papillary Conjunctivitis (GPC)

GPC is increasingly more common with the advent of extended-wear soft contact lenses and other foreign bodies such as suture materials and ocular prosthetics. There is an increase of symptoms during the spring pollen season; symptoms include itching. Signs include a white or clear exudate upon awakening which chronically becomes thick and stringy and the patient may develop papillary hypertrophy ("cobblestoning") especially in the tarsal conjunctiva of the upper lid, which has been described in 5–10% of soft and 3–4% of hard contact lens wearers (Fig. 3). The contact lens polymer, preservatives such as thimerosal and proteinaceous deposits on the surface of the lens have all been implicated as causing GPC, but this concept remains controversial. Common symptoms include intense itching, decreased tolerance to contact lens wear, blurred vision, conjunctival injection and increased mucous production. Treatment involves

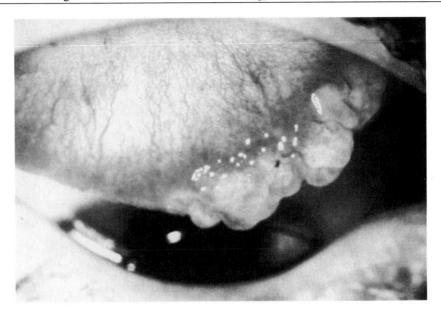

Fig. 3. Giant papillary conjunctivitis in a contact lens patient. Note the giant papillae on inversion of the upper eye lid. Photograph courtesy of Tom Landgraf.

corticosteroids, antihistamines, mast cell stabilizers; frequent enzymatic cleaning of the lenses; or changing the lens polymers. Disposable contact lenses have been proposed as an alternative treatment for giant papillary conjunctivitis. It will usually resolve when the patient stops wearing contact lenses or when the foreign body is removed.

Bacterial Conjunctivitis

Ocular irritation, conjunctival redness, and a mucopurulent discharge that is worse in the morning characterize acute bacterial conjunctivitis. The absence of itching should indicate an infectious cause of conjunctivitis such as bacterial or viral. In bacterial conjunctivitis the eyelids usually become matted to each other; this is primarily noted in the morning when the patient awakens. There is large accumulation of polymorphonuclear cells on the surface of the eye that causes the discharge to become discolored (yellowish green) (Fig. 4). Scraping and culturing of the palpebral conjunctiva can assist in the diagnosis and treatment with the appropriate topical antibiotic regimens.

Some forms of bacterial infection such as inclusion conjunctivitis that has been associated with chlamydial infections are associated with a preauricular node. Common findings of inclusion conjunctivitis include a mucopurulent discharge and follicular conjunctivitis lasting for more than 2 wk. A Giemsa stain of a conjunctival scraping may reveal intracytoplasmic inclusion bodies and will assist in confirming the diagnosis. In addition, such prolonged ocular infections are commonly associated with a conjunctival response that reveals grayish follicles on the upper palpebra. The condition can be chronic, and treatment consists of lid margin scrubs, warm compresses and antibiotics. In general, a topical, broad-spectrum antibiotic, such as sulfacetamide, erythromycin or a combination of polymyxin B, bacitracin and neosporin, is appropriate. Cultures are necessary only if the conjunctivitis is severe; it would be best if they were carefully

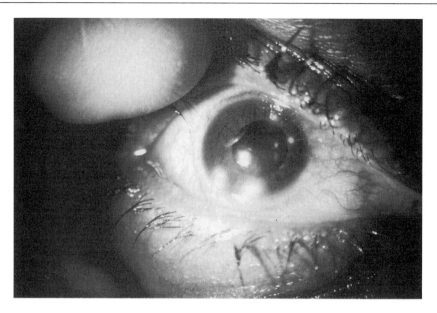

Fig. 4. Bacterial conjunctivitis most likely due to *Staphylococcus*. Note the purulent discharge. Photograph courtesy of Barbara Jennings.

examined by an ophthalmologist. The condition should be followed carefully to ensure that the eye improves.

Topical gentamicin and tobramycin are indicated if Gram-negative organisms are suspected or seen on Gram stain. It should be noted that all of these antibiotics have the potential to elicit an allergic reaction. A careful history for drug allergies, a time limit for therapy and re-evaluation will minimize complications. Topical ciprofloxacin or ofloxacin offers coverage for a wide spectrum of infecting agents, but should be used only when there is the likelihood for therapeutic failure or the conjunctivitis is thought to be due to multiple infecting organisms or *Pseudomonas* sp. Treatment of inclusion conjunctivitis should be aggressive, since there is the potential for the cornea to perforate in a short time. Both topical and systemic antibiotics should be used. The patient should be observed for other sexually transmitted diseases.

Viral Conjunctivitis

Viral conjunctivitis usually has an acute onset, is unilateral and lasts a week, but it frequently becomes bilateral. A major clinical symptom that differentiates this from allergic conjunctivitis is burning and the absence of itching. Adenoviral infections are among the most common viral ocular infections and are extremely contagious. The viral infection produces an inferior follicular response and a serous discharge. It may also involve the cornea as a punctate keratopathy or superficial ulcerations (herpes simplex or herpes zoster infections).

Common findings of viral conjunctivitis include a watery discharge, conjunctival injection, chemosis and enlargement of the preauricular (pretragal) lymph nodes. Patient history also assists in the diagnosis. Viral conjunctivitis is usually transmitted between family members or among school children. As in chronic bacterial infections, gray elevated vascular areas known as lymphoid follicles may also be present.

> It is important to distinguish sensations of burning and irritation
> from true pruritus to differentiate keratoconjunctivitis sicca from
> allergic eye disease.

A more serious form of viral conjunctivitis is that caused by herpes simplex, which is one of the leading infectious causes of blindness in Western countries. The viral infection produces an inferior follicular response and a serous discharge and can occur without any other sign of a herpetic infection. The pain associated with herpetic infections is excruciating. The pain can occur days before the lesions appear. The absence of pruritus should guide the clinician away from a diagnosis of allergic eye disease and toward an infectious complication. It may also involve the cornea in the form of punctate keratopathy or the classic "dendritic" superficial ulcerations. The possibility of herpes keratitis is one of the most compelling reasons for a primary care physician to examine the cornea with fluorescein staining. Treatment of nonspecific viral conjunctivitis is largely supportive and requires no drug therapy. Topical vasoconstrictors may provide symptomatic relief, and they may decrease conjunctival injection. If the corneal epithelium becomes compromised and there is a risk for secondary infection, prophylactic antibiotics may be indicated.

Proptosis

Eyes that protrude past the capacity for the lids to close can become extremely dry. Without proper lubrication and protection, loss of vision can result. One of the most common conditions causing proptosis is Graves' ophthalmopathy with or without hyperthyroidism. Symptomatic treatment includes ocular lubricants, especially at night. The underlying cause of proptosis should be defined.

Keratoconjunctivitis Sicca

Keratoconjunctivitis sicca (KCS) is a dry eye syndrome commonly associated with an underlying systemic autoimmune disorder such as Sjögren's syndrome, rheumatoid arthritis or HIV infection. Clinically it occurs more commonly in postmenopausal women, but has also been shown to be increased in AIDS patients. Tear production decreases with age—60% fewer than at the age of 18. The eye produces approximately 400 drops of tears per day. It is characterized by an insidious and progressive lympho-cytic infiltration into the main and accessory lacrimal glands. Patients initially complain of a mildly injected eye with excessive mucous production. Symptoms include a gritty, sandy feeling in the eyes as compared to the itching and burning feeling many patients complain of with histamine release into the eye. As the cornea becomes involved a more scratchy and painful sensation as well as photophobia may appear. The corneal epithelial injury can be detected with punctuate staining with fluorescein. The symptoms worsen throughout the day as the limited portion of the aqueous tear film evaporates. Exacerbation of symptoms also occurs in the winter months while heating systems decrease the relative humidity in the household to less than 25%. Schirmer's test demonstrates decreased tearing, generally with 0–1 mm of wetting at 1 min and 2–3 mm at 5 min. Normal values for the Schirmer test are more than 4 mm at 1 min and 10 mm at 5 min. The most common cause of dry eye syndrome not associated with an autoimmune disorder is long-term use of medications with anticholinergic properties that cause decreased lacrimation. Many drugs with antimuscarinic properties include the first-generation antihistamines, phenothiazines, tricyclic antidepressants, atropine and scopolamine. Other agents that are associated with a sicca syndrome include the retinoids, β-blockers and chemotherapeutic agents. Treatment includes addressing the underlying pathology, discontinuing the offending drug if possible and generous use of artificial tears or ocular lubricants. For severe symptoms, insertion of punctal plugs may be indicated.

OCULAR EXAMINATION

The ocular examination begins with the eyelids and lashes. One should look for evidence of lid margin erythema, telangiectasia, thickening, scaling and/or lash collars. The sclera and conjunctiva are then examined for the presence of redness (injection). Certain characteristics that can assist in pinpointing the diagnosis are characterized below.

Subconjunctival hemorrhages spontaneously occur after coughing, sneezing or straining as a result of spontaneous rupture of a conjunctival or episcleral capillary. A painless focal area of solid redness surrounded by normal white sclera on all sides characterizes it. It commonly resolves without any intervention.

Scleritis tends to develop progressively over the course of several days and is associated with several systemic autoimmune disorders, particularly rheumatoid arthritis and Wegener's granulomatosis. Major signs and symptoms of scleritis include moderate to severe ocular pain, tender and inflamed conjunctiva and thickened and injected sclera.

Uveitis is a significant ocular condition that requires immediate ophthalmological evaluation. One of the signs of this disorder is circumcorneal injection (ciliary flush), which is often described as a ring of redness that completely encircles the edge (limbus) of the cornea. Pupil size is also extremely helpful in formulation of the diagnosis of a red eye. In iritis, the affected pupil is usually smaller and sluggish. In acute-angle closure glaucoma attacks, the pupil is usually mid-dilated and sluggish or fixed.

The cornea is examined next. A corneal opacity, seen as a whitish infiltrate, is often a sign of a bacterial corneal ulcer. Corneal ulcer is an ophthalmological emergency. Fluorescein stains help to differentiate among punctate epithelial defects (diffuse punctate staining), herpes simplex keratitis (dendrite-like shaped staining) and abrasion (large solid area of staining seen after trauma).

OPHTHALMIC PROCEDURES AND TESTING

Primary health care providers should also be familiar with some ophthalmic procedures and test to assist in completing detailed and thorough history and physical examination in order to assist them in confirming a diagnosis of ocular allergy. More importantly, these various tests help to differentiate between the many disorders that mimic allergic disorders of the eye.

The *Schirmer tear test* is the most commonly used and easily performed test for the evaluation of dry eye. Tear production is assessed by the amount of wetting seen on a folded strip of sterile filter paper after it is placed into the conjunctival sac. The patient is seated with the room lights dimmed and is then asked to "look up" as the lower eyelid is gently pulled downward. Excess moisture and tears are dried along the eyelid margin and conjunctiva with a sterile cotton-tipped applicator. The *rounded* end of the test strip is bent at the notch ~ 90–120 degrees and is hooked into the conjunctival sac at the junction of the middle and lateral one third of the lower eyelid margin. The patient's eyes remain closed throughout the examination. The test strips are removed after 5 min. The length of the moistened area from the notch to the *flat* end of the sterile strip is measured using a millimeter ruler or the scale imprinted on the test-strip package. Some of the test strips have a leading edge of tear film that changes color, thus improving the reading of the results. The Schirmer I test (without anesthesia) measures both basal and reflex tearing, whereas the Schirmer II test (with anesthesia) measures only the basal secretion of tearing and is performed as outlined above, but with topical anesthesia instilled.

Fluorescein is a water-soluble dye used to examine the cornea and conjunctival surfaces. It stains the denuded epithelium. It is placed into the eye either with a sterile fluorescein sodium ophthalmic strip (Fluor-1-Strip) or with a dropper in liquid form. A cobalt blue filter is needed to best appreciate the fluorescein-staining pattern of the conjunctiva and cornea. This filter produces a blue hue against the intense green color of the fluorescein dye. The patient is asked to blink several times to spread the fluorescein uniformly and evenly over the entire corneal and conjunctival surface. Soft contact lenses must be removed prior to fluorescein instillation to prevent their permanent staining. At least 1 h must pass after completion of the examination before the soft contact lenses can be replaced in the eyes.

Conjunctival scraping can also assist in differentiating various forms of red eye. After the administration of a topical local anesthetic, the palpebral conjunctiva (under the upper lid) is gently scraped several times with a spatula for cytological examination. The sample is spread on a slide and stained with May-Grunwald, Giemsa or another orthochromatic stain to identify eosinophils or neutrophils. The absence of inflammatory cells does not rule out the diagnosis of allergic conjunctivitis, but the presence of eosinophils strongly suggests it.

Conjunctival and eyelid cultures are obtained using a sterile cotton-tipped applicator moistened in thioglycolate broth. The lower palpebral conjunctiva is lightly wiped with the applicator stick for 5 s as the patient is asked to look up. Moistened swabs are preferred as they pick up and release bacteria better than do dry swabs. The sample is then placed into the transport medium.

Ocular provocation testing can be likened to "skin testing" of the eye. Known quantities of specific allergen are instilled onto the ocular surface and the resulting allergic response is measured. This technique is commonly performed by allergists in a research study, especially in the assessment of new drugs against ocular allergies.

OCULAR DRUG FORMULATIONS

Solutions and suspensions are the most common formulation of ocular medications. Like other medications, ocular drugs contain inactive ingredients, including preservatives, agents to increase viscosity, antioxidants, wetting agents, buffers and agents to adjust tonicity. Preservatives control growth of microorganisms that may be introduced into the solution accidentally. Some of these agents can stain contact lenses or have a high incidence of hypersensitivity reactions. Ocular ointments are ideal for prolonged

> **The Topical Preparations for Therapy of Allergic Eye Disease**
>
> - Vasoconstrictors
> - Antihistamines
> - Nonsteroidal anti-inflammatory agents
> - Mast cell stabilizers
> - Costicosteroids
>   All of these are safe and can be used by a primary care physician without concern except for corticosteroids. The use of corticosteroids should be under the direction of a primary eye care provider.

contact of the drug with the eye. Ointments can cause blurry vision; the patient should be informed of the possibility of a temporary decrease or blurring of vision. Drugs formulated into ocular gels also serve as vehicles for prolonged contact of the drug with the eye. Sometimes the use of multiple ocular medications is necessary, in which instance, drops should be administered no less than 5 min apart to allow for adequate drug-tissue contact time and to prevent one drug from diluting the other. When using an ointment and solution, apply the solution before the ointment, since it can retard the entry of subsequent ocular drops.

DRUGS USED IN THE TREATMENT OF OCULAR ALLERGIC DISORDERS

The primary stage of treatment focuses on avoidance, which provides modest symptom improvement. This form of intervention can be implemented with the use of over-the-counter forms of artificial tears. These are safe for all ages. Refrigeration of all ocular products further improves their soothing qualities. The use of cold compresses is extremely soothing by decreasing nerve C fiber stimulation for mild-to-moderate symptoms. Many patients are concerned about the extensive superficial vasodilation; this is easily treated with ocular decongestants.

The secondary stage of treatment is focused on the use of antihistamines (oral and topical). Antihistamines primarily affect ocular pruritus. There are various forms of antihistamines, including levocabastine, emedastine, azelastine, and olopatadine. (Azelastine is not yet approved for use in the United States.) Many of these agents may have dual functions as an antihistamine and as a mast-cell–stabilizing agent or inhibition of other inflammatory mediators. Treatment of ocular allergies is largely based on the severity of symptoms. The various treatments for ocular allergy primarily associated with mast-cell–mediated reactions include avoidance of allergens and use of cold compresses, lubrication (artificial tears), decongestants (vasoconstrictors), antihistamines, nonsteroidal anti-inflammatory drugs, mild topical steroids and immunotherapy. There was a paucity of treatment options, especially after the removal of topical cromolyn sodium from the market, but since 1996 the physician's armamentarium for the treatment of ocular allergy has increased dramatically.

Antihistamines: In the conjunctiva, H_1 stimulation principally mediates the symptom of pruritus whereas the H_2 receptor appears to be clinically involved in the vasodilation. Although topical antihistamines can be used alone to treat allergic conjunctivitis, combined use of an antihistamine and a vasoconstricting agent is more effective than either agent alone. There are three H_1 antihistamines for ocular use, including an alkylamine (pheniramine maleate) and two ethylenediamines (pyrilamine maleate and antazoline phosphate) that are available in combination with a vasoconstrictor, either phenylephrine or naphazoline. Oral antihistamine use in the treatment of allergic conjunctivitis is commonly linked in studies to its effect on allergic rhinitis. However, many of these studies have poorly reflected their impact on the ocular component.

Levocabastine was identified from a series of cyclohexylpiperidine derivatives as a potent antihistamine agent having rapid and long-lasting activity. Levocabastine has pronounced selective H_1 receptor activity, 6½ times more potent than astemizole with minimal to nonexistent binding to dopamine, adrenergic serotonin or opiate receptors. Interestingly, recent focusing by industry on isomers to improve potency of pharmacotherapeutic agents has also shown that the levo isomer of this compound has greater binding affinity and specificity than the dextro isomer; therefore, only the levo isomer is used in the preparation, which is a suspension, in the treatment of allergic conjunctivitis.

Azelastine is presently under investigation for the indication of allergic conjunctivitis. Azelastine is a second-generation H_1 receptor antagonist that was first shown to be clinically effective in relieving the symptoms of allergic rhinitis following oral or intranasal administration.

Emedastine is a relatively selective histamine H_1 antagonist, with no apparent effect on adrenergic, dopaminergic, or serotonin receptors. Relief of the signs and symptoms of allergic conjunctivitis have been demonstrated in patients treated for 6 wk with emebastine in an environmental study.

After many years of clinical use, the possible mechanisms of action of cromolyn sodium are still unknown, although there are many hypotheses. At first it was thought that the material had an effect on phosphodiesterase or cyclic AMP, but most recently it appears that cromolyn may act on B-lymphocytes switching from mu (IgM) to epsilon (IgE) heavy chains. This is a novel potential mechanism for the prevention of mast cell–mediated disorders. Sodium cromoglycate was originally approved for more severe forms of conjunctivitis (giant papillary conjunctivitis, atopic keratoconjunctivitis and vernal conjunctivitis). Many physicians have used it for the treatment of allergic conjunctivitis with an excellent safety record, although the original studies reflecting its clinical efficacy were marginal for allergic conjunctivitis when compared to placebo. The efficacy of the medication appears to be dependent on the concentration of the solution used: a 1% solution, no effect; a 2% solution, a possible effect; a 4% solution, a probable effect. Lodoxamide, approved in the winter of 1993, is a mast cell stabilizer. It has recently been approved for the treatment of all forms of vernal conjunctivitis in a concentration of 0.1% four times a day.

Olopatadine is both an inhibitor of mast cell–mediator release and an H_1 receptor antagonist. Many consider this to be both a topical antihistamine and mild anti-inflammatory agent, and it is presently the largest prescribed ocular allergy agent in the United States. However, the primary efficacy is based on ocular challenge studies and not active clinical studies of allergic conjunctivitis.

Pemirolast potassium, a pyridopirimidine compound that is approved in Japan for use in the treatment of bronchial asthma, allergic rhinitis and allergic/vernal conjunctivitis, was recently approved in the United States for patients with seasonal

> **When to Refer to a Specialist**
>
> Patients should be referred to an allergist/immunologist or ophthalmologist when:
> - There are other, more severe symptoms in addition to ocular itching
> - Pharmacotherapy proves ineffective
> - Symptoms are increasing despite pharmacotherapy
> - Presentation is atypical
> - The physician feels the condition warrants referral:
>   for an intraocular examination by an ophthalmologist
>   for a full evaluation by an allergist/immunologist
>   at the patient's request, in accord with the physician's management strategy

allergic conjunctivitis. Although its mechanism is not entirely understood, it appears from available data that pemirolast prevents mast cell degranulation and subsequent release of histamine (and 5-hydroxytryptamine in some species), perhaps through inhibition of phospholipid by-products involved in intracellular signal transduction.

When topically administered medications such as antihistamines, vasoconstrictors or cromolyn sodium are ineffective, milder topical steroids are a consideration. Topical corticosteroids are highly effective in the treatment of acute and chronic forms of allergic conjunctivitis; regretfully, they are required for control of some of the more severe variants of conjunctivitis, including atopic keratoconjunctivitis, vernal conjunctivitis and giant papillary conjunctivitis. The local administration of these medications is not without possible localized ocular complications, however, including increased intraocular pressure (glaucoma), viral infections and cataract formation. Fluorometholone, 0.1%, eye drops are often selected as useful in treatment of external ocular inflammation. Two modified steroids have been investigated recently for their efficacy in allergic conjunctivitis. Rimexolone and another modified corticosteroid, loteprednol etabonate, are highly effective in treatment of allergic conjunctivitis and are only rarely associated with a significant rise in intraocular pressure.

More data are being released on immunotherapy. The efficacy of allergen immunotherapy is well established, although it appears that allergic rhinitis responds better than allergic conjunctivitis to treatment.

Future developments in the treatment of ocular allergy include research into the use of immunophilins such as cyclosporine. Cyclosporine A is a fungal antimetabolite that can be used as an anti-inflammatory agent. It has been shown to inhibit mast cell mediators such as histamine and mast cell-leukocyte cytokine-induced cascades. It reduced the number of neutrophils, eosinophils and lymphocytes infiltrating the conjunctiva 24 h after challenge with compound 48/80, a well-known mast cell–degranulating agent. In addition, FK-506, a hydrophobic macrolide lactone, is of special interest in ophthalmology because it may be effective in the treatment of a variety of immune-mediated diseases such as corneal graft rejection, keratitis, scleritis, ocular pemphigoid and uveitis. Its potential use is now being focused on allergic conjunctivitis (Table 4).

In some cases, the primary health care provider must consider patients with contact lenses. Since 25% of the general US population have allergies, and more than 20 million patients wear contact lenses, the overlap of these two issues is large. Individuals who

Table 4
Treatment Options for the Various Forms of Allergic Conjunctivitis
and for Occasional/Intermittent (Acute) Symptoms of Ocular Allergy

Primary

1. Avoidance of allergens: Effective and simple in theory, but typically difficult to practice. There is commonly more than 30% symptom improvement.
2. Cold compresses: Decrease nerve C fiber stimulation; effective for mild to moderate symptoms; reduce superficial vasodilation.
3. Preservative-free tears: Effective inexpensive OTC treatment that is extremely soothing; even more soothing if products are refrigerated; safe for all ages and can be used as needed without concern

Secondary

1. Topical antihistamine: Topical application of antihistamine more effective than systemic in relief of itching; have a quick onset.
   - Levocabastine: Approved for children 3 yr and older
   - Emedastine: Approved for children 12 yr and older
2. Decongestants: Have limited duration of action; no effect on itching
3. Topical antihistamine/decongestant combination: Limited agents that are OTC that relieve redness and minimally affect itching (pheniramine-naphazoline, antazoline-naphazoline)
4. Oral antihistamines: Systemic antihistamine treatment should be accompanied by eyedrops, as systemic agents may cause drying, and thus further irritation, of the eyes.
   - Sedating antihistamines (e.g., diphenhydramine, chlorpheniramine): Oral agents mildly effective for itching; common anticholinergic effects may cause dry eyes, nose, mouth and throat; sedation; excitability; dizziness; disturbed coordination
   - Nonsedating antihistamines (e.g., loratadine, fexofenadine): Oral agents mildly effective for itching may not effectively resolve ocular symptoms; may be associated with dry eyes, which can potentially worsen signs and symptoms of allergy
5. Topical mast cell stabilizers
   - Cromolyn: Used prophylactically
   - Lodoxamide: Relatively potent; relatively rapid onset of action; provides effective relief of symptoms; has additional eosinophilic effect; approved for use for diseases with corneal changes
6. Topical nonsteroidal anti-inflammatory agents
   - Ketorolac: Approved for treatment of ocular itching; stinging/burning on instillation experienced by up to 40% of patients
7. Topical antihistamine/mast cell stabilizer
   - Olopatadine: more effective at relieving symptoms; twice-a-day dosing because of long duration of action
8. New topical agents under development
   - Azelastine (topical antihistamine/mast cell stabilizer)
   - Ketotifen* (topical antihistamine/mast cell stabilizer)
   - Pemirolast* (Mast cell stabilizer)
   - Cyclosporine (anti-inflammatory immunomodulator)
9. Topical corticosteroids: Relieve inflammatory symptoms of itching, redness, and edema; appropriate for short-term use in severe conditions (atopic keratoconjunctivitis, ‡ giant papillary conjunctivitis, vernal keratoconjunctivitis) and in recalcitrant cases of perennial allergic conjunctivitis; contraindicated in herpes simplex or ocular viral, fungal or mycobacterium infection; may permit secondary infection or cause intraocular hypertension, glaucoma, or cataracts; intermediate therapy (more than 1 wk) should be monitored by an eye-care professional
   - Loteprednol: Low-potency steroid approved for allergic conjunctivitis
   - Rimexolone: Low-potency steroid approved for allergic conjunctivitis
10. Allergy skin testing: To identify and possibly improve environmental measures
11. Immunotherapy: If avoidance and pharmacotherapeutic measures fail

* Recently approved.

suffer from the more chronic forms of ocular allergy—atopic keratoconjunctivitis, viral conjunctivitis and giant papillary conjunctivitis—should refrain from using contact lenses. In some cases of giant papillary conjunctivitis a "lens-free holiday" will help in the resolution of symptoms. The application of topical medications in contact lens wearers poses many issues, including permanent staining of the contact lens by the preservative and alteration of drug distribution while wearing the contact lens. Individuals should not wear their contact lens while placing topical medications into their eyes. They should place the medication into the eye first, wait 10 min and then place their contact lenses.

SUGGESTED READING

Bielory L. Allergic Disorders of the Eye. In Rich R (ed.) *Principles and Practices of Clinical Immunology* Mosby Year Book, Inc. St. Louis, 1996, Chapter 63, pp. 976–987.

Bielory L (ed.). Ocular allergy. *Immunology and Allergy Clinics of North America.* WB Saunders, 1997, volume 17.

Zecca T, Bielory L. Allergic disorders of the eye. Chapter 17. In Fitzgerald F, Lieberman P, (eds.). Current Practice of Medicine, 3rd ed., *Current Medicine*, Philadelphia, 1999, pp. 183–189.

Bielory L. Allergic disorders of the eye. Chapter 16. In Bone R, Lieberman P, (eds.). Current Practice of Medicine. 2nd ed. *Current Medicine*, Philadelphia 1998, pp. 133–140.

12 Urticaria and Angioedema

Albert F. Finn, Jr., MD

CONTENTS

INTRODUCTION
CLASSIFICATION AND ETIOLOGICAL CONSIDERATIONS
EVALUATION
PATHOPHYSIOLOGY OF URTICARIA AND ANGIOEDEMA
TREATMENT OF URTICARIA AND ANGIOEDEMA
CONCLUSION
SUGGESTED READING

INTRODUCTION

Patients exhibiting hives and associated soft tissue swelling are common in the outpatient setting. These complaints brought to the primary care physician generally will result in a diagnosis of urticaria and angioedema. The patients refer to the urticaria and angioedema by various descriptive terms, such as hives, welts or an itchy rash. Indeed, the lesions that are described by patients with a variety of terms can have a diverse appearance. Categorically, urticarial lesions are pruritic and have a center portion that is elevated. The elevated center is often surrounded by an erythematous halo. This prototypical lesion morphologically has a central wheal with a surrounding flare. However, the configuration of the lesions can be quite different, with some lesions typically being round and circumscribed, while others can be serpiginous or diffuse. Characteristically, the lesions should blanch with pressure, and they generally resolve within 24 h, leaving no residual change to the skin. Lesions that do not blanch, result in pigmentation or scarring of the skin, or are not pruritic should be assessed for other dermatological processes or vasculitis.

Swelling of the subcutaneous tissue, or angioedema, commonly accompanies urticaria. This swelling generally results from the same pathophysiology. However, the actual process is occurring deeper in the tissue. As a result, the erythema that is seen surrounding superficial lesions is not observed, though the swelling can be visualized. Angioedema generally occurs on the extremities and digits as well as areas of the head, neck, face and, in males, genitalia. Patients often describe it as being painful in comparison to urticaria, which is described as itchy.

From: *Current Clinical Practice: Allergic Diseases: Diagnosis and Treatment, 2nd Edition*
Edited by: P. Lieberman and J. Anderson © Humana Press Inc., Totowa, NJ

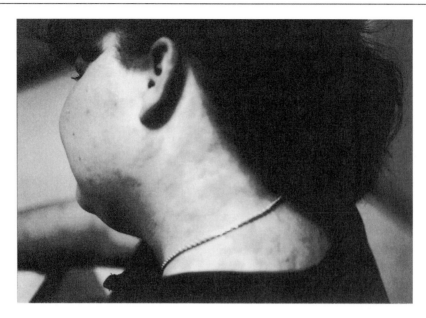

Fig. 1. Chronic urticaria, which can affect quality of life on a daily basis.

A primary care physician will see many patients with urticaria and angioedema, which affect up to 15–20% of the general population, more commonly women. The majority of outbreaks are acute and self-limiting. Less than 10% of urticarial eruptions will become a chronic process. When urticarial lesions develop, they are associated with angioedema in as many as 50% of cases. Approximately 10% of the cases have only angioedema in the absence of urticaria, and the remaining 40% have solely urticaria.

Acute urticaria is a daily problem that primary care physicians handle frequently and effectively. The etiology is often elusive. However, its acute and self-limited character limits morbidity. Chronic urticaria and angioedema tend to be a much more vexing problem, often disabling and interfering with the patient's quality of life (Fig. 1). Recently, research suggests an autoimmune etiology for a subpopulation of those with chronic urticaria and angioedema, which could result in different approaches to the treatment of these patients.

CLASSIFICATION AND ETIOLOGICAL CONSIDERATIONS

Urticaria and angioedema are classified by several characteristics. The most common classification scheme is based on duration. Urticaria that lasts less than 6 wk is deemed acute, and episodes that persist beyond 6 wk are classified as chronic. Designation of acute or chronic urticaria by duration is important, as it portends underlying pathophysiology and should guide both the prognosis and the therapeutic interventions.

Acute urticaria is very common in both children and adults. The acute type is a self-limited process that occurs when mast cells in the skin degranulate. This process is an isolated event and often occurs following exposure to an allergen. It is mediated by IgE, which is affixed to the surface of mast cells in the skin. When the allergen advances via the bloodstream to the mast cells in the skin, IgE is crosslinked, and the mast cells degranulate. This degranulation results in the release of a host of mediators of inflammation, including histamine, products of arachidonic acid metabolism, and cytokines. This acute event will result in increased vascular permeability and local edema, which is visible as the wheal. The patient will experience itching of the skin and swelling of the dermal tissue. Allergens that can result in acute urticaria include foods, antibiotics such as penicillin, and venoms from bee or fire ant stings. Virtually any antigen that can be disseminated systemically, and for which there is an IgE response, has the potential to cause diffuse hives. If an allergen can penetrate the skin locally, hives will develop at the site of exposure. This might happen, for example, following exposure to latex from latex gloves. These individuals develop acute "contact" urticaria in the geographic distribution of the glove. If sufficient latex is absorbed through the skin and reaches the circulation, generalized urticaria can occur.

Acute urticaria can result from nonspecific stimulation of mast cells as well. This occurs when a physiochemical process degranulates mast cells in the absence of an allergen. Thus, IgE on the surface of mast cells is not directly involved. An example in which mast cells can be degranulated directly is exposure to certain radiocontrast media (RCM). This type of exposure to RCM during a radiographic procedure will change the osmolality of the environment in which the mast cell resides and can result in degranulation. Complement may also be directly activated by these agents, and C5a anaphylatoxin can contribute to mast cell degranulation. These patients will develop acute urticarial eruptions that can progress to anaphylaxis with hypotension and bronchospasm. The use of low-ionic radiocontrast media has lessened the occurrence of this acute urticarial event. Other etiological factors that should be considered in individuals with acute urticaria include coincident viral illnesses. Acute viral prodromes in children are associated commonly with nonspecific urticarial eruptions. However, often these patients are also taking penicillin, which can confound the issue. Noteworthy, while many medications can result in a specific IgE-mediated degranulation of mast cells, codeine and other opioid-derived medications can cause nonspecific degranulation of mast cells via opioid receptors. This acute urticarial eruption does not require IgE and is not a specific allergic process, though it does result in an urticarial eruption and is treated similarly.

In certain individuals, urticaria and angioedema are the result of agents that alter the metabolism of arachidonic acid. The occurrence of hives and angioedema is of an acute nature and is often self-limiting. Once again, this interaction occurs in the absence of a specific response with the involvement of IgE. Therapeutic agents included in this category are aspirin and nonsteroidal anti-inflammatory drugs (NSAIDs). Rarely, these responses to NSAIDs can be fulminant and life-threatening.

Thus, when a child or an adult has an isolated event of a short duration of urticaria, the clinician must attempt to identify a specific cause or exposure. In the child, typical allergens causing acute urticaria include medications such as antibiotics. A common inciting group is penicillin or other β-lactams regularly used for respiratory tract infections. Food is another common cause of acute urticaria in children, with the leading allergens being derived from egg, milk, soy, peanut or wheat. In adults, foods more commonly encountered that result in allergic urticaria include shellfish and tree nuts (walnuts, hazelnuts, pecans, etc.). Virtually any food can result in an allergic reaction. However, historical evidence will usually reveal that a particular food resulted

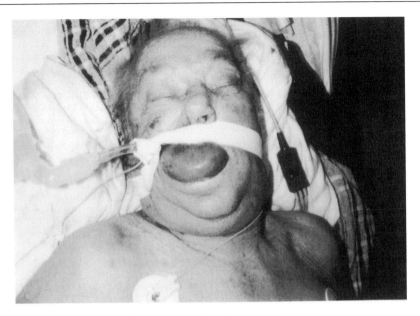

Fig. 2. Glossal angioedema from use of NSAIDs.

in the outbreak of hives shortly after ingestion. In addition, repeated ingestion of that food will result in repeat episodes of acute urticaria. One should be very suspect of an individual who believes that he is allergic to a certain food even though he has ingested it on other occasions without typical urticarial or allergic symptoms.

In children, always consider the possibility that an acute viral illness is responsible for the urticarial eruption. If the child is also taking an antibiotic for a presumed bacterial infection, determine whether the eruption is from an underlying viral etiology or exposure to one of the antibiotics for which skin testing reagents are available. In making this determination, skin testing for penicillin allergy, for example, might be worthwhile, in contrast to the unsubstantiated conclusion that the child is "penicillin allergic."

The widespread acceptance of NSAIDs for musculoskeletal symptoms and their availability as an over-the-counter medication have resulted in many episodes of urticaria and angioedema following their use (Fig. 2). Careful review of all recently used medications could help assess this etiologic consideration. Note that adults are not the only individuals who use NSAIDs; this group of medications is commonly used by the public in the treatment of febrile illnesses for children. Further, aspirin enjoys popularity because of its benefit in preventing heart disease and can be the cause of an acute urticarial eruption. Thus, careful questioning regarding over-the-counter preparations must be pursued in adults and children alike.

Chronic urticaria and angioedema, by definition, result in a skin process of greater than 6 wk in duration. Patients with this classification of urticarial disease tend to be a far more troublesome group with severe, protracted and often disabling disease. Typically, they make multiple visits to their primary care physicians because of lack of efficacy from therapeutic regimens. This group of patients does require a more intense effort on behalf of the clinician to rule out (at least initially) the possibility of recurrent episodes of acute urticaria. Once it has been determined that this protracted

---

Acute Urticaria and Angioedema

- Less than 6 wk in duration
- Short-lived and self-limiting
- More common in children
- Associated with isolated exposure to allergens (foods, drugs, bee sting, latex)
- Associated with exposure to agents resulting in nonspecific reaction (radiocontrast dye, NSAIDs, codeine)

---

episode of urticaria is not a result of repetitive exposures to an allergen or agent that results in recurrent acute urticaria, the diagnosis of chronic urticaria and angioedema may be established.

Patients with chronic urticaria and angioedema typically are observed for IgE-mediated causes (allergies) that result in their recurring hives. However, this is generally unrewarding, as true allergy, i.e., IgE-mediated hypersensitivity, is rarely the etiologic factor responsible for chronic urticaria. Food-elimination diets and skin testing to foods, while generally negative, often help to convince the patient and the clinician alike that foods are not contributing to this process. When positive, eliminating the suspected offender should quickly reveal whether it is relevant to the patient's symptoms. Only strongly positive reactions should be seriously considered. In addition, a thorough review of the patient's medications will disclose whether any agents might be causing a chronic urticarial eruption, though this is uncommon. The use of angiotensin-converting–enzyme inhibitors (ACEIs) can result in recurrent episodes of angioedema. However, urticarial skin lesions are not observed. The swelling is thought to be due to increased bradykinin levels because kininase normally inactivates bradykinin and ACEIs interfere with the normal activity of kininase. This is an example of a metabolic or pharmacological cause of swelling that is not immune.

Once the diagnosis of chronic urticaria and angioedema has been established, and they are believed not to be secondary to allergens such as foods or drugs or recurrent exposure to nonspecific agents such as codeine or NSAIDs, the possibility of underlying systemic disease must be entertained. Atypical aspects of the gross appearance of the hives should heighten concern that a systemic process could be involved. Lesions that do not blanch or are associated with petechiae or purpura suggest vasculitis. Lesions that result in pigment changes, scarring or blistering, or in which individual lesions persist longer than 36 h, suggest systemic diseases that could be resulting in lesions that resemble hives.

Once the evaluation has been completed and the chronic hives do not appear to be associated with any other systemic disease, the lesions are, by exclusion, deemed idiopathic. In the past, greater than 95% of all chronic urticaria was suspected to be of idiopathic classification, assuming that physical causes of hives such as dermatographism had been excluded. Recently, information has resulted in an improved understanding of the cause of chronic idiopathic urticaria. Evidence from research suggests an autoimmune etiology in a large number of the cases that have been previously deemed idiopathic urticaria. Recent data suggest that perhaps 35–45% of individuals with chronic idiopathic urticaria actually do have an underlying autoimmune disease.

Chronic Urticaria And Angioedema

- Greater than six weeks in duration
- Often refractory to commonly used therapeutic regimens
- Rarely associated with foods or drugs resulting in IgE-mediated hypersensitivity
- Rule out recurrent acute episodes due to nonspecific mast cell degranulators (opioid derivatives, NSAIDs) and physically-induced hives
- Chronic angioedema without urticaria could be secondary to ACE inhibitors.
- Chronic angioedema without urticaria can also be associated with complement abnormalities seen in lymphoproliferative disorders, such as lymphoma or connective tissue diseases.
- 35–40% or more of cases are due to an autoimmune process.
- Any atypical lesion requires investigation for vasculitis, coincident systemic disease or other dermatological disorders.

Physical urticaria includes a group of urticarial eruptions and angioedema that occur secondary to a physical stimulus. They can be of the acute or chronic type with respect to their duration, but typically are present for many months and in that sense are chronic. They result from a specific thermomechanical or physical stimulus. These stimuli include exposure to cold or hot temperatures, tensile movement of the skin, application of pressure to the skin, exposure to light of various wavelengths and the induction of a cholinergic response with sweating. Practitioners often encounter physical urticaria that is described as dermatographism. This results when scratching of otherwise normal-appearing skin produces a linear hive that lasts less than 2 h (Fig. 3). This is true of all physically induced hives, with the exception of pressure-induced urticaria, and distinguishes this group of patients from the aforementioned groups with chronic urticaria in which individual lesions last greater than 4 h and often 8–24 h. Dermatographism can follow or coexist with acute or chronic urticaria. Mast cell degranulation occurs when the skin is disturbed by the physical stimulus of tensile force. Other mechanical stimuli that can result in urticaria or angioedema include pressure and vibration. Pressure applied to the skin and subcutaneous tissue often can cause the development of hives at the point of pressure or the development of swelling several hours later. The specific stimulus of vibration also can result in angioedema. Individuals who use mechanical devices that result in vibrations, such as jackhammers and vortexes in laboratories, describe soft tissue swelling. Individuals who ride motorcycles report development of swelling and/or hives on their inner thighs.

Thermal stimuli can result in urticaria and angioedema. Exposure to cold is a common stimulus for the development of hives on the face and hands. Patients will describe hives on the parts of their bodies that are exposed to cold water or cool air. If they have significant exposure to cold water over a sufficient portion of their bodies, they can develop hypotension, which may lead to a life-threatening episode. Swimming is a classic example. Heat applied to the skin can also result in urticaria. This is a rare disorder termed local heat urticaria. More commonly, systemic overheating or

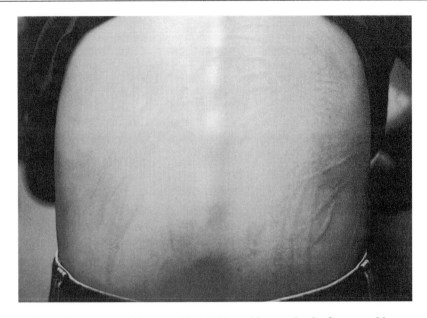

Fig. 3. Dermatographism resulting in linear hives on back after scratching.

exercise results in a cholinergic response of sweating with the development of urticaria. Cholinergic urticarial lesions have a characteristic appearance in that they are punctate (1–5 mm) and intensely pruritic. They resolve within an hour following removal of the stimulus or cessation from exercise. Note, however, that an entity deemed exercise-induced anaphylaxis occurs when an individual develops multiple manifestations of mast cell degranulation, including urticaria, bronchospasm and cardiovascular collapse, in association with exercise. The distinguishing feature that separates cholinergic urticaria from exercise-induced anaphylaxis is that individuals with cholinergic urticaria develop their hives reproducibly following an increase in core body temperature from exposure to a warm climate, exercise or hot showers. They react within 5–10 min. Individuals with exercise-induced anaphylaxis must undergo a major physiological challenge of exercise such as jogging to develop symptoms, and do not develop hives solely when exposed to a warmer environment, i.e., hot showers or passive sweating. Further, it does not occur reproducibly with every challenge; the exercise often has to occur for a protracted period, and the hives are large. On the other hand, respiratory symptoms or hypotension are rarely, if ever, seen with cholinergic urticaria (Table 1).

Other physical stimuli have been noted to result in urticarial eruptions. Cases in which individuals develop urticaria when the skin is exposed to water are deemed aquagenic. Furthermore, several cases have been described in which a combination of physical stimuli can result in urticarial eruptions. For example, hives that develop following exercise in a cold environment are classified as cold-induced, cholinergic urticaria. Pressure-induced urticaria is an exception: the lesions develop 4–6 h after the stimulus, and the appearance of the hives resembles those of chronic urticaria visually and histologically. The term chronic *idiopathic* urticaria presumes seemingly spontaneously occurring hives or swelling in the absence of a physical stimulus or identifiable allergen.

Table 1
Physical and Physiological Stimuli That Can Result
in Urticaria and Angioedema (Physical Urticaria)

Thermal stimuli	Cold: idiopathic cold urticaria Heat: cholinergic urticaria, local heat urticaria
Mechanical stimuli	Dermatographism Delayed pressure urticaria/angioedema Vibratory urticaria/angioedema
Light-induced urticaria	Solar urticaria, types I–VI
Exercise stimuli	Cholinergic urticaria Exercise-induced anaphylaxis (with urticaria)

EVALUATION

First and foremost, in establishing a diagnosis the primary care clinician knows the importance of a complete history and physical examination of the patient. The patient with urticaria or angioedema typically is assigned the correct diagnostic classification following the history and physical examination. This information establishes whether the disease process is acute or chronic. Hives or swelling persisting beyond 6 wk will be assigned to the chronic designation. Questioning will reveal whether those cases with a duration of greater than 6 wk represent recurrent episodes of acute urticaria following inadvertent ingestion or exposure to allergens. A history will reveal whether a child has had an acute viral prodrome and/or is taking antibiotics for a presumed bacterial infection. Furthermore, a careful history will reveal medications or over-the-counter preparations that can result in urticaria. Review of the patient's dietary history is paramount in determining whether foods in the diet or food additives are the culprit. Finally, a discussion with the patient regarding activities and any relationship of hives or swelling with exposure to physical stimuli or exercise might reveal physical urticaria as the diagnosis. Mild dermatographism or pressure-induced urticaria can be present in patients with chronic urticaria; other physically induced hives are always separate. If the urticaria has persisted beyond 6 wk and does not appear to be recurrent episodes of acute urticaria, the primary care clinician must pursue other issues in the patient's history. The patient needs to be questioned about traveling to areas that could have endemic parasitic disease (eosinophilia is a clue to this). The review of systems also must pursue complaints that reflect the possibility of underlying systemic disease. Symptoms of importance include fevers, night sweats, unintentional weight loss, changes in vision, mouth sores, swollen lymph nodes, nausea, vomiting, abdominal pain, genitourinary discomfort or joint discomfort. A careful and complete physical examination should be performed. Specific attention should be focused on mucosal lesions, adenopathy, thyromegaly, abnormal chest findings on auscultation, hepatosplenomegaly, synovitis and joint effusions.

Commonly, an episode of acute urticaria in a child or an adult is secondary to the ingestion of a specific food or medication. The history will reveal this connection, and treatment will be empiric for symptom relief. The evaluation should be expanded to confirm or refute any food and medication allergy. Skin tests often confirm the suspicion that a dietary component is responsible for the allergic reaction. In equivocal cases, the gold standard for establishing a food allergy is a double-blind, placebo-controlled food challenge. However, this should be recommended and performed only by an individual who is trained in this procedure. Life-threatening allergic reactions can be induced on challenging individuals with foods or medications to which they have an IgE-mediated process. Penicillin and other β-lactams frequently are responsible for acute IgE-mediated eruptions. This diagnosis can be confirmed through skin testing to investigate IgE-mediated processes to both the major and minor determinants of penicillin. Skin testing to cephalosporins can be done as well. Skin testing is especially helpful for the patient in whom it is unclear whether the infectious process or the antibiotic is responsible for the urticarial eruption. Again, this procedure does carry significant risk for side effects and should be performed only in a controlled setting by individuals who are trained and experienced in the diagnosis and treatment of allergic reactions. Further laboratory workup might not be indicated in the patient in whom a diagnosis of urticaria has been established following the history and physical examination.

The evaluation of chronic urticaria and angioedema is fundamentally different from that of acute urticarial disease. Other coincident disease must be considered in the patient who discloses a history of greater than 6 wk of urticaria and angioedema, Generally, the history and physical will have excluded the possibility of a clear relationship between a specific food or medication and the development of hives or swelling. The history should reveal whether the individual has hypertension or heart disease and is presently taking an angiotensin-converting enzyme inhibitor that might be resulting in chronic angioedema. Historical evidence of musculoskeletal disease and the possible need for NSAIDs might suggest a nonspecific mast cell degranulation following the alteration of arachidonic acid metabolism in mast cells. Travel to underdeveloped countries and gastrointestinal complaints might provide evidence of an underlying parasitic infection. Similarly, a history of blood transfusion, intravenous drug abuse or jaundice might establish the possibility of viral hepatitis causing an urticarial eruption. Any atypical aspects to the gross appearance of the lesions described by the patient might indicate other systemic disease. Following a careful history and physical examination, laboratory studies might be helpful in the patient with protracted disease. Laboratory studies that can be considered include a complete blood count with differential, urine analysis and determination of the erythrocyte sedimentation rate. Underlying hepatic or renal disease might be reflected in abnormalities found in serum chemistries. If petechiae or purpura is present, antinuclear antibody and cryoglobulin determinations might be helpful. Thyroid function tests, including serum thyroxine (T_4) and thyroid-stimulating hormone (TSH), as well as antiperoxidase and antithyroglobulin antibody, should be performed. Approximately 25% of individuals with chronic idiopathic urticaria have abnormal thyroid laboratory results. Other autoimmune serological findings might be useful for the individual in whom there is suspicion of an underlying autoimmune disease. Finally, IgG anti-IgE receptor antibodies have been described in approximately 35–45% of patients with chronic idiopathic urticaria. This antibody crosslinks the IgE receptor, activates complement and together lead to mast cell degranulation. However, at this time, anti-IgE receptor antibodies are exclusively used in research efforts and are not clinically available.

Evaluation and Workup of Urticaria and Angioedema

Acute Urticaria/Angioedema
- History and physical
- Consider skin testing or double-blind, placebo-controlled food challenge for possible food allergy.
- Consider penicillin skin testing with major and minor determinants for possible β-lactam allergy.
- Skin biopsy not recommended (will show only dermal edema)

Chronic Urticaria/Angioedema
- History and physical examination
- Laboratory studies to be considered (CBC, UA, ESR, thyroid function tests, ANA, serum chemistries, antimicrosomal antibody, antithyroglobulin antibody)
- Skin biopsy if lesion is atypical or if there is suspicion of underlying systemic disease

---

Skin biopsy can be a helpful tool in patients with atypical skin lesions that have a questionable appearance and are suggestive of vasculitis. Histopathological study of an acute urticarial lesion reveals dermal edema with a minimal cellular infiltrate. Physically-induced hives (except delayed-pressure urticaria) have no infiltrate at all. This results primarily from the release of histamine, which causes vasodilatation and increased vascular permeability. However, chronic urticaria does reveal a prominent perivascular mononuclear cell infiltrate (CD_4-positive lymphocytes and monocytes) with increased numbers of mast cells and variable numbers of neutrophils and eosinophils. While this is similarly nonspecific as compared to the dermal edema seen with acute urticaria, the cellular infiltrate does reflect chronicity of the process and release of chemotactic substances in sufficient concentration and of sufficient duration to attract blood cells. The vessel wall is, however, intact. There is no necrosis of cells or deposition of immune complexes. Thus, it is clearly distinguishable from true vasculitis.

The most important reason for performing a skin biopsy is to eliminate the possibility of any coincident systemic disease that would have a different prognosis or require a different therapeutic approach. Invasion of the dermal blood vessels with neutrophils in combination with leukocytoclasis, nuclear debris, and deposition of either complement or immunoglobulins suggests vasculitis. This finding should prompt further investigation to differentiate the possibility of cutaneous vasculitis from a systemic disorder in which there is a cutaneous vasculitis component.

PATHOPHYSIOLOGY OF URTICARIA AND ANGIOEDEMA

Mast cells and basophils have high-affinity receptors for IgE on their surfaces. If an individual develops a specific IgE response to an antigen, re-exposure to that antigen has the potential of crosslinking IgE on the mast cell or basophil, causing cellular degranulation. Degranulation of mast cells and basophils results in histamine release as well as prostaglandin D_2 and leukotriene C_4 from mast cells, plus other mediators of inflammation. If the mast cells are located in the skin, the patient will develop urticaria.

Table 2
Cytokines Reported to Activate or Prime Basophils for Histamine Release

Interleukin - 1
Interleukin - 3
Granulocyte-macrophage colony–stimulating factor
Connective tissue–activating protein III
Neutrophil activating peptide - 2
Macrophage inflammatory protein-1 α and -1 β (MIP-1α, MIP-1β)
Monocyte chemotactic and activating factor/monocyte chemoattractant protein-1
    (MCAF or MCP-1)
Regulated upon activation, normally T-cell expressed and secreted (RANTES)
Monocyte chemotactic and activating factors-3 and -4 (MCP-3, MCP-4)

However, if there is more generalized degranulation of mast cells and basophils, the patient can develop bronchospasm and cardiovascular collapse. Thus, the crosslinking of IgE by an allergen, such as penicillin, or a food allergen, such as peanut, results in the degranulation of mast cells or basophils and causes acute urticaria. In patients with chronic urticaria, there is no specific allergen that can be identified that crosslinks specific IgE on the surface of mast cells or basophils. In this light, research efforts have been focused on discovering a factor or factors that could cause histamine release from dermal mast cells. Over the past two decades, a number of substances have been identified that have been termed histamine-releasing factors (HRF). These HRF-type substances have been proven to release histamine and other mediators from basophils in the absence of any specific allergen. Sources for the HRF substances have included platelets and white blood cells. The finding that white blood cells, specifically lymphocytes, elaborate substances with the potential to release histamine became relevant when considering the biopsy finding of a perivascular mononuclear infiltrate in chronic urticaria. In fact, immunohistochemistry does reveal a predominance of T-lymphocytes in and around blood vessels of the skin from patients with chronic urticaria. Therefore, the mononuclear cells found in proximity to dermal blood vessels might be elaborating HRF substances that, in turn, could cause mast-cell histamine release from resident mast cells or infiltrating basophils. Once these cells degranulate, the histamine and other mediators found within their granules can result in urticaria and angioedema. Note, however, that most of the HRF substances identified to date cause basophil degranulation but not mast-cell degranulation.

Histamine-releasing ability was first established as a property of interleukin-1 (IL-1); however, it is not very potent. Continued efforts by various investigators next revealed HRF properties associated with interleukin-3, granulocyte-macrophage colony–stimulating factor, connective tissue–activating protein III, and neutrophil activating–peptide 2. (These cytokines are outlined in Table 2.)

In most cases, these agents have been shown to effectively cause histamine release from basophils with mixed results in mast cell preparations. Whether these agents cause significant histamine release from cells seen in biopsies of patients with chronic urticaria has not been established. However, these histamine-releasing factors have been demonstrated in iatrogenically induced blisters formed over urticarial lesions in patients with chronic idiopathic urticaria. The most potent of these factors are contained within

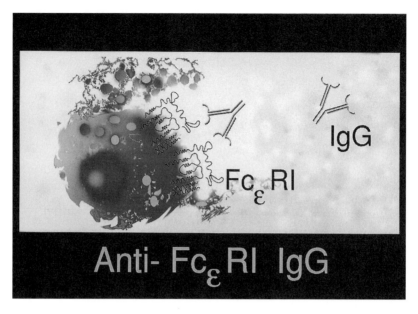

Fig. 4. High-affinity IgE receptor found on mast cells and basophils.

a group of chemotactic cytokines known as β-chemokines. These include from Table 2 the following: MCP-1, RANTES, MCP-3, MCP-4, and MIP-1 α and β.

Previously, the association of thyroid disease (specifically Hashimoto's thyroiditis) with chronic idiopathic urticaria had been demonstrated in approximately 12% of patients. These individuals were found to have elevated titers of either antimicrosomal or antithyroglobulin antibodies. This finding was further studied at our clinical facility, The National Urticaria Research and Treatment Center, Inc., Charleston, S. C., and the presence of antithyroid antibodies has been shown to be higher in patients with severe chronic idiopathic urticaria. As many as 20–25% of patients with recalcitrant hives have been found to have increased antimicrosomal (peroxidase) and antithyroglobulin antibodies even if they are euthyroid. This higher incidence of elevated autoimmune thyroid serological findings could reflect an association more common in severe disease or a difference in current methods for measuring thyroid autoantibodies. Regardless, this association of autoimmune thyroid disease serves to heighten interest in the possibility of an autoimmune mechanism in chronic urticaria and angioedema. To date, a causal relationship between autoimmune thyroid disease and chronic idiopathic urticaria has not been established. Recent efforts pursuing histamine-releasing factors have identified an immunoglobulin of the IgG isotype that causes mast cell secretion. This immunoglobulin has been identified as an autoantibody against the high-affinity IgE receptor found on mast cells and basophils. It is capable of causing degranulation from dermal mast cells. Various methods used in several laboratories have confirmed the capability of this IgG autoantibody to elicit histamine release from mast cells and basophils. These methods have included the induction of degranulation from rat basophil leukemic cells transfected with the α subunit of the IgE receptor, degranulation of human basophils, and degranulation of cutaneous mast cells. Further, the specific target of this IgG autoantibody is the α subunit of the high-affinity IgE receptor found on basophils and mast cells (Fig. 4). Studies have demonstrated this anti-IgE receptor

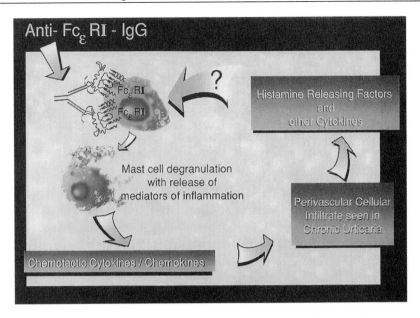

Fig. 5. Autoantibody (IgG) specific for the α-subunit of the high-affinity IgE receptor on mast cells and basophils.

autoantibody (Fig. 5) in approximately 35–45% of patients with the diagnosis of chronic idiopathic urticaria.

With this evolving insight into the autoimmune activity present in patients with chronic idiopathic urticaria, a growing consensus supports the idea that the histopathological lesions are secondary to autoantibody-dependent activation of cutaneous mast cells. Most recent data suggest complement activation and liberation of C5a, which itself is chemotactic and can degranulate cutaneous mast cells. This would result in the release of histamine, prostaglandin D_2, leukotriene C_4, enzymes, cytokines and chemokines from mast cells, followed by release of cytokines and chemokines from vascular endothelial cells. These products, particularly C5a and chemokines, would encourage the influx of cells as seen on biopsy. Furthermore, cells that accumulate in the dermis around blood vessels do have the potential to elaborate and secrete other histamine-releasing factors that might, to some degree, contribute to ongoing mast-cell degranulation. However, the extent to which this IgG autoantibody, complement and other histamine-releasing factors contribute to the histological appearance of the urticarial lesions seen in chronic idiopathic urticaria has not been determined to date.

TREATMENT OF URTICARIA AND ANGIOEDEMA

In the primary care setting, the common encounter is with that patient who develops acute urticaria following the ingestion of a food or medicine to which he is allergic. The patient with an acute allergic reaction often develops urticaria with or without angioedema. If the allergic response extends beyond the skin, bronchospasm, laryngeal edema or hypotension from cardiovascular collapse might occur. However, in the case of urticaria and angioedema, the patient is treated first by avoidance of that agent. If the patient is hemodynamically stable, the acute urticaria will resolve over the next 12–24 h if there is no further allergen exposure.

Treatment of Acute Urticaria and Angioedema

- Avoidance of food, drug or other allergen
- Symptomatic relief (H₁ antihistamines, oatmeal baths)
- Short course (no more than several days) of corticosteroid for severe or protracted episodes and to prevent late-phase response
- Epinephrine to be considered only for acute intervention of severe attacks. *Use carefully in the older patient.*

Some degree of relief can be immediately provided with the use of oatmeal baths. Alcohol-containing beverages should be avoided, as they will cause vasodilation, which can worsen the pruritus. An extensive battery of antihistamines is available for symptomatic relief. First-generation H_1 histamine blockers do have the significant side effects of sedation and mucosal drying. Recently developed second-generation antihistamines (e.g., cetirizine [Zyrtec™]; fexofenadine [Allegra™]; loratadine [Claritin™]) are less soporific and have been demonstrated to be safe and effective in the treatment of urticaria. If the acute urticarial eruption is persistent or especially pronounced, a short course of systemic corticosteroids could lessen the intensity or duration of the episode.

Systemic corticosteroids must be used judiciously, as they are associated with significant side effects. However, a course of systemic steroids for acute urticaria need not be longer than several days. Exceedingly high doses of systemic steroids or protracted courses are not justified, as this is a short-lived allergic reaction, and the steroids are primarily aimed at preventing any late-phase response. Subcutaneous epinephrine may be employed when acute urticaria and angioedema progress toward frank anaphylaxis. Adrenergic agents should be employed carefully in older patients who might have cardiovascular or cerebrovascular disease predisposing them to myocardial or cerebral ischemia.

Physical urticaria can be similarly treated with antihistamines. However, physical urticaria can be of protracted duration. The first approach to physical urticaria should be avoidance or lessening of the stimulus causing the urticaria or angioedema. In the individual in whom a thermal stimulus is causing the urticaria or angioedema, exposure to extremes of temperatures should be avoided. In those patients with cold-induced urticaria, appropriate clothing should be used to minimize exposure to cold climates. Individuals should avoid holding cold objects, such as soft-drink cans and should wear cotton inserts under vinyl gloves when preparing cold food. They must avoid swimming or bathing in cold water, as profound hypotension can develop, which could be potentially life threatening. Individuals with urticaria and angioedema secondary to pressure should wear loosely fitting clothing. They should avoid the use of tight shoes or sitting for long periods, which can result in angioedema of the buttocks. Women with pressure-induced urticaria and angioedema should not carry pocketbooks or luggage with a strap that might apply pressure to the shoulder. The use of tools that require the application of pressure, such as drills or sanders, should be avoided. Mechanical tools that induce vibration, such as orbital sanders or jackhammers, should be avoided in individuals with vibratory urticaria and angioedema. Those patients with cholinergic urticaria that is induced by warm environments or exercise causing sweating must limit activities leading to this cholinergic response. Finally, individuals with dermatographism should try to minimize any scratching of their skin, for it will result in linear urticaria. Antihistamines are very helpful, and nonsedating ones should be tried first. If insufficient relief is obtained, the older sedating ones can be utilized. The drugs of choice are: for cold urticaria, cyproheptadine (Periactin™) 16–32 mg daily in divided doses (four times a day); for cholinergic urticaria, hydroxyzine (Atarax™) 100–200 mg daily in divided doses (four times a day); and for dermatographism, any of these or diphenhydramine (Benadryl™) 100–200 mg daily in divided doses (four times a day). These are adult doses for severe disease and should be adjusted downward for milder disease and for children.

Long-term care for chronic urticaria and angioedema can be challenging. Antihistamines are the initial mainstay of treatment. H_1 antihistamines will result in symptomatic relief, though they are often less than optimal. Since chronic urticaria/angioedema is a chronic disorder, the long-term use of sedating antihistamines can be problematic. Often, H_1 antihistamines can be combined with H_2 antihistamines in the more severe cases. Approximately 15% of histamine receptors found on endothelial cells are of the H_2 subtype, and studies have suggested that the combination of H_1 and H_2 antihistamines in treating chronic urticaria is beneficial. The antidepressive agent doxepin has been found to be effective in the attenuation of symptoms found in chronic idiopathic urticaria. It does have significant antimuscarinic and antiserotoninergic properties in combination with its antihistaminic activity. However, it is very sedating, and its use generally is limited to nighttime hours. The use of sedating antihistamines must be accompanied by warnings to the patient that these agents do cause sedation, and appropriate precautions must be taken. Nevertheless, high doses spread out four times a day, e.g., 25–50 mg hydroxyzine, lead to tolerance of the soporific effects if taken regularly in the vast majority of patients.

Since up to 25% of patients with chronic idiopathic urticaria have coincident thyroid abnormalities, an interest has developed regarding thyroid replacement. In patients with chemical or clinical hypothyroidism, replacement therapy is the standard of care. However, in individuals in whom there is no evidence of clinical or chemical hypothyroidism, thyroid replacement has not been demonstrated uniformly to be beneficial to the chronic urticarial disease. The use of thyroid supplementation does have significant side effects, including development of clinical hyperthyroidism, osteopenia and cardiac arrhythmias. In this light, present recommendations are that individuals with the presence of elevated autoimmune thyroid antibodies should be monitored for the development of chemical or clinical hypothyroidism. This monitoring should include measurement of thyroxine (T_4) and thyroid-stimulating hormone (TSH) approximately every 6–12 mo. A small percentage of individuals who do have autoimmune thyroiditis will become hypothyroid over time. If this percentage is higher in individuals with chronic idiopathic urticaria and autoimmune thyroiditis has not been determined.

Corticosteroids by the systemic route will attenuate the symptoms of chronic urticaria and angioedema. These effects are generally short lived, and the patient's symptoms generally recur following discontinuation of the steroid. As this is a chronic disorder, there is little rationale to the ongoing use of systemic steroids if they will result in significant side effects. Systemic steroids will result in a cushingoid appearance, weight gain, glucose intolerance, hypertension, hyperlipidemia, osteopenia and easy

---

Chronic Urticaria/Angioedema

- H_1 antihistamines (e.g., nonsedating—cetirizine, fexofenadine, loratadine or sedating diphenhydramine, hydroxyzine)
- H_2 antihistamines (e.g., cimetidine, ranitidine, famotidine)
- Short course of systemic corticosteroid (no longer than 1–2 wk)
- Consideration of alternate-day, low-dose steroid and other immunomodulators in severe, refractory disease

---

bruising. With this in mind, the regular or protracted use of systemic corticosteroids is routinely avoided. However, the histopathology of lesions seen in chronic urticaria does reflect an inflammatory aspect with a significant cellular component.

Short bursts of systemic steroids will attenuate the cellular influx. However, the degree to which they affect any autoimmune process that is associated with an anti-IgE receptor antibody is not clear. While systemic corticosteroids have not been demonstrated to affect pathogenic titers of autoantibodies in other disease states or inhibit mast cell degranulation, they do have the potential to modulate secretion of cytokines and/or histamine-releasing factors that could contribute to the local inflammatory response seen in the skin, including the migration of lymphocytes, monocytes, eosinophils and basophils. However, to reiterate, no studies have been performed to establish steroid regimens as preferred in the long-term treatment of chronic urticaria, and as such, the prolonged use of systemic corticosteroids should be avoided. Thus, alternative therapies are being pursued on a case-by-case basis in the most severe forms of chronic urticaria and angioedema. For example, corticosteroids are advocated on an alternate-day basis, e.g., 20 mg prednisone every other day with a slow, gradual decrease in dosage. Regimens of this sort are well tolerated for weeks or even months, but with care being taken to avoid inordinate weight gain or other steroid side effects. Conceptually, the use of plasmapheresis could be considered if an IgG autoantibody is believed to be responsible for the mast cell degranulation. However, plasmapheresis has been demonstrated to have variable success in disease states associated with autoimmune processes. In addition, if significant amounts of the inciting IgG autoantibody were removed, the effect would be short lived, as IgG levels in plasma would be reconstituted from other extravascular sites and the plasma cells would continue synthesis. Controlled studies will be helpful to ascertain the utility of systemic steroid regimens, immunomodulators and plasmapheresis in the long term for management of chronic urticaria and angioedema that is secondary to an autoimmune abnormality.

CONCLUSION

The primary care physician will encounter many cases of urticaria and angioedema. The most common presentation will be of an acute episode following ingestion of a food to which the individual is allergic or use of a medication to which the individual has developed an allergy. The primary treatment will be empiric with avoidance of the allergen and the use of H_1 antihistamines. A short course of systemic steroids should be reserved for the most severe cases. Generally, the patient will be warned of the predisposition to further allergic reactions, which can be more severe in intensity. An evaluation can include skin testing for foods, penicillin or cephalosporins if deemed necessary. A Medic-Alert bracelet is often useful to emergency health care providers, should the patient be at risk for life-threatening attacks in the future. A self-injectable epinephrine syringe (EpiPen™, Ana-Guard™) is appropriate if future life-threatening episodes are possible.

Physically induced hives are suspected based on the history and can be confirmed by challenge, e.g., exercise to the point of sweating for cholinergic urticaria, scratching the skin for dermatographism, or a 5-min application of ice on the forearm for cold urticaria. The treatment employs antihistamines in dosages differing with the severity.

The more troublesome cases of urticaria and angioedema are those of the chronic classification. These patients often have persistent or severe disease that is refractory to antihistamine therapy. They might require maximum doses of both H_1 and H_2 antihistamines. An evaluation can be extended to ensure that underlying systemic disease is not responsible for the mast cell degranulation. With information recently developed regarding the autoimmune aspects of chronic idiopathic urticaria, the use of immunomodulators might be appropriate in select cases. The most commonly utilized is alternate-day low-dose prednisone. The possibility of coincident thyroid disease should be investigated in all individuals with chronic idiopathic urticaria, as up to 25% of these individuals will have the presence of thyroid autoantibodies. In addition, many of these individuals will develop overt clinical or chemical hypothyroidism. Studies presently focused on the relevance of the anti-IgE receptor antibody are expected to be illuminating. The contribution of this autoantibody to the fundamental pathogenesis could reveal future therapeutic directions that will be helpful in the long-term management of these patients. Until such time that the relevance of the anti-IgE receptor antibody as well as other histamine-releasing factors to the pathogenesis has been determined, the use of immunomodulators, immunosuppressives or plasmapheresis cannot be recommended routinely. Finally, no consensus suggests the uniform benefit of thyroid supplementation in individuals who have elevated thyroid autoantibodies but are chemically and clinically euthyroid. Further study of populations of patients with chronic idiopathic urticaria and coincident autoimmune thyroid disease will need to be performed to evaluate their progression to overt hypothyroidism. It should be emphasized that if an autoimmune origin proves to be correct for 35–45% of patients with chronic urticaria, the remaining 55–65% are still "idiopathic." But the cause appears most likely to be an endogenous abnormality affecting the skin rather than a response to an exogenous substance not yet identified.

SUGGESTED READING

Alam R. Chemokines in allergic inflammation. *J Allergy Clin Immunol* 1997;99:273–277.

Dayan CM, Daniels GH. Chronic autoimmune thyroiditis. *N Engl J Med* 1996;335:99–107.

Finn A, Kaplan AP, Fretwell R, Qu R, Long J. A double-blind, placebo-controlled trial of fexofenadine HCl in the treatment of chronic idiopathic urticaria (CIU). *J Allergy Clin Immunol* 1999;103:1071–1078.

Hide M, Francis DM, Grattan CEH, et al. Autoantibodies against the high-affinity IgE receptor as a cause of histamine release in chronic urticaria. *N Engl J Med* 1993;328:1599–1604.

Kaplan, AP. Urticaria and angioedema. In: *Allergy*. Philadelphia; WB Saunders, 1997, pp. 573–592.

Monroe EW. Nonsedating H_1 antihistamines in chronic urticaria. *Ann. Allergy* 1993;71:585–591.

Monroe, EW, Fox RW, Green AW. Efficacy and safety of loratadine in the management of idiopathic chronic urticaria. *J Am Acad Dermatol* 1998;19:138–139.

O'Donnell BF, Lawlor F, Simpson J, et al. The impact of chronic urticaria on the quality of life. *Br J Dermatol* 1997;136:197–201.

Paradis L, Lavoic A, Brunet C, et al. Effects of systemic corticosteroids on cutaneous histamine secretion and histamine-releasing factor in patients with chronic idiopathic urticaria. *Clin Exp Allergy* 1996;25:815–820.

Pierson WE. Cetirizine: A unique second-generation antihistamine for treatment of rhinitis and chronic urticaria. *Clin Ther* 1991;13:92–99.

Soter NA. Acute and chronic urticaria and angioedema. *J Am Acad Dermatol* 1991;25:146–154.

Tong, LF, Balakrishan G, Kochan JP, et al. Assessment of autoimmunity in chronic urticaria. *J Allergy Clin Immunol* 1997;99:461–465.

13 Atopic Dermatitis

Stacie M. Jones, MD *and A. Wesley Burks,* MD

CONTENTS

INTRODUCTION

Atopic dermatitis (AD) is a complex, multifactorial disorder that was first described in the medical literature over 100 years ago. Although clinicians and researchers agree that this disorder is caused by many factors, the role of allergic disease has remained at the forefront of clinical research. In the late 19th century, Besnier provided a detailed description of a chronic, pruritic dermatitis beginning in infancy and showing associations with asthma and rhinitis. The term *prurigo Besnier* was subsequently used to describe these patients. In 1902, Brocq coined the term *neurodermatitis* to refer to a chronic, pruritic skin condition seen in patients with apparent nervous disorders. Coca (1933) was the first to denote the familial occurrence of hay fever, asthma and eczema and introduced the term *atopy* to describe the inherited nature of human hypersensitivity disorders. In 1933, Wise and Sulzberger condensed the past terminology into the descriptive term we use today—*atopic dermatitis.*

From: *Current Clinical Practice: Allergic Diseases: Diagnosis and Treatment, 2nd Edition*
Edited by: P. Lieberman and J. Anderson © Humana Press Inc., Totowa, NJ

Key Clinical Features of Atopic Dermatitis

- A chronic, eczematoid dermatitis with 90% of cases beginning before age 5
- Characteristic distribution pattern that varies with age
- Intensely pruritic
- 50–80% of patients will suffer from allergic respiratory disorders later in life.

NATURAL HISTORY

Prevalence

Although AD is known to be a common skin disorder, the true prevalence is unknown and has been the subject of much debate among physicians and clinical investigators in many fields of medicine. The incidence in pediatric populations has been estimated to range from 1.1 to 4.3%; however, comprehensive, longitudinal surveys have not been performed to date. In addition, most investigators agree that this condition is affected by many factors such as geographic location and climate, thereby making prevalence studies difficult. It is well recognized that AD is more prevalent in industrialized countries compared to nonindustrialized countries or tropical regions.

Disease Course

AD is a chronic disease of infants, children and young adults. Onset of disease is typically during early infancy. Sixty percent of affected individuals manifest characteristic lesions during the first year of life. Ninety percent of individuals will be affected by age 5 yr. The remaining individuals will typically manifest disease during late childhood or adolescence. It is rare for symptoms to begin during adulthood and should be a clue to question the accuracy of diagnosis.

The clinical course is variable and unpredictable. Some infants and children will have a mild course with spontaneous remission by 2–3 yr of age. Others will have more persistent disease with a chronic unremitting course throughout childhood and even into adulthood. Still others will have a waxing and waning course highlighted by unexplained remissions of varying degrees followed by equally unexplained exacerbations.

Characteristic Distribution

AD is typically divided into three clinical phases based on age of onset. The infantile phase is from birth to 2 yr of age. The onset in this group is typically after 2 mo of age, but onset during the first few weeks of life may be seen. The childhood phase is between 2 and 11 yr. The adolescent and adult phase begins at age 12 yr and proceeds through adulthood. Each of these phases has a typical distribution of skin lesions that can prove useful in diagnosis (Fig. 1).

The infantile phase is characterized by erythematous, pruritic, exudative, maculo-papular lesions that contrast to the more dry, lichenified lesions seen later in childhood and adult life. In infancy these lesions first appear on the cheeks, forehead, and scalp. Progression then occurs to involve the trunk and extensor surfaces of the extremities.

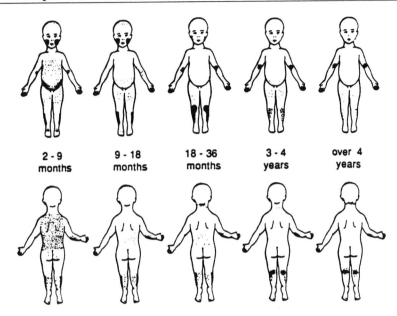

Fig. 1. Distribution of atopic dermatitis in relation to age. (Adapted from Sedlis. *J Pediatr* 1965; 66 (2):235.)

As the infant grows older the distribution of lesions may change to involve the entire extremity surface or the more typical flexural distribution of childhood.

During the childhood phase, lesions of atopic dermatitis are typically dry and involve a more flexural distribution of the extremities. The face, with the exception of the lips and perioral region, is less commonly affected by the age of 4–5 yr. The hands can be especially difficult areas to control in this age group. Intense pruritus and secondary scratching can produce a very anxious, hyperactive child.

The adolescent and adult phase is most commonly manifested as lichenified, pruritic macular lesions involving the face, neck, upper trunk and flexural regions of the extremities. Many young women in their 20s experience hand involvement (i.e., hand eczema) as the first or only manifestation of AD. As previously noted, the onset of disease later in life is very uncommon and should be a clue to search for other etiologic factors or diseases.

PATHOGENESIS

Role of Allergens

There is a strong correlation of atopic dermatitis with other atopic conditions such as asthma and allergic rhinitis. As many as 50–80% of children with AD will develop allergic respiratory disease later in life. In addition, many clinicians note the peculiar tendency of AD and asthma to alternate in their courses in some patients. This observation is unexplained and inconsistent with episodes of both diseases occurring simultaneously on occasion. Because of earlier historical observations of AD associated with other atopic diseases, investigators have explored the role of various allergens as causal factors in these diseases (Table 1).

Table 1
Common Allergens in Atopic Dermatitis

Aeroallergens	Food allergens	Microorganisms
Pollens	Milk	Bacteria
Molds	Egg	*Staphylococcus aureus*
Dust mite	Peanuts	Streptococci
Animal dander	Soy	Fungi/Yeasts
Cockroach	Wheat	*Pityrosporum ovale/orbiculare*
	Shellfish	*Trichophyton* species
	Fish	Other yeast species (*Candida, Malassezia*)

AEROALLERGENS

Pollens were the first aeroallergens reported in association with AD. Ragweed pollinosis has been of particular interest, with clinicians citing case reports of patients with seasonal exacerbation of AD and of clearing in a pollen-free environment. In the 1950s Tuft performed intranasal challenges with ragweed pollen and noted rhinorrhea and itching of affected skin areas in AD patients. More recently, investigators have shown positive prick skin tests and patch tests to common pollens in patients with seasonal distribution of their AD. In a study of children, 90% of AD children tested with epicutaneous patch testing developed eczematous lesions in one or more AD predilection sites when tested with dust mite, cockroach, mold and grass mix. Others have shown positive immediate skin tests to birch pollen in AD patients who had worsening of their disease during the birch pollen season.

Mold allergens have also been implicated as causal factors in patients with AD. Tuft induced symptoms of dermatitis in his patients following inhalation challenge with Alternaria when compared with talc powder or pine pollen. Rajka has also demonstrated eczematous lesions in two of five atopic individuals with AD following inhalation of mold extract.

The largest body of scientific and clinical data regarding aeroallergens and atopic diseases exists in reference to dust mite allergy. Sensitivity to dust mite was first examined in patients with asthma. Reports soon followed of improvement in AD when patients were placed in a dust-free environment and subsequent aggravation of symptoms after exposure to dust. Extensive studies of dust mite antigen and atopic disease association have been performed. They and others have shown positive prick skin testing and patch testing to dust mite antigen in patients with AD. In a recent epidemiological survey, the homes of patients with moderate to severe AD showed a higher dust mite concentration than homes of controls. Elevated serum levels of dust mite–specific antibody and increased basophil sensitivity have also been shown in AD patients when compared with controls. Several groups of investigators have also demonstrated an increased lymphocyte response and specific cytokine profile (e.g., TH_2-type profile with IL-4, IL-5) production in patients with AD and evidence of dust mite allergy. Perhaps the best clinical evidence for dust mite allergen playing a role in the AD condition of some patients comes from reports of patients showing improvement when living in a dust-free environment and having flares of disease upon return to an environment of exposure to dust mite.

> ### Key Features of the Pathogenesis of Atopic Dermatitis
>
> - Immediate hypersensitivity may be key to pathogenesis in the majority of patients.
> - Exacerbations clearly related to contact with aeroallergens or the ingestion of foods to which a patient is allergic.
> - Many patients have IgE-mediated allergic responses to microorganisms growing on the skin.
> - Nonimmunological factors, such as climate and nonspecific irritants, may play a role.

Two other types of aeroallergens are felt to play a role in the pathogenesis of AD—animal dander and cockroach allergens. Both of these allergen groups have been studied in association with asthma and allergic rhinitis and are felt to be important factors in certain susceptible individuals. Less scientific information is available with regard to AD; however, anedoctal clinical experience would support their causative roles. Of the animal danders, cat and dog dander are implicated most commonly in atopic disease states. Cat dander allergy, in particular, can manifest as severe in some atopic individuals, especially those with asthma. Cockroach allergens have been recognized more recently in atopic disease, especially in endemic areas and climates. In a study of atopic children, many of them had positive prick and intradermal skin tests to animal dander and cockroach, indicating the possible relevance of these allergens in atopic disease. More study is needed to define further the role of animal dander and cockroach allergens in AD.

Foods

Adverse reactions to foods have been reported in the medical literature since the early 1900s when Smith reported the case of a man with "buckwheat poisoning." In 1918 Talbot was one of the first physicians to observe an improvement in a patient's eczema while on a milk and egg restriction diet. Tuft (1950s) considered food allergy to be the most important pathogenic factor in infants and young children with AD, yielding to inhalant allergies in older children and adults. Since that time many investigators have studied children with AD and food hypersensitivity. In general, they have shown that dietary manipulation has resulted in dramatic improvement in many patients with AD, especially young children.

Bock and colleagues were the first to establish the use of double-blind, placebo-controlled food challenges (DBPCFC) to assess patients with suspected food hypersensitivity. Because there is poor correlation between allergen-specific IgE antibodies (skin tests or radioallergosorbent tests [RAST]) and clinical symptoms related to food hypersensitivity, oral food challenges (both open and blinded) have been crucial in assisting many investigative groups in the study of food hypersensitivity and AD. Sampson first reported findings of food hypersensitivity in 26 children with AD. These findings were confirmed during a study in our institution in which 46 children with AD were studied with DBPCFC. Positive challenges were detected in 33% of patients, with 91% reacting to only one or two foods. These groups have shown a direct correlation between hypersensitivity to foods (Table 1) and the development of AD. In addition, these groups have consistently reported improvement in AD in food protein–sensitive patients while on food elimination diets.

Perhaps the largest body of information regarding AD and food hypersensitivity has been provided by Sampson and coworkers. To date they have evaluated 450 children with AD for food hypersensitivity by performing 1400 initial DBPCFC to suspected foods. Egg, milk, peanut, soy and wheat accounted for 87% of positive food challenges, with egg sensitivity being the most prevalent. Cutaneous symptoms were seen in 75% of positive challenges. The most common cutaneous manifestation consisted of a pruritic, erythematous morbilliform rash involving the AD predilection sites. Other symptoms noted during positive challenge included respiratory (stridor, wheezing, nasal congestion, rhinorrhea and sneezing) and gastrointestinal (nausea, vomiting, abdominal cramping and/or diarrhea). All patients found to be allergic to particular foods were placed on an appropriate avoidance diet of that food. Virtually all patients reported improvement in symptoms, either noted as complete resolution or marked clearing.

In a more recent study in our institution we sought to further delineate the role of food hypersensitivity in AD and to determine if patients with AD who had food hypersensitivity could be identified by screening prick skin tests using a limited number of food allergens. Patients with AD attending the Arkansas Children's Hospital Pediatric Allergy Clinic were enrolled. After a detailed medical history and physical examination, the patients underwent allergy prick skin testing to a battery of food antigens. Patients with positive prick skin tests underwent DBPCFC; 165 patients were enrolled and completed the study; patients ranged in age from 4 mo to 21.9 yr (mean 48.9 mo); 98 (60%) patients had at least one positive prick DBPCFC. A total of 266 DBPCFC were performed. 64 patients (38.7% of total) were interpreted as having a positive challenge; seven foods (milk, egg, peanut, soy, wheat, cod/catfish, cashew) accounted for 89% of the positive challenges. Utilizing screening prick skin tests for these seven foods we could identify 99% of the food allergic patients correctly. This study confirms that the majority of children with AD have food allergy that can be diagnosed by a prick skin test for the seven foods.

Sampson and colleagues have presented studies of mediator release that provide further evidence that food-specific IgE-mediated mechanisms play a role in the pathogenesis of AD. They have demonstrated increased plasma histamine levels in AD patients following a positive food challenge, increased spontaneous histamine release from basophils in patients with AD and food hypersensitivity, spontaneous release of a cytokine (histamine-releasing factor) from mononuclear cells in these patients and increased cutaneous hyperirritability to a variety of minor stimuli. These mediators and the associated cutaneous hyperirritability were all noted to be diminished to normal levels after 6–9 mo of food allergen avoidance.

In an earlier study examining the natural history of patients with AD and food hypersensitivity, Sampson reported that 26% of patients lost their clinical hypersensitivity during the first year of allergen avoidance, and 11% lost reactivity during the second year. Therefore, Sampson and others have shown that most children tend to "outgrow" their food hypersensitivity to most foods early in life. Some of these children also show subsequent resolution of their AD while others manifest aeroallergen sensitivity that seems to perpetuate the AD cycle.

Through the years, much attention has been focused on the role of maternal dietary restriction during pregnancy and lactation in the prevention of AD and food hypersensitivity. The most current and comprehensive information to date comes from a study that followed 288 American children from birth through age 4 yr and 125 of these children through age 7 yr. Some mothers and infants were randomized to a prophylactic group consisting of maternal avoidance of cow's milk, eggs and peanuts during the third trimester of pregnancy and during lactation; use of a casein hydrolysate formula for supplementation or weaning; avoidance of all solid foods for 6 mo; and avoidance of defined allergenic foods for up to 24 mo. Others provided a control or "untreated" group in which no prophylaxis was implemented. After 7 years the only atopic parameters affected between groups were the prevalence of food allergy and milk sensitization prior to age 2 yr. No difference was seen in the prevalence of AD, asthma, allergic rhinitis, food sensitization, or positive skin tests to inhalant allergens. Other studies in children have shown a direct correlation between the number of solid foods introduced before age 6 mo and the prevalence of AD at age 2 yr. These and other studies indicate the potential role of food allergens in the development of AD and the potential benefits of early allergen avoidance in some high-risk infants.

MICROORGANISMS

The role of microorganisms in the pathogenesis of AD has received much attention in recent years. Their potential role as complicating skin pathogens has long been recognized as important, but more recently their role as "allergens" perpetuating the allergic response has been of particular interest. It is postulated that the altered skin barrier seen in patients with AD provides a portal of entry for various pathogens to gain access to the immune system, thus activating mast cells, basophils, Langerhans' cells and other immune cells (Fig. 2). The primary classes of microorganisms involved include bacteria and yeasts.

The most extensively studied and widely recognized microorganism of importance in the disease process of AD is *Staphylococcus aureus* (*S. aureus*). *S. aureus* skin colonization of both affected and normal skin has been shown to be increased in patients with AD compared to controls. Some investigators have demonstrated colonization in over 90% of lesions in some individuals with AD. In addition increased IgE-specific antistaphylococcal antibodies have been demonstrated in sera of patients with AD. More recently investigators have focused on the role of staphylococcal exotoxins in the disease cycle of AD. These studies have focused on the role of stimulating T-cell–dependent IgE production and subsequent enhancement of the allergic response. Evidence for an IgE-mediated mechanism has been supported by Neuber's reports of increased CD23 (low-affinity receptor for IgE) expression in cells from AD individuals following stimulation with *S. aureus*. Leung and coworkers have reported specific IgE antibodies to staphylococcal exotoxins produced from staphylococcal organisms grown from the skin of 32 of 56 AD patients. Basophils from 10 AD patients with IgE antibodies to these exotoxins released histamine in response to specific staphylococcal exotoxins. Basophils from normal individuals or from patients with AD but without IgE anti-exotoxin antibodies failed to release histamine after exotoxin stimulation. Other data show that low concentrations of toxic shock syndrome toxin-1 (TSST-1) are able to stimulate mononuclear cells from AD patients to produce IgE in a T-cell–dependent

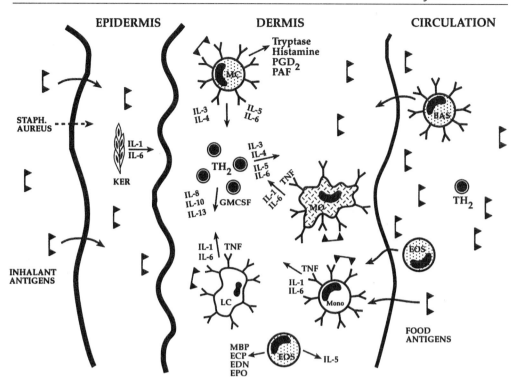

Fig. 2. Schematic representation of the immunopathological events in atopic dermatitis. Allergens transported via circulation or through fissures in the skin enter the epidermis and dermis and activate local inflammatory cells. These cells secrete a variety of mediators and cytokines that perpetuate the cutaneous inflammatory response. TH_2 = T lymphocytes capable of secreting IL-3, IL-4, IL-5, IL-6, IL-8, IL-10, IL-13, GMCSF; KER = keratinocytes; MC = mast cells; LC = Langerhans' cells; EOS = eosinophils; Mono = monocytes; BAS = basophils, MΦ = macrophages. (Adapted from Sampson, HA. *Acta Derm Venereol* 1992;176:34–37.)

fashion. These groups and others have also suggested that these exotoxins may function as "superantigens," thereby perpetuating the immune response by stimulating T-cell proliferation independent of the usual allergic mechanisms. To further emphasize the role of *S. aureus* in the AD process, it has been clearly demonstrated that patients with AD show a better clinical response when treated with combinations of antistaphylococcal antibiotics and topical steroids than with steroids alone. Other bacteria, such as streptococcal species, may also be important, but little clinical or investigative information exists to document their role.

Various species of yeast organisms have been implicated as causal factors in the pathogenesis of AD. *Pityrosporum ovale* and its gestational counterpart, *P. orbiculare*, are lipophilic yeasts that may inhabit the skin of all individuals, with a predilection for the neck, face and upper trunk. Colonization is more commonly seen in older children and adults than in infants and younger children. Many investigators have shown a strong correlation between active AD lesions and specific antibodies to *P. ovale*. The antibodies have been demonstrated via prick skin testing and serum analysis via RAST. Wessels showed the presence of *P. ovale*–specific IgE antibodies in 49% of AD patients. In addition, patients with head, neck and upper trunk distribution of AD lesions and evidence of specific antibodies to *P. ovale*, have been reported to show clinical improvement following ketoconazole therapy. Mononuclear cells from AD patients have been shown to demonstrate a higher proliferative response and atopic cytokine pattern to *P. orbiculare* stimulation than nonatopic controls. Although not conclusive, these data suggest the pathogenic role of *Pityrosporum* species in some patients with AD and emphasize the need for consideration when refractory AD is seen in the typical head and neck distribution, especially in older children and adults. A possible role of other yeasts, such as *Candida albicans*, *Trichophyton* and *Malassezia furfur*, has been implicated in the pathogenesis of AD. Specific IgE antibodies to *M. furfur* have been detected in 70% of sera from *M. furfur*–sensitized patients with AD. More extensive study is needed to draw firm conclusions regarding the role of these yeasts in the pathogenesis of AD.

Role of Environmental Factors

AD is a complex, multifactorial disease. The course of the disease is influenced by many primary and secondary factors that are often difficult to tease apart. Environmental factors frequently act as "triggers," causing exacerbations of disease, yet they are not primary causes of the underlying disease.

CLIMATE

Several environmental factors can influence the course of disease in AD. One of the most important, yet often obscure, factors is climate. Individuals will respond differently to various climatic influences. Most authors report disease intensification during the winter months and patients having the most comfort during the months of summer. Rajka has reported that improvement during the summer may be due to better sebum and sweat secretion, UV rays from sun exposure, exposure to water during swim activities, reduced exposure to indoor allergens (i.e., dust mite and molds), less exposure to infection and less psychosocial stressors during summer vacations. He also mentions that some of these same influences may in fact aggravate the skin condition of other patients. Clinical researchers have noted the impaired sweating mechanism in patients with AD, making excess sweating and strong heat adverse factors in those individuals. UV light exposure without appropriate skin protection can also be harmful. Although indoor allergen exposure may be minimized during summer months, outdoor allergen exposure (i.e., grass pollens) may be exacerbating in some regions. As a general rule, cold dry weather is more aggravating to patients with AD secondary to the drying effect. Hot humid weather may also be aggravating as a result of increased perspiration and the increased potential for secondary skin infection. Extremes or sudden changes of any climatic condition (i.e., temperature and humidity) can be aggravating to patients with AD, most likely secondary to an impaired ability for immediate skin adaptation. Several reports have emphasized the beneficial effect of sunny climates such as California or Florida or dry, warm climates as found in Arizona. As previously stated, these factors are only secondary in the large majority of patients and are vary individually.

IRRITANTS

Factors other than primary irritants (i.e., allergens and infection) may complicate the course of AD. Clothing fabrics can influence the comfort level and the amount of pruritus experienced by AD patients. Wool fabrics clearly provide the most irritation and should be avoided in patients with AD. Synthetic fibers such as nylon and polyester may also be poorly tolerated by some individuals. Cotton is generally the fabric that provides the most comfort and least pruritic potential, and its use should be emphasized to patients.

Certain laundry detergents, bleaches, soaps and household cleaning chemicals act as irritants for patients with AD. Mild laundry detergents without bleach are generally better tolerated. Washing clothing through a rinse cycle twice usually ensures removal of the detergent and may be beneficial in some sensitive patients. Mild skin soaps should also be used for bathing by AD patients. They are generally less drying, less irritating and less likely to induce pruritus. Skin should be protected from household cleaners by wearing protective gloves or clothing. The skin barrier is frequently altered in AD and will not withstand the general intrusions that normal skin can endure.

Some foods can also act as triggers of irritation and pruritus. Certain fruits and vegetables, such as tomatoes and citrus fruits, are especially irritating in some individuals. These foods are not primary allergens, but rather irritants causing pruritus secondary to their acidic composition.

PSYCHOSOCIAL FACTORS

Most clinicians agree that psychosocial factors influence the disease process of AD and further agree that these factors remain secondary and not primary in disease etiology. Emotional upset, stress, job or school tension and unstable or unsupportive home environments all can contribute as exacerbating factors. Some investigators have stated that these psychological influences may lead to autonomic dysregulation, abnormal vascular responses and mediator release, all of which act to trigger an adverse response. In addition, the chronic pruritus seen in all patients with AD, especially those with severe disease, will cause sleep disturbance, hyperirritability and emotional distress, which contribute to the vicious cycle. Although not primary causes of disease, these issues must be addressed in caring for patients with AD to provide maximal symptomatic relief during periods of disease exacerbation. These issues are especially important in children and adolescents and may occasionally require psychological as well as medical intervention.

OCCUPATION

Choice of career or occupation may strongly influence the disease state for some adult patients with AD. Surveys have reported AD more frequently in occupations in which exposure to dust, wool, textiles or chemicals is common. The dry, hyperirritable skin of AD is prone to cracking, scaling and infection following exposure to irritants. For this reason, patients in a workplace of high exposure have frequent or persistent flares of disease. Studies have reported that 65–75% of AD patients report hand eczema, often related to nonspecific irritants in the workplace. The consequences of hand dermatitis and exacerbation of AD may be quite serious in some individuals, requiring a change of duties or occupation to minimize exposure to irritants.

GENETIC ASSOCIATIONS

Like other atopic conditions, AD has a strong genetic predisposition. As many as 60–80% of patients with AD have a family history of a first-degree relative with

---

Key Features of Diagnosis

- There is no single diagnostic marker; therefore, the diagnosis is dependent on a global evaluation.
- Morphology, distribution, pruritus and associated atopic diseases are noteworthy features of history and physical examination.
- Laboratory findings of peripheral eosinophilia, increased serum IgE, positive allergy skin tests and positive food challenge can be markers of disease.

AD, asthma or allergic rhinitis. In studies of twins, Rajka reported a much higher concordance for atopy in monozygotic twins, whereas AD alone revealed only a 50% concordance in both monozygotic and dizygotic twins. Rajka's data cast doubt on the strictly hereditary influence, yet underscore the importance of the combination of hereditary and environmental factors in the disease process. Numerous reports have suggested HLA associations among families with atopic disease in general and AD specifically. These data are not definitive at present and suggest that a single set of genes is not responsible for atopic disease inheritance. Multiple patterns of disease inheritance such as autosomal dominance, autosomal recessive and multifactorial inheritance have been found, emphasizing the obvious complexity of genetic influence on the disease process. Throughout all these studies, however, it is maintained that individuals from atopic families are at greater risk for development of atopic disease in some form.

CLINICAL MANIFESTATIONS

History

AD typically begins early in life, most commonly with skin lesions developing in the first 6 mo. Although this pattern is typical, alterations in presentation frequently occur. A careful history can therefore be useful in making the diagnosis of AD. As noted previously, a family history of atopic disease may provide a clue to the etiology of a patient's skin disease. As many as 80% of patients with AD have a positive family history of atopy. A comprehensive history with regard to possible exacerbating triggers can also be helpful. These triggers may include foods, seasonal allergens, environmental conditions, irritants, emotional distress, and occupational exposures. A careful history will often uncover an exacerbating factor that is unapparent to the patient or the physician. The most prominent and persistent feature detected by historical evaluation is intense pruritus associated with a chronically relapsing course of skin disease.

Physical Findings

Although typical distribution of lesions can be detected during various stages of development (Fig. 1), no firm diagnostic pattern is seen among all patients. The diagnosis of AD therefore relies on information compiled from all aspects of the clinical history, physical examination and laboratory data. Hanafin and Rajka have provided useful guidelines to assist in diagnosing AD (Table 2).

Table 2
Guidelines for the Diagnosis of Atopic Dermatitis.

Must have three or more basic features

Pruritus
Typical morphology and distribution:
    a. Flexural lichenification or linearity in adults
    b. Facial and extensor involvement in infants and children
Chronic or chronically relapsing dermatitis
Personal or family history of atopy (asthma, allergic rhinitis, AD)

Plus three or more minor features

Xerosis
Ichthyosis/palmar hyperlinearity/keratosis pilaris
Immediate (type I) skin test reactivity
Elevated serum IgE level
Early age of onset
Tendency toward cutaneous infections (especially Staphylococcus aureus and herpes simplex)/
    impaired cell-mediated immunity
Tendency toward nonspecific hand or foot dermatitis
Nipple eczema
Cheilitis
Recurrent conjunctivitis
Dennie-Morgan infraorbital fold
Keratoconus
Anterior subcapsular cataracts
Orbital darkening
Facial pallor/facial erythema
Pityriasis alba
Anterior neck folds
Itch when sweating
Intolerance to wool and lipid solvents
Perifollicular accentuation
Food intolerance
Course influenced by environmental/emotional factors
White dermographism/delayed blanch

Data from Hanafin and Rajka. *Acta Derm Venereol* 1980; suppl. 92:44

The rash of AD typically begins as an erythematous, papulovescicular eruption that, with time, progresses to a scaly, lichenified maculopapular dermatitis. Weeping, crusting lesions of the head, neck and extensor surfaces of the extremities are common in infancy (*see* Fig. 1). These lesions may involve the entire body surface, yet the diaper area may be spared. The scalp is often affected in infants with some having features of concomitant scalp seborrhea. Because of intense pruritus and scratching, traumatic injury occurs over time, providing a portal of entry for secondary bacterial infection. The early erythematous lesions will frequently discolor after a while and become dry, hyperpigmented lesions as seen in chronic dermatitis of the older child. Older children and adults have a more flexural distribution of lesions (*see* Fig. 1). Lesions are typically dry, lichenfied maculopapular lesions. These lesions commonly remain intensely pruritic with resultant scratching, traumatic skin injury and secondary infection. Hyperpigmentation of chronic lesions is seen with areas of hypopigmentation from older, healed AD lesions. Dry skin, ichthyosis, hand eczema, and chronic chelitis may also be prominent features of the disease. Skin lichenification may be persistent long after "active" dermatitis lesions resolve.

Clinicians have long recognized that patients with AD have a generalized "pallor" to their skin. This has been attributed to an abnormal vascular response that can be demonstrated by the abnormal "blanching" response seen in these patients. This delayed blanching response can be seen in both affected and normal skin of AD patients, as demonstrated by application of pressure or cold on the skin. In addition, these patients will frequently demonstrate "white dermographism." When the skin of an AD patient is stroked with a blunt object, a red line will form and then will be rapidly replaced by a white line without an associated wheal. Under the same conditions, normal skin will develop a red line due to capillary dilatation, an erythematous flare caused by arteriolar dilatation, followed by a wheal secondary to the leaky, dilated capillaries. These abnormal vascular responses of AD have also been implicated in the temperature instability and poor regulatory responses seen in some patients.

Another prominent physical finding in patients with AD is an impaired sweating mechanism. Several investigators have documented this phenomenon, with patients demonstrating less sweating under periods of stimulation. In addition, patients frequently complain of increased pruritus during periods of sweating. Increased transepidermal water loss has also been noted in patients with AD. This has been attributed to fewer sebaceous glands and less total lipid content of AD skin. All of these findings contribute to the clinical manifestations of dry skin and increased pruritus.

LABORATORY FINDINGS

Laboratory tests provide few clues to the diagnosis of AD. Several parameters can be helpful in eliciting triggering agents and underlying causes of disease, but none is diagnostic.

Hematological Findings

Peripheral blood eosinophilia is commonly seen in patients with AD. Eosinophils usually comprise 5–10% of the total white blood cell count in AD patients. The degree of eosinophilia typically does not correlate with the degree of disease severity and is generally not a useful parameter to follow disease activity. Eosinophil mediators, such as major basic protein (MBP) and eosinophil cationic protein (ECP), have been found in the circulation and biopsy specimens of patients with AD. Eosinophil cationic protein has been found in increased amounts in the circulation of AD patients with disease activation compared to AD patients with inactive disease or with normal controls. Additionally, soluble IL-2 receptor (IL-2R) and the eosinophil-specific vascular adhesion molecule, E-selectin, have both been seen in higher circulating levels in patients with AD than in controls and appear to correlate with disease severity in preliminary study. These parameters (ECP, IL-2R, E-selectin) have therefore been proposed as useful markers for disease activity. More information in larger, controlled trials is needed to determine if these parameters are actually valid means of following the disease status in AD.

Serum IgE Antibody

Many investigators have found a correlation between elevated serum IgE concentrations and the presence of AD. Juhlin reported that 82% of AD patients observed had elevated serum IgE levels. In two subsequent surveys, Johnson and O'Loughlin reported the incidence of elevated IgE in AD to be 43% and 76%, respectively. Both noted that increased levels were seen more commonly in patients suffering from more severe disease and in those with concomitant atopic respiratory disease. In addition, these investigators reported a significant number of patients with typical AD and normal IgE concentrations. Other groups have also found elevated IgE levels in nonatopic individuals. At present, most investigators agree that the finding of an elevated serum IgE concentration is a secondary, not a primary, phenomenon. Serum IgE determinations in patients with AD provide little practical benefit in the diagnosis or management of AD.

Skin Test Reactions

Prick and intradermal skin tests to various aeroallergens and food allergens are commonly used in the assessment of AD and provide the most sensitive test for allergen detection. Controversy exists among allergists and dermatologists with regard to the clinical relevance of positive tests. Some investigators have reported that as many as 80% of individuals with AD will have positive specific IgE to a variety of allergens. This finding has been explained by some groups to be nonspecific and only an indicator of a generalized atopic state. Others report the clinical significance of specific IgE antibody and skin test reactivity in some patients with AD and report the observation of clinical improvement while instituting specific allergen avoidance. Knowledge of the allergens eliciting positive skin test reactions can be used as a clinical guide for the management of disease and detection of exacerbating conditions. These tests must be interpreted with caution. The presence of a positive skin test to an aeroallergen or a food allergen may not have strict clinical relevance and must be analyzed in light of the clinical history. For aeroallergen sensitivity, findings of seasonal distribution of other associated disease, such as allergic rhinitis and asthma, may provide additional clues for interpreting positive skin tests and instituting appropriate avoidance procedures. In the case of food allergen sensitivity, Sampson found prick skin tests to have an excellent negative predictive accuracy of 82–100%, but a poor, highly variable, positive predictive accuracy of 25–75% when compared to blinded food challenge. Positive results must be correlated with the clinical history and dietary assessment and then confirmed with a trial of an allergen-elimination diet and subsequent food challenge.

RAST

RAST provide another, less sensitive, method of evaluating the presence of IgE antibody to specific allergens in the serum. RAST can be performed on patients with AD in whom the extent of body surface involvement and severity of the dermatitis prohibit skin testing. These tests are less reliable than skin testing, especially when assessing for food allergen sensitivity. Like prick skin tests, Sampson found that RAST had an excellent negative predictive accuracy approaching 100% but a poor positive predictive accuracy of 0–57% when compared to blinded food challenge. These findings limit their usefulness but may still provide clinical clues, especially when negative results are found. In a preliminary study by Sampson, the CAP-RAST™

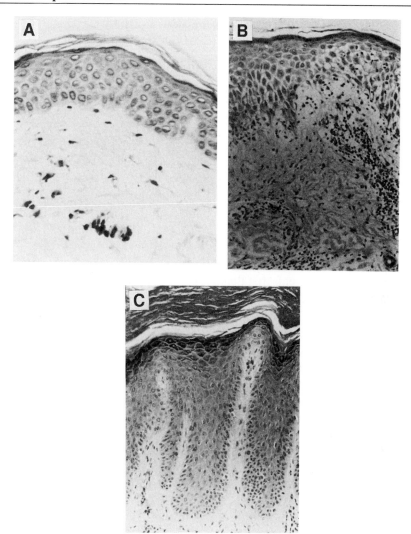

Fig. 3. Skin biopsy specimens of normal skin (**A**), acute lesions of AD (**B**), and chronic lesions of AD (**C**)

has been found to have better predictive values for at least some of the major food allergens, including milk, eggs and peanuts. The study indicated that if the patient had a CAP-RAST™ value above a certain point, there was either a 90 or 95% likelihood that the patient would have a positive food challenge. The cutoff value was different for each of the food allergens.

HISTOPATHOLOGY

The appearance of AD lesions on routine histological specimens is not pathogno-monic and can frequently be seen in a variety of inflammatory skin disorders, such as contact dermatitis, acute photoallergic dermatitis and inflammatory pityriasis rosea. The histopathological changes detected depend on the stage of the lesion (Fig. 3). These stages are typically divided into acute and chronic.

The acute AD lesion (Fig. 3B) is characterized by hyperkeratosis, parakeratosis and hyperplasia of the epidermis, with absence or diminution of the granular cell layer. In addition, spongiosis, secondary to intercellular and intracellular edema of keratinocytes, is prominent. A marked mononuclear cell infiltrate, composed primarily of lymphocytes and occasional monocytes, is seen around the dermal venous plexes. Normal numbers of mast cells, basophils, eosinophils and Langerhans' cells are found in the acute lesions.

Chronic lesions of AD (Fig. 3C) are characterized by marked hyperkeratosis of the epidermis with elongation of the rete ridges, prominent parakeratosis and papillomatosis of the dermis. Only minimal amounts of spongiosis are detected. There is a marked inflammatory infiltrate in both the perivenular and intervascular areas that consists of monocytes, macrophages and lymphocytes. Increased numbers of mast cells and Langerhans' cells can also be detected, but eosinophils are rarely found. Demyelination and fibrosis of the cutaneous nerves can be seen at all levels of the dermis.

Immunohistochemical staining using monoclonal antibodies in specimens from acute and chronic skin lesions, reveals that the predominant lymphocytic infiltrate consists of T-cells bearing the CD3, CD4 surface antigens (i.e., helper/inducer T-cell phenotype) and only occasional CD8 positive surface antigens (i.e., cytotoxic/suppressor T-cell phenotype). There are no natural killer cells or B cells in the lymphocytic infiltrate. In addition, most cells express major histocompatibility complex (MHC) class II surface antigens, indicating an "activated" state. Increased numbers of Langerhans' cells (i.e., CD1a and HLA-DR antigen-positive cells) are detected in lesional biopsies, especially chronic lesions. These Langerhans' cells and associated infiltrating macrophages display IgE molecules bound to their surface. Epidermal keratinocytes located in the dermis of lesional skin also show evidence of activation with increased surface expression of MHC class II antigens and expression of the adhesion molecule, intracellular adhesion molecule-1 (ICAM-1). These cells are felt to be of importance with regard to antigen presentation and processing and subsequent lymphocyte activation and trafficking.

Although biopsy specimens from lesional skin of AD show few eosinophils, large amounts of major basic protein (MBP) is deposited in the chronic skin lesions. MBP is a cationic protein released by activated eosinophils and has been found to have cytolytic activity in lesional skin of patients with AD, as well as in respiratory biopsies from asthmatics. In addition, MBP has been shown capable of stimulating mast cell and basophil degranulation. Other investigators have found increases of other eosinophil mediators (i.e., eosinophil cationic protein and eosinophil-derived neurotoxin) in the biopsy specimens and skin blister fluid of patients with AD following allergen challenge. These findings support the important role of eosinophils and their mediators in the pathogenesis of AD.

IMMUNOPATHOLOGY

Although the full understanding of the immunopathology of AD remains to be elucidated, various immune abnormalities can be routinely detected in these patients. Findings include increased serum IgE, abnormal delayed-type skin reactivity to common antigens (i.e., tetanus antigen), decreased incidence of contact dermatitis (i.e., poison ivy dermatitis) and increased susceptibility to cutaneous viral infections

---

Immunological Abnormalities

- Uncontrolled synthesis of IgE with T-cell profile of immediate hypersensitivity (TH$_2$ cells predominate)
- Decreased delayed hypersensitivity with increased susceptibility to cutaneous viral infections
- High spontaneous basophil histamine release

---

such as herpes simplex, verruca vulgaris, molluscum contagiosum, and vaccinia. In vitro experiments also show a decreased lymphocyte response to mitogens (i.e., phytohemagglutinin) and recall antigens (i.e., tetanus) and a defective cytotoxic T-cell response. Reduced chemotaxis of monocytes and polymorphonuclear leukocytes has also been reported in AD. These data indicate that a combination of mechanisms may be important in the immunopathogenesis of AD (Fig. 2).

Role of IgE in AD

Support for an IgE-mediated mechanism in AD is suggested by the following findings typical of AD: elevated serum IgE concentration, positive immediate skin tests and RAST to a variety of food and aeroallergens, association with other atopic diseases (i.e., asthma and allergic rhinitis) and a positive family history for atopy in 80–90% of patients. In addition, bone marrow transplant data have documented the ability to transfer IgE antibody, specific allergen sensitivity and AD to previously nonatopic bone marrow recipients. Although the histological appearance of AD lesions suggests a type IV, cell-mediated hypersensitivity reaction due to the cellular infiltrative pattern, recent information on the allergic late-phase reaction (LPR) has shown a distinctive cellular infiltrate that is consistent with that seen in AD. Following allergen challenge, IgE-bearing mast cells bind allergen and become activated, releasing cytokines and mediators that perpetuate the allergic response. This immediate or early reaction occurs within 15–60 min of allergen challenge and is characterized by erythema, pruritus and increased capillary permeability. Approximately 4–8 h after the initial allergen challenge, the LPR begins with infiltration of eosinophils, neutrophils, lymphocytes and monocytes into the site of inflammation. At 24–48 h, lymphocytes and monocytes predominate the cellular infiltrate. This infiltrate seen during the LPR following antigen challenge is similar to the infiltrate noted in the lesions of AD.

Clinical and laboratory correlates have been made in numerous studies in patients with food hypersensitivity and AD. Following positive food challenge, Sampson and colleagues have shown a rise in plasma histamine, without a change in complement activity, basophil number or total basophil histamine content. Skin biopsy specimens obtained 4 and 14 h after challenge revealed eosinophil infiltrate and deposition of major basic protein. They concluded that food allergen–induced mast cell activation was shown to trigger both an early and a late-phase reaction in the skin of patients with AD.

IgE molecules have also been found to participate in the inflammatory response via mechanisms other than direct mast cell activation. Sampson has shown that children with AD and food hypersensitivity have high spontaneous basophil histamine release in vitro when compared with normal controls or AD patients without food hypersensitivity. Mononuclear cells from these patients also secreted high levels of histamine-releasing factor (HRF). These levels were associated with cutaneous hyperreactivity to a variety of minor stimuli. After an appropriate food elimination diet was implemented for approximately 1 yr, spontaneous basophil histamine releasability and production of HRF fell to baseline levels and correlated clinically to less cutaneous hyperreactivity. In addition, passive transfer of this releasing factor could be demonstrated in nonatopic controls. Basophils from nonatopic individuals were stripped of all IgE molecules and sensitized with IgE from food-allergic patients. This rendered the "normal" basophils capable of secreting histamine in response to HRF.

The observation that Langerhans' cells and macrophages infiltrating into the dermis of AD skin lesions bear IgE surface molecules provides an important link to understanding the immunopathology of AD. These IgE-bearing cells also express the low-affinity receptor for IgE (CD23) and presumably function in antigen processing and presentation. Mudde and coworkers demonstrated that in vitro, IgE-bearing Langerhans' cells from dust mite allergic patients were capable of capturing house dust mite allergen for antigen presentation, whereas IgE-negative cells from normal controls or atopic controls who were not dust mite allergic were unable to capture the allergen. Once activated, these cells have been shown to produce cytokines, such as IL-1 and tumor necrosis factor (TNF), that are important in lymphocyte attraction and activation at the inflammatory site. In Mudde's study, IgE-positive cells were shown to activate lymphocytes after specific allergen challenge, whereas IgE-negative cells did not result in lymphocyte activation. In addition to mast cells, these cells likely function as a bridge between initial allergen contact and processing and subsequent lymphocyte activation and perpetuation of the immune response.

Role of T cells in AD

The role of T-lymphocytes in the pathogenesis of AD has been the subject of many investigative studies during the last 15–20 yr. The concept that T-cells play a critical role in IgE regulation has been elegantly demonstrated in the murine model. Recently, evidence for this same type of interaction has been found in human studies. Cytokines produced by activated lymphocyte clones regulate the immune response. In the murine model, T helper (TH) cells are divided into two distinct subpopulations based on the cytokine profile secreted. T helper type 1 (TH$_1$) cells produce IL-2, IL-3, IL-10 and IFN-γ and function in cell–mediated immunity responses (i.e., infection and delayed-type hypersensitivity). T helper type 2 (TH$_2$) cells produce IL-3, IL-4, IL-5, IL-6, IL-8, IL-10, IL-13 and GM-CSF and function in hypersensitivity responses. These same profiles have been seen in human studies, but with some degree of overlap.

It has been demonstrated that IL-4 acts as an isotype switch factor that commits B-cells to produce IgE. Furthermore, B-cells from patients with AD have been shown to spontaneously produce higher levels of IgE than normal controls. These B-cells also have increased expression of the low-affinity IgE receptor (CD23) on their surface. In vitro data have also shown that IL-4 not only increases IgE production but up-regulates the expression of CD23. Numerous investigators have shown an imbalance in cytokine profiles in patients with AD. These patients typically have a TH$_2$-like cytokine profile with increased secretion of IL-4 and IL-5, in particular. Human T-cell clones from such patients demonstrate decreased production of IFN-γ and increased production of IL-4, resulting in an ability to induce IgE synthesis. This reciprocal relationship between IFN-γ and IL-4 and subsequent induction of IgE synthesis has been documented by several groups. Many have shown that production of IFN-γ or its addition to cell culture will inhibit IgE production and will down-regulate the expression of CD23. Van der Heijden and coworkers have also demonstrated a high frequency of IL-4–producing allergen-specific T cells in lesional skin from AD patients. Van Reijsen noted the same allergen-specific clones from lesional skin with 70% demonstrating a TH_2 phenotype. Both groups suggested that percutaneous sensitization to aeroallergens (e.g., dust mite) may occur and that activation of TH_2-type allergen-specific T cells may be responsible for the high levels of specific IgE found in 80% of AD patients. These data suggest that atopic patients, and those with AD in particular, have an inability to produce IFN-γ and therefore have a predominance of TH_2-type cells, resulting in increased IL-4 production, increased IgE synthesis and continuation of the allergic immune response. Recent data have also suggested that this TH_2-like cytokine profile can be demonstrated from CD8+ (T suppressor) T-cells, in addition to CD4+ (T helper) T-cells in AD patients when compared to nonatopic controls.

Some groups have suggested a model of sequential T helper cell activation in AD involving both TH_2- and TH_1-type T-cells. These investigators have noted more abundant expression of IFN-γ in some chronic AD lesions, suggesting the possible role of TH_1-type cytokines in maintaining the inflammatory response of AD. Of further interest is the apparent differential expression of certain cytokines in acute versus chronic AD skin lesions. Increased expression of IL-16 has been noted in acute AD skin lesions only. IL-16 has chemotactic activity specific for CD4+ (T helper) cells; therefore, it may play a role in the initiation of skin inflammation in AD via enhanced recruitment of CD4+ T-cells. Differential expression of IL-13 and IL-12 has also been demonstrated in acute vs chronic AD skin lesions, respectively. These data provide further evidence for a TH_2 phenotype (i.e., IL-13) in acute lesions leading to inflammation. In contrast, the increase in IL-12 in chronic lesions suggests a possible role for IL-12 producing cells in modulating chronic inflammation, possibly via preferred activation of TH_1-type cells instead of TH_2-type cells. Of additional interest is the role of memory T-cells in recognizing skin-related allergens. Memory T-cells display the cutaneous lymphocyte-associated antigen (CLA) that acts as a skin homing receptor for T-cells recognizing skin-related allergens. In vivo studies have demonstrated activation and increased expression of CLA+ T-cells in patients with AD compared to controls. These CLA+ T-cells demonstrate an increased production of the TH_2-type cytokine, IL-13, and induction of IgE antibodies, indicating their potential pivotal role in the allergic inflammation of AD. Obviously, the immunological aspects of AD are very complex, but provide an intriguing look at interactions between the skin and the immune system that are being continually updated by experts in both fields.

DIFFERENTIAL DIAGNOSIS

Many types of primary skin disorders, metabolic disorders and immunological diseases have associated skin conditions that resemble AD (Table 3). Certain characteristics of these conditions help to distinguish them from AD.

Skin Diseases

Seborrheic dermatitis is is the most common skin disorder confused with AD. It is characterized by a greasy yellow or salmon-colored scaly dermatitis that begins within

Table 3
Differential Diagnosis for Atopic Dermatitis

Skin diseases
    Seborrheic dermatitis
    Nummular eczema
    Contact dermatitis
    Psoriasis
Metabolic disorders
    Phenylketonuria
    Acrodermatitis enteropathica
    Celiac disease/dermatitis herpetiformis
Immunological diseases
    Wiskott-Aldrich syndrome
    Nezelof syndrome
    DiGeorge anomaly
    SCID
    Selective IgA deficiency
    Hyper-IgE syndrome
Other disorders
    Leiner's disease
    Langerhans' cell histiocytosis disease

the first few weeks of life, usually before the typical age of onset of AD. Lesions are primarily distributed on the scalp, cheeks and postauricular areas, but may also occur on the trunk, perineum and intertriginous regions of the hands and feet. In contrast to AD, significant pruritus is generally not a feature of seborrhea.

Nummular eczema is a disorder characterized by well-circumscribed, circular lesions occurring primarily on the extensor surfaces of the extremities in areas of dry skin. Lesions begin as vesicles and papules that coalesce to form the discrete nonexudative, coin-shaped lesions. Lesions are only mildly pruritic. This disorder is not typically associated with atopy or increased serum IgE.

Contact dermatitis, both irritant and allergic, can be seen in infants and young children. The skin eruption of irritant dermatitis varies with etiological agent, but is commonly seen on the cheeks, chin, extensor surfaces of the extremities and the diaper area. Irritant dermatitis is typically less pruritic than AD and improves with removal of the irritant, i.e., soaps, detergents, abrasive bedding. Allergic contact dermatitis is characterized by a pruritic, erythematous papulovesicular eruption that involves exposed areas of contact. This dermatitis is uncommon during the first few months of life and can frequently be delineated by a careful history.

Psoriasis is a primary skin disorder that is most commonly seen in older children and adults, but may be seen on occasion in younger children. Fully developed lesions are distinctively different in appearance from those of AD. Lesions are usually erythematous and covered by a silvery scale. Distribution is primarily on the scalp, extensor surfaces of the extremities and the genital region. Nail involvement is commonly seen with pitting or punctate deformities of the nail surface.

Metabolic Disorders

Phenylketonuria is an inherited disorder caused by inability to metabolize phenyl-alanine secondary to a defect in the enzyme phenylalanine hydroxylase. Affected individuals have fair complexion and blond hair. If untreated, seizures and mental retardation result. Approximately 25% of these individuals have an eczematous-like rash associated with their disease.

Acrodermatits enteropathica is a lethal autosomal recessive disorder with clinical symptoms resulting from profound zinc deficiency secondary to an undefined defect in zinc absorption. The condition is characterized by dermatitis, failure to thrive, diarrhea, alopecia, nail dystrophy, severe gastrointestinal disturbances and frequent infections. Dermatitis lesions are vesciculobullous and are distributed in a symmetrical pattern in the acral and periorificial regions. Treatment of choice is elemental zinc replacement.

Celiac disease is a malabsorption disorder secondary to sensitivity to gliadin, the alcohol-soluble portion of gluten found in cereal grains. An eczematous dermatitis, dermatitis herpetiformis, has been reported to occur in some patients. Dermatitis herpetiformis is a highly pruritic skin rash that is characterized by a chronic papulo-vescicular eruption on the extensor surfaces and buttocks. This disorder is associated with celiac disease in up to 85% of patients. Treatment for celiac disease is life-long dietary avoidance of gluten-containing foods.

Immunological Diseases

Wiskott-Aldrich syndrome is an X-linked disorder characterized by the triad of thrombocytopenia, recurrent infections and eczema. Patients have impairment of both humoral and cellular immune function. Increased serum IgE is frequently found. The distribution of the eczematous rash is different from that typically seen in AD and is less responsive to usual medical management.

Nezelof and DiGeorge syndromes are disorders of T-cell immunity. Both have been associated with eczematous rashes and elevated serum IgE concentrations in some patients. The cause of the rash is unknown, but it is likely associated with the underlying immune dysfunction.

Severe combined immune deficiency (SCID) is a disorder of profound humoral and cellular immune deficiency. In the first 6 months of life, infants frequently have failure to thrive, recurrent infections, diarrhea and dermatitis. Like other immune deficiency syndromes, the eczematous-appearing rash is in an atypical distribution and less responsive to conventional therapy.

Selective IgA deficiency is the most common immune deficiency disorder, affecting approximately 1 in 400 individuals. It is characterized by decreased mucosal immunity, resulting in recurrent sinopulmonary, gastrointestinal and genitoureteral infections. Some patients remain asymptomatic while others manifest evidence of disease. IgA deficiency may be seen in association with atopic disease in some patients. These patients may develop asthma, allergic rhinitis or atopic dermatitis. The dermatitis is more typical of AD, both in character and distribution.

Hyper-IgE syndrome is an immune deficiency disorder characterized by markedly elevated serum IgE concentrations primarily in association with recurrent, severe staphylococcal abscesses of the skin and lungs. A chronic, pruritic dermatitis is commonly seen, but does not occur in the same distribution or have the same course as AD. Immunological abnormalities have been found in both humoral and cellular function.

Other Disorders

Leiner's disease (erythroderma desquamativum) is a disorder that usually begins during the first few months of life and is characterized by severe generalized seborrheic dermatitis, intractable diarrhea, recurrent infections (usually Gram-negative organisms), and marked wasting and dystrophy. The dermatitis involves an intense erythema of the entire body and extensive large, yellow, greasy scales affecting large portions of the body surface. These scales are desquamative, and large skin areas may slough. IgE levels are typically normal and eosinophils are not present. The exact etiology of this disease is unknown but a familial form exists and has been associated with dysfunction of the fifth component of complement (C5).

Langerhans' cell histiocytosis disease is a lethal disorder that is a spectrum of diseases affecting the reticuloendothelial system. A subset of that spectrum, previously known as Letterer-Siwe disease, involves a dermatitis that displays features of both seborrhea and AD. The eruption usually begins on the scalp and postauricular areas as a scaly, erythematous rash resembling seborrhea. The rash progresses to involve the trunk with dark, crusted papules that may be associated with petechiae or purpuric papules.

COMPLICATIONS

Infection

Secondary infection of the skin is the most common complication of AD. Infection can be caused by a variety of bacterial, viral and fungal organisms. The most frequent infections occur with bacterial organisms, most commonly Staphylococcus aureus. As previously stated, some investigators have demonstrated an increased colonization of the skin of patients with AD, with over 90% of lesions showing colonization in some patients. These organisms gain access to the deeper skin layers because a loss of skin integrity in AD permits secondary infection. Although S. aureus is the most common culprit causing impetiginous lesions, β-hemolytic streptococci are also common. Infected skin lesions may be difficult to detect because of the similarity of appearance of chronic AD and secondary infection. Infected lesions may appear more erythematous, pruritic and crusting with areas of open excoriations. Deep pyogenic infections such as furuncles, abscesses and cellulitis are unusual in AD. Systemic antibiotics are the treatment of choice and frequently provide significant relief of symptoms and aid in clearance of skin lesions.

Viral infections are a particularly troublesome complicating factor in some patients with AD. Patients have an unusual susceptibility to certain types of viral infections. The most common organisms found are those of herpes simplex (eczema herpeticum), verruca vulgaris (common warts), molluscum contagiosum and vaccinia (eczema vaccinatum). Kaposi's varicelliform eruption is a particularly severe, explosive infection caused by herpes simplex or vaccinia infection. Viral lesions are typically vesiculopustular in appearance and occur in clusters on both affected and unaffected skin, but with a predilection toward affected skin. The lesions of molluscum contagiosum are papular, centrally umbilicated lesions surrounded by a pale halo. All viral lesions can be seen on any portion of the body. Infection may be localized or result in systemic toxicity (i.e., herpes and vaccinia). Appropriate antiviral therapy may be indicated on a long-term basis to combat these infections, some of which can become latent and recur later (i.e., herpes simplex). In addition to the mentioned viral infections, patients with AD may be at increased risk for developing severe infection following exposure to varicella.

Fungal infections can also complicate the course of AD. Trichophyton rubra and Pityrosporum ovale or orbiculare are the most commonly implicated organisms. Candida albicans and Malassezia furfur have also been implicated in some reports, but strong evidence for those yeasts being a source of infection does not exist at present. Infection with P. ovale/orbiculare is typically seen in the adolescent or adult patient with AD in whom a typical head and neck distribution of lesions is noted. Topical and systemic antifungal agents may be necessary to control infection.

Ocular Conditions

Ocular abnormalities may be seen in patients of all ages with AD. The most common and potentially severe complication is the development of anterior subcapsular cataracts in some patients with AD. The incidence has been reported to be between 5 and 16%, with most cataracts occurring between 10 and 30 yr. Rarely, posterior subcapsular cataracts may occur, but this is more commonly seen in the patient treated with systemic corticosteriods.

Other ocular conditions seen in association with AD include conjunctivitis, keratitis and keratoconus (elongation of the corneal surface). Conjunctivitis is frequently a year-round complication of AD, but may also be seen in a seasonal distribution in association with allergic rhinitis in patients with aeroallergen hypersensitivity. Vernal conjunctivitis, characterized by a "cobblestone" pattern of papules on the inner eyelid, may be especially troublesome, requiring prompt treatment to prevent corneal abrasion. The association of AD and keratoconus is unexplained, yet of concern in approximately 1% of patients with AD. Corneal erosions may also be seen in patients with secondary herpetic infections that go undiagnosed and untreated.

Skin Conditions

Pityriasis alba and keratosis pilaris are two benign skin conditions that are commonly seen in patients with AD. Pityriasis alba is characterized by patchy areas of depigmentation of the skin, primarily occurring on the face and extensor surfaces of the extremities. Keratosis pilaris is a follicular hyperkeratosis characterized by fine papular lesions surrounded by dry skin that primarily occur on the buttocks and extensor surfaces of the upper arms and thighs. Both conditions may be seen in other skin disorders and in patients with otherwise normal skin. Their causes are unknown, but both remain only as benign nuisances.

TREATMENT

At present there are no known cures for AD, and current therapy is largely symptomatic. Certain therapeutic measures can be instituted that will dramatically reduce symptoms and control the overall skin condition (Table 4).

Table 4
Treatment for Atopic Dermatitis

Environmental control
    Climatic control
    Nonabrasive clothing and bedding (cotton)
    Minimization of emotional stress
    Avoidance of irritants
    Avoidance of aeroallergens

Dietary control
    Specific food allergen restriction

Skin care
    Minimize trauma
    Avoidance of harsh soaps/detergents
    Hydration
    Lubrication

Antipruritics
    Hydroxyzine
    Diphenhydramine
    Other nonsedating antihistamines

Corticosteroids
    Topical
        1% Hydrocortisone ointment to facial lesions
        Medium potency ointment to body lesions
    Systemic (rare use only)

Tar preparations

Antibiotics
    Antistaphylococcal/antistreptococcal
    Antifungal (rare use only)

Phototherapy

Immunomodulatory therapy

Environmental Control

Environmental control measures, in the form of minimizing both allergen exposure and pruritic stimuli, should be instituted in all patients with AD. Minimization of extreme fluctuations of temperature and humidity results in less pruritus. Sweating will induce pruritus in many patients with AD; therefore, a moderate temperature environment should be maintained. Clothing should be loose and free of wool. Cotton fabrics are generally the best tolerated. Coarse fabrics in clothing and bedding should be avoided. Complete rinsing of detergents, soaps and bleach from clothing and bedding will also minimize their irritant potential. Occupational aggravating agents such as chemicals, irritants and solvents should be avoided by older patients with AD. Minimization of emotional stress will also lessen the potential for pruritus.

Avoidance of known aeroallergens should be instituted when possible. The most easily avoided allergens are dust mites and animal danders. Dust mite–sensitive patients should institute full dust mite–avoidance procedures consisting of the following: plastic or hypoallergenic covers encasing mattresses and pillows, removal of all feather pillows and stuffed animals from the patient's room, frequent high-temperature washing of the bedding and removal of carpeting and draperies from the patient's room when practical. Animals (especially cats and dogs) should be removed from the home, and contact should be minimized. Practical avoidance of other aeroallergens (e.g., avoidance of cut grass) should be attempted.

Dietary Restriction

In patients with food hypersensitivity, food allergen avoidance results in improvement of AD. Sampson and coworkers have shown that following a strict avoidance diet of relevant food allergens patients experience symptomatic relief of pruritus and clearing of skin rash. Because of the high false-positive rate of prick skin testing and RAST for food allergens, an elimination diet followed by a blinded (single- or double-blind) or open food challenge should be performed to confirm clinical reactivity to a particular food, unless a convincing history of anaphylaxis is obtained. A possible exception to this rule may be applicable when an elevated CAP-RAST is obtained that demonstrates a greater than 90–95% likelihood that a patient will have a positive food challenge. The CAP-RAST can be applied only to milk, egg and peanut at this time. Extensive elimination diets should not be prescribed on the basis of skin test positivity alone because of the obvious nutritional complications. The period of dietary restriction is allergen dependent, but generally should last for 1–2 yr before reintroduction or rechallenge with the implicated food.

Skin Care

General measures to reduce skin trauma due to scratching should be instituted. Appropriate bedding and clothing can help minimize itching. In infants and children, gloves and socks can be used to reduce scratching, especially during sleep. Fingernails should be trimmed to minimize skin trauma from scratching.

Skin hydration is an extremely important measure in controlling the rash and pruritus associated with AD. Although some clinicians feel that frequent or routine bathing is contraindicated in AD, may others institute frequent bathing as part of the treatment protocol. Bathing hydrates the chronically dry skin of AD and may reduce the likelihood of bacterial superinfection, which will reduce pruritus and activation of lesions. In addition, swimming has long been recognized by patients with AD as soothing therapy. Patients should bathe in lukewarm water for 30 min once or twice a day (depending on the severity of disease). Burow's solution, oatmeal or oils (i.e., Alpha-Keri) may be added to the bath water to further reduce pruritus. Hydrating body wraps with water-soaked towels may be used in addition to bathing to maximize hydration of severely affected areas. Showers are inadequate in the management of AD because of the lack of hydration obtained. Mild soaps (i.e., Dove or Basis) should be used for cleansing. Harsh soaps may be drying and serve to increase pruritus.

Lubricants should be applied to the skin immediately following bathing and other times during the day with a minimal application of twice daily. Lubricants will counteract dryness and "seal in" the hydration obtained from the prolonged bathing experience. Lubricants should be free of alcohols and perfumes, both of which can be irritating and drying. Effective lubricants include Vaseline, Unibase (oil-in-water preparation), Eucerin or Aquaphor (water-in-oil preparations) plus others.

Antipruritics

Of major importance in the successful treatment of AD is interruption of the itch–scratch cycle. In addition to the methods mentioned previously, antihistamines and occasionally sedatives provide valuable relief of symptoms. Hydroxyzine (2 mg/kg/d divided every 6 h or given at bedtime; maximum adult dose 600 mg/d) and diphenhydramine (5 mg/kg/d divided every 6 h or given at bedtime; maximum adult dose 400 mg/day) have been shown to dramatically reduce itching and reduce sleep disturbance in patients with AD. Other nonsedating antihistamines (e.g., loratidine and cetirizine) may also be useful for daytime use to relieve pruritus when a sedating medication is prohibitive. In young children with severe disease, short-term sedation with chloral hydrate (50 mg/kg/d given at bedtime) may be needed until control of symptoms can be obtained. Topical application of doxepin cream also provides relief of pruritus, but poses a greater risk for side effects because of its systemic absorption. Doxepin should be used with close observation in all patients, especially children and patients with large skin surface areas affected.

Corticosteroids

Corticosteroids are used in AD to control inflammation. These preparations are very effective in controlling skin lesions of AD, but should be used wisely. There is little role for systemic corticosteroids in the management of AD except in the most severe cases. When used, oral corticosteroids should be prescribed for only a limited time and should be tapered judiciously. The skin disease will typically clear quickly with the use of oral corticosteroids, but frequently relapse once their use is discontinued. In addition, the side effects associated with use of systemic corticosteroids are well known and generally preclude their use.

Topical corticosteroid use in AD is the mainstay of therapy. The potency of topical steroids used is dependent on the severity of the skin disease and the location of skin lesions. In general, topical steroid potency is related to the vehicle and the chemical preparation. Gel preparations penetrate more effectively, but are drying and therefore not of great benefit in AD. Ointments penetrate well and enhance hydration, but feel occlusive and may be poorly tolerated during periods of high temperature (i.e., summer). Creams and lotions are less potent and penetrate less effectively than gels or ointments, but are more comfortable to some patients. Except in mild cases, ointments should be used because of their higher penetrance and potency. The lowest strength that gives adequate results should be used. Halogenated corticosteroid preparations, such as 0.1% betamethasone (Valisone), 0.025% fluocinolone (Synalar) and 0.1% or 0.025% triamcinolone (Aristocort, Kenalog) have potent anti-inflammatory properties and can be used sparingly on affected body lesions. These preparations should not be used on the face and neck. Hydrocortisone cream or ointment, 1%, can be used sparingly on the face and neck, but stronger preparations should be avoided. Topical steroids should be applied twice daily after application of lubricating creams or ointments as discussed. These preparations will penetrate the lubricant and reach the affected skin. Although generally safe from systemic absorption, diffuse application of topical steroids over long periods can have the adverse effects of striae, atrophic thinning of skin, ulcerations, hirsutism, acne, and telangectasia. In addition, cases of adrenal suppression secondary to use of topical steroids have been reported. Although these complications are rare with prolonged use of low-potency topical steroids, their use in children and adults with severe disease should be monitored.

Tar Preparations

Coal tar preparations have been used for many years in the management of AD. Although topical corticosteroids have generally replaced the routine use of these keratolytic agents, they are still effective in the management of chronic, lichenified skin lesions that respond poorly to corticosteroids. The mechanism by which coal tar preparations work is unknown, but clinical evidence has shown that they have both anti-inflammatory and antipruritic effects. These preparations are will tolerated, but prolonged use may lead to folliculitis and photosensitivity. Shampoos containing tars are especially useful in the patient with scalp involvement, i.e., as in both AD and seborrhea.

Antibiotics

As previously stressed, patients with AD have a high degree of bacterial colonization of both affected and unaffected skin. The risk and occurrence of bacterial superinfection of the AD skin is therefore high, most commonly with Staphylococcus aureus and streptococcal organisms. In addition, Leung and others have shown that some patients with AD produce specific IgE antibodies to various exotoxins produced from S. aureus. Because of these factors, antistaphylococcal and antistreptococcal antibiotics should be used liberally in the AD patient with documented or suspected bacterial superinfection. Skin cultures can be helpful in documenting the type of organism present and the antibiotic sensitivities of the organism. From a clinical standpoint, exudative, crusted or excoriated lesions should raise the clinical index of suspicion for secondary bacterial infection. Appropriate antibiotic therapy should be instituted for 10–14 d. In cases of limited distribution of infected skin lesions, topical antibiotic therapy with preparations such as Bactroban ointment may be adequate. For most cases, systemic antibiotics will be required to eradicate the infection. An increased skin care regimen with more frequent bathing may also help to reduce the bacterial load.

A few reports have addressed the issue of secondary infection caused by fungal infections, such as Pityrosporum ovale, in which investigators have advocated the use of topical agents such as Sebulex or Selsun shampoo, to fight fungal growth. Others have recommended the use of oral antifungal agents when fungal organisms are documented or highly suspected. Experience to date is relatively empiric and not well established.

Phototherapy

Ultraviolet light therapy with UV-A rays has been offered to some AD patients for control of lesions. Rajka has reported favorable results in a small series of AD patients when phototherapy was provided to eczematous skin lesions and maintenance therapy was sustained. This method of therapy has been proposed for the patient who is poorly responsive to conventional therapy or in whom severe AD is present. Rajka also notes that phototherapy may be beneficial in children with severe disease requiring systemic steroids to reduce the potential side effects of long-term corticosteroids. Most commonly, UV therapy must be given at least weekly and sustained over long periods to prevent relapse. This regimen raises the issue of adverse effects of long-term UV light exposure, such as induction of malignant disease and chronic skin changes. Most clinicians feel that the risk/benefit ratio is too high to encourage this form of therapy for the average AD patient. Phototherapy should therefore be reserved for the complicated case that is poorly responsive to other forms of therapy.

Immunotherapy

Although allergen immunotherapy has been useful in some atopic conditions (i.e., allergic rhinitis), its role in the treatment of AD has been limited. In clinical practice, immunotherapy will frequently exacerbate the condition of AD rather than provide relief. Some clinicians advocate the use of immunotherapy, especially in older patients with significant aeroallergen hypersensitivity, but recommend initiating therapy with a much smaller dilution of allergen extract than in standard therapy for allergic rhinitis. The dose of extract needed to induce tolerance is often greater than the dose tolerated by the patient with AD, thereby precluding its use in most patients.

Immunomodulatory Therapy

As previously discussed, AD is associated with abnormalities of the immune system, especially with regard to cytokine production and IgE regulation. In particular, many investigators have shown a predominance of TH_2-type lymphocytes, which produce excess amounts of IL-4 and therefore up-regulate IgE production. These patients are noted to have little IFN-γ production in comparison. Some of these same investigators have also shown that IFN-γ suppresses IgE production in vitro and has effects on immune effector cell function. Several immunomodulatory agents, including recombinant IFN-γ. cyclosporine A and tacrolimus (FK506) have been used in clinical trials of AD.

A recent, double-blind, placebo-controlled, multicenter trial was conducted to examine the effects of recombinant IFN-γ (rIFN-γg) administration to patients with chronic AD. Patients treated with IFN-γ had a significant reduction in symptoms and a mean reduction in circulating eosinophils when compared to the placebo-treated group. A previous trial of 23 patients also showed a significant fall in IgE synthesis in rIFN-γ treated patients. In another trial of 15 patients (adult and pediatric) treated for a minimum of 22 mo, patients had a significant reduction in mean body surface involvement of AD from 61.6% at baseline to 18.5% at 24 mo.

Topical tacrolimus (FK506), a potent immunosuppressant marketed to treat solid-organ transplant rejection, has been evaluated in clinical trials. Most recently, Boguniewicz and colleges reported their findings from a double-blind, controlled trial of tacrolimus treatment for 22 days in children ages 7–16 yr. The mean improvement from their three treatment groups (77%) was significantly better than in controls (26%) with no serious side effects noted. The authors concluded that tacrolimus was a safe, effective treatment for children with refractory AD when used in their short-term treatment protocol. Similar results were seen for both adult and pediatric patients in a recent study by Alaiti and colleagues.

Cyclosporine A, a potent T-cell suppressant, has been evaluated extensively in two recent clinical trials. In the first, 42 patients were treated for one or two 6-wk treatment periods and observed for 2 yr. A 58% reduction was noted in symptoms and AD scoring with 95% of follow-up cases still in remission after 2 years. In the second study, 100 adults with AD were treated for a maximum of 48 wk in an open trial. Most (65%) patients showed complete resolution or significant reduction in their symptoms and lesions, yet most reported relapse after cessation of therapy. Tolerability of cyclosporine therapy was rated good or very good in 85% of patients.

These studies provide examples of potential immunomodulatory therapy that will likely become of more importance as our understanding of the immunopathogenesis of AD expands. Further long-term evaluation of therapeutic efficacy and safety is needed, especially in pediatric populations. Other newer medications, such as phosphodiesterase inhibitors and leukotriene modifiers, may have clinical relevance for the treatment of AD in the future. Currently, information on these medications is limited to in vitro analysis and anecdotal reports.

Alternative Medical Therapy

As alternative therapeutic approaches to medical care have become more popular in the United States and other western countries, interest has developed regarding the application of some of these therapies for patients with AD. Chinese herbal therapy (CHT) has been evaluated in several trials, most of which are not population or placebo controlled. Xu and colleagues reported a reduction of inflammatory cells and markers (e.g., low-affinity IgE receptor [CD23], plus others) in 10 patients treated for 2 mo. These authors concluded that CHT is efficacious for patients with AD. Other case reports and small series using different CHT have drawn the same conclusions. Obviously, this form of therapy for AD needs to be evaluated by blinded, controlled trials in larger studies before it can be recommended for use. In addition, in some reports, CHT has been associated with significant adverse symptoms, such as cardiomyopathy, highlighting the fact that at this time CHT should not be used without caution and close observation.

Another alternative therapy, known as bioresonance or biophysical information therapy (BIT), has been reported as beneficial for AD in case reports and uncontrolled trials. To more rigorously test the efficacy of BIT for AD, Schoni observed 32 children with AD in a double-blind trial. Results showed no benefit of BIT in patients with AD compared to controls, leading the authors to dismiss the role of BIT as alternative therapy for AD.

Psychotherapy

AD is a very aggravating chronic disease that can be emotionally challenging for patients and families alike. Emotional distress and problems can trigger episodes of pruritus and worsen the AD. In addition, young patients and their families may have difficulty understanding and coping with this chronic condition and may need help to establish parameters for discipline without adding to the emotional tension of an already aggravated child. Older children and adolescents may also experience body image problems related to the obvious skin abnormalities. For all of these reasons, some patients and their families will benefit from social service support and/or psychological counseling to address these issues. This is particularly important in the patient with severe chronic disease.

PROGNOSIS

Currently there are no prospective, longitudinal studies evaluating the prognosis and disease remission of AD. Vickers retrospectively evaluated 2000 children with AD after 20 yr and noted an overall clearance rate of 84%. Vowles likewise evaluated 84 patients after 13 yr and found only 45% resolution of disease. These and other studies reflect the difficulty in assessing prognosis with reports of disease resolution ranging from 37 to 84% in various retrospective surveys. In addition, no specific disease factors are predictive of the disease severity or course. Some patients are noted to have spontaneous resolution of their disease during infancy and early childhood. Improvement may also be seen during puberty in some patients, but exacerbations noted in others. Cases in adults will often resolve or significantly improve after the second decade of life. As is common with atopic diseases, some cases of AD resolve, but patients develop other forms of atopy such as allergic rhinitis and asthma. Until a well-designed, prospective, longitudinal survey of AD is conducted, predictions of disease outcome will remain purely speculative and based on clinical experience. These factors reiterate the need for consistent long-term follow-up and management to best serve the needs of patients with AD.

SUGGESTED READING

Burks WA, James JM, Hiegel A, Wilson, G, Wheeler JG, Jones SM, et al. Atopic dermatitis and food hypersensitivity reactions. *J Pediatr* 1998;132:132–136.

Hanafin JM. Atopic dermatitis. *J Allergy Clin Immunol* 1984;73:211–222.

Hanafin, JM. Atopic dermatitis. In: Middleton, Reed, Ellis, Adkinson, Yunginger, Busse, eds. *Allergy: Principles and Practice*. St. Louis, Mosby–Yearbook, 1993, pp. 1581–1604.

Leung DYM. Immunopathology of atopic dermatitis. *Springer Semin Immunopathol* 1992;13:427–440.

Leung, DYM. Atopic dermatitis: Immunobiology and treatment with immune modulators. *Clin Exp Immunol* 1997;107(suppl 1):25–30.

Rajka, G. Essential Aspects of Atopic Dermatitis. Berlin, Springer-Verlag, 1989, pp. 1–261.

Sampson HA. Pathogenesis of atopic dermatitis. *Clin Exp Allergy* 1990;20:459–467.

Sampson HA. Food sensitivity and the pathogenesis of atopic dermatitis. *J R Soc Med* 1997;90(suppl 30):2–8.

14 Contact Dermatitis and Other Contact Reactions

Jere D. Guin, MD

CONTENTS

WHAT IS CONTACT DERMATITIS?

Contact dermatitis typically is an eczematous reaction, usually to a substance applied to the skin surface. It may have an allergic cause, or it may be irritant (nonallergic). The archetype of the allergic form is poison ivy dermatitis, while soap dermatitis is a typical example of irritant contact dermatitis. Of course, there are many forms of allergic contact dermatitis that differ prominently from poison ivy reactions, and irritant dermatitis is extremely diverse in cause and often in presentation. Both irritant and allergic contact dermatitis are very common. They often complicate other forms of eczema, which can be confusing to the inexperienced. However, recognition is critical to success in managing such patients.

From: *Current Clinical Practice: Allergic Diseases: Diagnosis and Treatment, 2nd Edition*
Edited by: P. Lieberman and J. Anderson © Humana Press Inc., Totowa, NJ

Key Features of Contact Dermatitis

- Contact dermatitis can be immune- or irritant-induced.
- Contact dermatitis is recognized in great part by its distribution.
- An eczema that fails to heal should suggest contact dermatitis.
- The appearance of contact dermatitis can range from a weeping, oozing lesion in the acute phase, to a thickened, lichenified rash in its chronic stages.
- Patch testing is the test of choice to identify the offending agent.
- Avoidance is the treatment of choice.

Irritant reactions are caused by (nonimmune) damage to cells in the epidermis from a variety of stimuli ranging from physical agents, such as friction, cold and sunburn, to chemical reagents, such as acids, bases, organic solvents and so on. The subject is quite complex, as the specific injury varies, and individuals may be exposed to multiple irritants in many occupations as well as at home. Fundamentally, agents that cause contact dermatitis on a basis other than allergy are by definition irritants. In occupationally induced contact dermatitis, irritant reactions account for about 70% of the total.

Allergic contact dermatitis is a delayed hypersensitivity response mediated by T-cells, with Langerhans' cells as the characteristic presenting cells. The number of cytokines and cell types involved in regulation of the response is beyond the scope of this chapter. For a more detailed explanation see Chapter 1.

Other "contact" reactions include allergic and nonimmunological contact urticaria, photoallergic and phototoxic dermatitis, protein contact dermatitis and systemic contact dermatitis, including some id reactions and some cases of dyshidrotic eczema.

Photoallergic dermatitis is essentially an allergic contact dermatitis in which the antigen must be activated by light, while phototoxic reactions are equivalent to light-induced irritant dermatitis. The former tends to be eczematous, whereas the latter frequently resembles a severe sunburn. Both are located in sun-exposed sites.

Contact urticaria may be either allergic (IgE mediated), or nonimmunological, in which a wheal occurs through inflammation without allergy. An example of the former is hives appearing on the hands of a chef allergic to shrimp, following the peeling of shrimp. An example of the latter is the erythema and swelling seen after local exposure to dimethyl sulfoxide or Trafuril.

HOW DOES ONE RECOGNIZE CONTACT DERMATITIS?

1. The first prerequisite for recognizing contact dermatitis is to suspect it. One should always consider the possibility of a contact reaction in anyone with an eczema. Even noneczematous conditions may have a contact reaction superimposed upon the pre-existing condition.
2. The eruption is typically eczematous, and as such it will normally show spongiosis histologically. Acute lesions demonstrate weeping, oozing, crusting and scaling, and chronic lesions tend to show thickening, hyperkeratosis, lichenification and scratch papules.

3. The pattern is man made. A good example is glove dermatitis (Fig. 1). Here one usually sees an eczema involving the palms and dorsum of the hands with a sharp cutoff above the level where the gloves are worn. Another suggestive picture is ear-lobe dermatitis (Fig. 2), in which the ears have been pierced and a weeping, oozing, crusting and itching eruption surrounds the puncture site.

4. A recognizable pattern may be present. This is often learned by experience, but almost all physicians in the United States recognize poison ivy dermatitis (Figs. 3–5) with its characteristic streaks caused by finger strokes and hand prints. Insole dermatitis to shoes (Fig. 6) characteristically involves contact sites on the plantar surface with sparing of the longitudinal arch and proximal toes and accentuation of pressure sites, such as over the metatarsal heads and the tips of the toes. In one case, the allergen is transferred from the hands, and in the other the eruption is seen where the causative object touches the skin (Fig. 7). One must be careful, however, in trying to identify a cause by pattern alone, as experts are often fooled. Therefore, patch testing is used for confirmation.

5. Eczema that fails to heal with treatment should make one suspect contact dermatitis. Those of us who subspecialize in contact dermatitis see this regularly. Sometimes the original problem is no longer present, and the patient proves to be allergic to a cosmetic lotion or topical medication that he or she applied to soothe the original dermatitis (Figs. 8 and 9). Sometimes a typical medication pattern is seen with eczema spreading around lesions from the applied substance, with fewer lesions at the periphery where less has been applied. In some cases of milder sensitivity, and especially corticosteroid allergy, one may see the original condition unchanged, but refusing to heal.

6. There is often a previous history of contact allergy or irritation. For example, one might look for contact dermatitis to an aminoglycoside in a nurse with previous allergy to neomycin.

7. A known allergy, irritation or predisposing condition is present. Atopics of all types typically are susceptible to certain irritants, e.g., soaps or propylene glycol. Persons with stasis dermatitis and chronic allergic contact dermatitis often develop sensitivity to agents used on the eruption.

8. There is often a history of the use of multiple agents, either prescribed or OTC. This is especially true in stasis dermatitis.

9. There may be a history of high-risk exposure, which is often associated with occupation or avocation. Hospital aides commonly develop irritant dermatitis from bathing patients, shampooing patients' hair, from scrubbing rooms, and so on. Dishwashers commonly develop irritant hand eczema. Construction workers are more likely to develop chromate allergy from exposure to cement and mortar. In some occupations, exposure is a complex mixture of irritation and allergy, not only to substances found on the job, but also to materials used for treatment and putative protection. For example, beauticians develop irritant dermatitis from shampoo and allergic contact dermatitis from glyceryl monothioglycolate in acid perms and p-phenlyenediamine in hair dye. They then commonly become allergic to the gloves used to try to protect their hands so they can continue to work!

HOW DOES ONE SEPARATE IRRITANT
FROM ALLERGIC CONTACT DERMATITIS?

This can be a very sticky, yet practical problem. There are no absolute rules, so one must use the weight of the evidence. Some helpful criteria are found in Table 1.

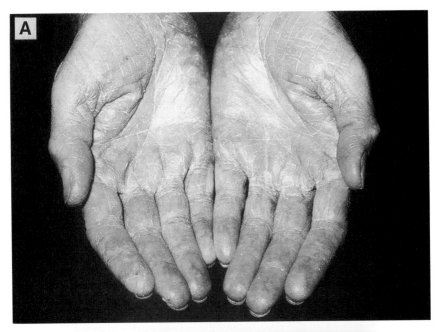

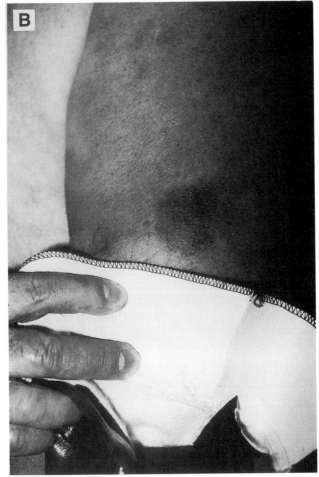

Fig. 1. (A) Glove dermatitis from rubberized work gloves. **(B)** Positive patch test to a piece of the glove.

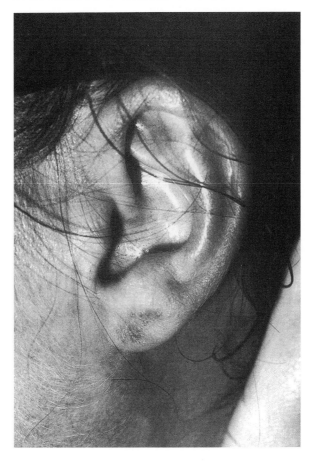

Fig. 2. Ear lobe dermatitis in a nickel-sensitive individual. The nickel spot test is helpful here as it allows the patient to test jewelry for free nickel before it is worn.

Irritant reactions tend to occur often within minutes, burn rather than itch and heal rapidly on avoidance. Irritant patch test responses typically are evident within a few minutes, although they may be cumulative or even delayed. They are often somewhat dose related, disappearing on dilution. They are often sharply marginated, and they occur on first exposure so that prior sensitization is unnecessary. Irritant reactions from soap, detergents and solvents are often shiny, dry and fissured.

Allergic contact dermatitis tends to itch more reliably than irritant dermatitis (but there are exceptions); the reaction may spread for days after the allergen has been removed; it is also less dose related; it occurs in susceptible persons (not everyone breaks out to even poison ivy); and it requires prior sensitization, Allergic contact dermatitis typically appears after 36–48 h, but can be earlier with strong allergy or in sites where absorption is rapid, e.g., the face.

Putative histological differences, and even sophisticated cytokine studies, have recently been questioned, so it may be difficult to separate irritant and allergic contact responses histologically. Patch testing may uncover unsuspected allergy in someone who seems to have an irritant dermatitis. Negative patch test results (sometimes wrongly) suggest an irritant cause. Reactions suggesting an irritant cause can be confirmed by serial dilution, since irritation more often disappears sharply with

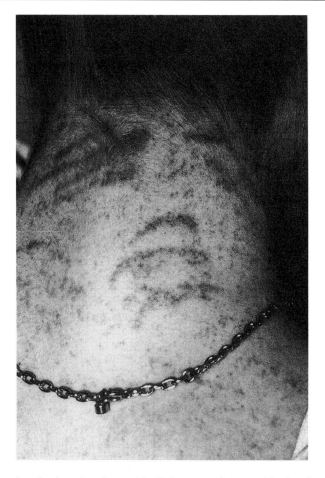

Fig. 3. Classic streaks of poison ivy dermatitis. This pattern is caused by hand transfer of a strong antigen.

decreased concentration. Some persons have both irritant and allergic contact dermatitis at the same time. Sensitization commonly occurs from irritants, and many allergens, e.g., poison ivy, are both irritant and allergic. Furthermore, the already tender skin from either cause is more susceptible to the other as a secondary event. *It is wise to have persons with irritant dermatitis avoid known allergens and those with allergic contact dermatitis avoid irritants.*

HOW CAN ONE SEPARATE CONTACT DERMATITIS FROM OTHER DERMATOSES IN DIFFERENT ANATOMICAL SITES?

Contact dermatitis can mimic many other skin conditions. A reasonable listing that can be used in differentiation is given in Table 2. The differential diagnosis in certain regions, especially the hands, deserves a bit more explanation.

The Hands

Hand eczema is a very special problem because the patient commonly has more than one cause for the eruption. Contact dermatitis of the hands is often irritant with

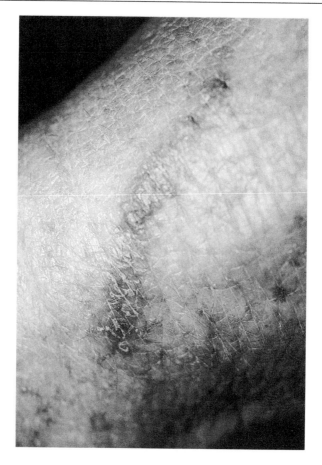

Fig. 4. Streak of poison ivy dermatitis.

dry scaly patches, which in some atopics are converted to a discoid eczema. Dermatitis under a ring is usually an irritation from soap. Occupational factors are important, since persons handling raw meat (slaughterhouse, chicken processing and fishery workers, butchers and chefs, for example), those engaged in wet work and mothers with small children are particularly vulnerable. Another often unsuspected cause is in mechanics, machine repairmen, and so forth, who try to remove insoluble metal dust, carbon and rubber dust with soap and abrasives, irritating the skin in the process. Often a nonsensitizing cream will remove such materials without irritation. Allergic contact dermatitis is covered in the (next) section on regional contact dermatitis.

Persons with a nummular or discoid pattern (Fig. 10) are often atopic individuals. Sometimes women who had atopic eczema as children but who have enjoyed a prolonged remission, break out anew from the stress of wet work and irritant exposure with the rearing of children.

Dyshidrotic eczema, or pompholyx (Fig. 11), is identified morphologically by its deep-seated single vesicles (at least initially) and the tendency for the vesicular eruption to form an apron pattern. It is commonly a dermatophytid, but systemic contact dermatitis, stasis eczema with id, infectious eczematoid dermatitis, nummular

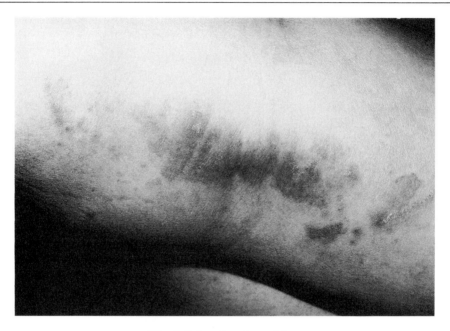

Fig. 5. Poison ivy dermatitis.

eczema and other causes can often be found if one looks carefully. Some cases are, however, idiopathic.

Hyperkeratotic hand eczema may occur from contact dermatitis. When it does, it is often difficult to know whether one is faced with a single or more than one condition. Perhaps the main things to rule out are certain skin diseases that characteristically occur in areas of trauma. This is often called the Koebner phenomenon in psoriasis, lichen planus, and the like. On the fingers and palms, psoriasis is often misdiagnosed as eczema because it is located in areas of contact such as the thumb and index and middle fingers, along with frictional areas of the palms. Psoriasis in this location usually does not itch, it fissures in winter, and it is usually associated with other findings characteristic of psoriasis such as pitting of the fingernails, onycholysis and lesions of the elbows, knees and scalp (especially in the nuchal area) and in the intergluteal fold. A positive family history should make one suspicious, but it is often negative. Lichen planus can also be located on the hands. Lesions of that disease elsewhere are usually more typical in morphology, and unlike most cases of psoriasis, a biopsy can be helpful. Certain drugs are often aggravating factors in psoriasis and lichen planus and may be the cause of the latter.

Lesions on the hands (and feet) can also be caused by infectious and parasitic conditions, including dermatophytosis, scabies and herpes simplex, which can all on occasion mimic contact reactions. The morphology and distribution help, and a KOH, Tzanck test and/or culture will confirm the diagnosis.

On the hands, allergic contact dermatitis is suspected especially when the grip and frictional areas of the palms are involved, but patch testing can be justified in most patients with hand eczema, as it helps establish the cause. A glove-like pattern is a giveaway for glove dermatitis. This is usually due to rubber, but it can also occur from leather and other materials. Occupational patterns (Fig. 12) are often seen in the grip

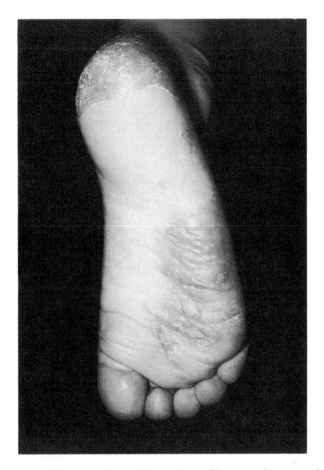

Fig. 6. Six-year-old girl with contact dermatitis to shoes. She reacted to potassium dichromate on patch testing, suggesting leather as a source.

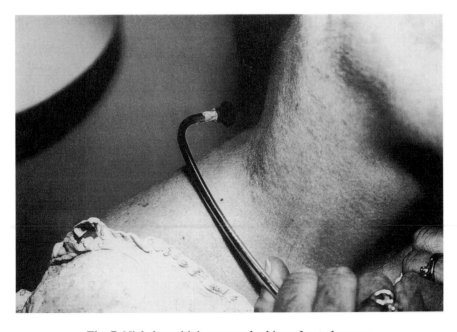

Fig. 7. Nickel sensitivity to metal tubing of a stethoscope.

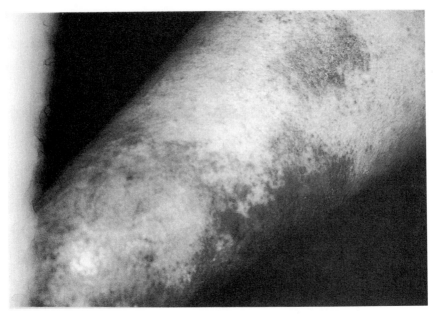

Fig. 8. Eczema that seems to spread where an ointment or lotion is applied suggests sensitivity to a medication. Patch testing was positive to neomycin, which was a component of the cream the patient had applied.

areas of the fingertips in florists and are due to Alstroemeria, in chefs due to garlic, in hairdressers due to glyceryl monothioglycolate in acid perms, and in industrial workers due to epoxy and other adhesives, to name a few. Sometimes a pattern can suggest a source, as with liquid soaps, which cause an eczema of the finger webs extending onto the palm at the base of the middle and adjacent fingers. Sometimes the contact dermatitis alters the appearance of the original condition, such as the fingertip eruption one sees from shampoo (which may be irritant or allergic) or the spreading eczema that occurs from reactions to medications. A diffuse dermatitis of the dorsum, sparing protected areas may be light induced. Remember, however, even typical presentations require patch-test confirmation.

Flexural Areas

In intertriginous areas, contact reactions are often from topically applied agents. Inframammary eruptions can be from the bra, especially from metals or rubber chemicals. In the hairy part of the axilla, deodorant ingredients must be ruled out, whereas in the periaxillary area clothing dermatitis may be present. In the differential diagnosis, various causes of intertrigo may be confusing, including candidiasis, seborrheic dermatitis, seborrheic psoriasis, tinea and Gram-negative superinfections, Hailey-Hailey disease is a familial condition inherited as an autosomal dominant, located usually on the neck, axillae or groin. Here a biopsy will make the diagnosis; the family history is often positive.

Elbows and Knees

Over the elbows, rubber dermatitis, topically applied lotions, OTC and prescribed medications, and clothing should be suspected. One must, of course, consider anything

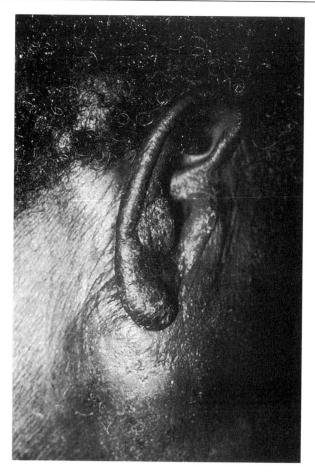

Fig. 9. Depigmentation following a reaction to ear drops containing neomycin. This patient was allergic to multiple aminoglycosides but not to streptomycin, which lacks the 2-deoxystreptamine ring.

on which the patient might lean. I have seen nickel-induced eczema in this location from metal contact. Even poison ivy–like dermatitis has occurred from furniture lacquered with varnish from the Japanese lacquer tree, a relative of poison ivy. In the differential diagnosis, psoriasis, dermatitis herpetiformis, frictional lichenoid eruption (in children), Gianotti-Crosti syndrome and papulovesicular acrodermatitis syndrome should come to mind, among other things. Systemic contact dermatitis and id reactions may also appear here.

Scalp

The scalp usually is not prominently involved even when hair-care products cause allergic contact dermatitis, since the hair is protective. What one usually sees is scalp involvement together with other areas. Shampoos commonly cause involvement in a rinse-off distribution anterior to and behind the ears, sometimes on the adjacent neck and forehead, and in persons who shampoo their own hair, the fingertips may be involved. Hair dye reactions cause severe involvement of the adjacent neck posteriorly,

Table 1
Differentiating Allergic and Irritant Contact Dermatitis[a]

	Allergic	Irritant
Appearance	Redness, vesicles, papules, oozing, crusting, lichenification	Redness, chapping, scaling, fissures, pustules
Population involved	Sensitive individuals (only one person at this job)	Anyone with adequate dosage (many doing the same job)
Onset following exposure	Varies with location (usually days)	Minutes to hours, but may be cumulative
Require for previous exposure	Yes	No
Dose dependency	Less	More Dilution tends to abolish the reaction
Typical symptoms	Itching	Burning, pain
Localization of patch test response	May spread beyond application site after removal of chamber	Often sharply marginated, limited to occluded area
Patch test, relevance	Positive and relevant	Negative or positive and not relevant

[a]Irritant and allergic reactions often coexist and can be difficult to reliably separate clinically or histologically. The criteria given are commonly used in evaluating patch test responses, but they are not absolute.

the ears superiorly and especially the forehead. Beauticians break out on the hands. Allergy to acid perms may cause a similar eruption in the near term and a chronic pattern where the hair touches, as the allergen is retained in the hair. One also should think of dermatitis herpetiformis in the scalp as well as follicular lichen planus, seborrheic dermatitis, seborrheic psoriasis, some types of folliculitis, and pityriasis rubra pilaris. Eruptions limited to the hairy scalp are seldom allergic contact dermatitis.

Eyelids

Allergic contact dermatitis on the eyelids may occur from nail polish, medications used in the eyes or on the lids, contact lens solution, makeups and the brush or applicator used to apply them, mascara, eyelash curlers, plants, and hand transfer, especially from black rubber, nickel, and so forth. Plant allergens may involve the eyelids, whereas photodermatitis, which can look similar, typically spares that location. In the differentiation, one must consider atopic dermatitis, seborrheic dermatitis, psoriasis, rosacea, neurodermatitis, irritant dermatitis, irritation from respiratory allergy, bacterial, herpetic and fungal infection, and even dermatomyositis.

Lips and Perioral Skin

Contact dermatitis of the lips includes lipstick dermatitis, caused by any of several ingredients, topical and dental medications, objects habitually chewed, e.g., metal

Table 2
Differential Diagnosis of Contact Dermatitis

Other Eczemas	Other Dermatoses
Atopic eczema	Cutaneous T-cell lymphoma
Nummular eczema	Psoriasis
Stasis eczema	Seborrheic dermatitis
Dyshidrotic eczema (pompholyx)	Zinc nutritional and vitamin deficiency
Asteatoic eczema	Glucagonoma syndrome
Infectious eczematoid dermatitis	Tinea
Lichen simplex chronicus	Candidiasis
ID reactions	Scabies
Juvenile plantar dermatosis	Herpes simplex
Frictional lichenoid eruption	Lichen planus
	Dermatitis herpetiformis
	Some bullous dermatoses, (Hailey-Hailey, pemphigus, etc)
	Disorders of cornification, etc
	Graft vs host reactions
	Immunodeficiency disease (Wiskott-Aldrich syndrome, etc)
	Phenylketonuria
	Drug reactions
	Syphilis
	Actinic prurigo, Polymorphic light eruption, noncontact phototoxicity
	Papular urticaria
	L.E., dermatomyositis, etc
	AIDS - related dermatosis

or plastic in pens and pencils or rubber in pencil erasers, musical instruments, e.g., reeds or wooden instruments, e.g., recorders or flutes, flavors, or dental braces (which can also be a source of irritation directly or from drooling). Other conditions to be considered include candidal cheilitis, cheilitis glandularis, cheilitis granulomatosia, lichen planus, lupus erythemtosus and actinic cheilitis, to name a few.

In the periorificial locations, contact dermatitis can occur from flavors and other ingredients of orally administered agents, e.g., toothpaste dermatitis at the commisure, hand transfer of black rubber chemicals and metal allergens, e.g., nickel and cobalt, medications used on self and others, and following a visit to the doctor or dentist, rubber dermatitis from the gloves or rubber dam used. One should also think of zinc and vitamin deficiencies as well as glucagonoma. Around the mouth one can also see an irritant reaction to chronic licking, and lichen planus can localize here.

Face

On the face one sees cosmetic sensitivity typically, and this may be irritant as well as allergic. However, there are many other causes. Hand transfer occurs from poison ivy and Compositae (weed) allergens as well as nail polish. Other materials contacted include sources of phototoxic and photoallergic dermatitis, sunscreens, contact with

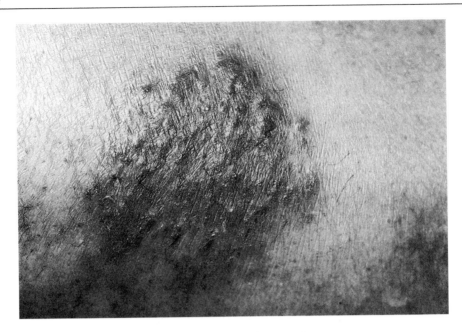

Fig. 10. Coin-shaped plaque of nummular eczema.

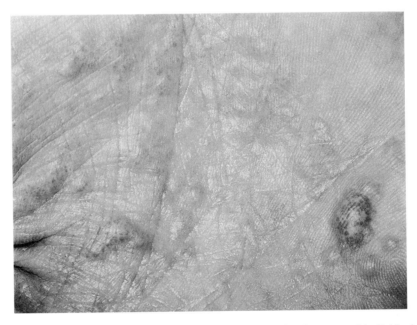

Fig. 11. Dyshidrotic eczema or pompholyx of the palm. Note the deep-seated individual vesicles suggesting an endogenous eczema.

a pillow or a child's favorite doll and, of course, the ubiquitous therapeutic agents including not only those prescribed, but also the long list of lotions and home remedies so often applied. The list is actually too long to include everything, so one should be circumspect.

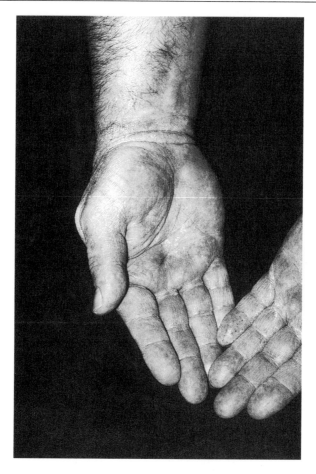

Fig. 12. Hand eczema in a factory worker handling carpet. Reactions on patch testing were from rubber chemicals. The source proved to be rubber backing on the carpet.

Trunk

On the trunk, clothing dermatitis is often the first thing considered, especially when the eruption is located around the axillae and is worse over the lower rib cage . Causes of clothing dermatitis include not only formaldehyde–releasing fabric finishes, but disperse dyes, detergents left in clothing (both irritant and allergic), medications used that contaminate clothing, metal snaps and supports, elastic fibers, and even epoxy used to cement pads or to mark labels. Waistband eruptions may be from detergents or from latex allergens or an antigen in bleached underwear, dibenzyl carbamyl chloride. Other dermatoses found on the trunk include most papulosquamous diseases and cutaneous T-cell lymphoma. Drug eruptions and systemic contact dermatitis can also be a problem here.

Feet

The feet typically break out to shoes and topically applied materials. The most common pattern of shoe dermatitis is insole dermatitis from either rubber chemicals or adhesive allergens in sponge rubber insoles of athletic shoes. This characteristically

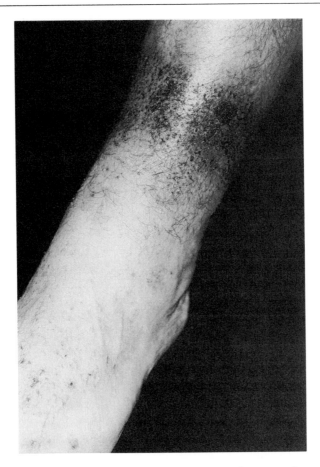

Fig. 13. Allergic reaction to diethylthiourea in a wet suit.

involves the plantar surface except for the proximal toes and the longitudinal arch. The pattern in shoe dermatitis depends upon the cause and the points of contact so one sees a different pattern with leather (chromate) sensitivity and rubber allergy other than the insoles. Differentiation includes dyshidrotic eczema, atopic dermatitis, id reactions, tinea, psoriasis, lichen planus, cutaneous T-cell lymphoma and palmoplantar pustulosis, among other things.

Lower Extremities

On the legs and thighs, contact dermatitis may be from nickel or phosphorus sesquisulfide in matches, rubber or dyes in stockings, detergents, fabric finishes and clothing (Fig. 13); even reactions from epoxy in knee pads have been reported. The differential diagnosis includes nummular, atopic and stasis eczema (Fig. 14), poison ivy dermatitis (Figs. 3–5), contact from medications (Figs. 8,9), other eczemas and many other dermatological diseases.

EXFOLIATIVE DERMATITIS

Exfoliative erythroderma may be caused by contact and other eczemas (especially atopic dermatitis). However, it may also be caused by malignant disease (especially

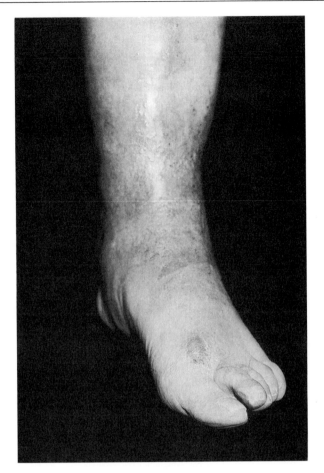

Fig. 14. Stasis dermatitis is often complicated by allergic contact dermatitis to substances applied for treatment or symptomatic relief. This patient was allergic to an OTC lotion.

cutaneous T-cell lymphoma), psoriasis, seborrheic dermatitis (especially in infants), pityriasis rubra pilaris, several different congenital ichthyoses, drug eruptions, pemphigus foliaceous, pemphigoid, scabies and other things. Here, a wise generalist will seek consultation early.

SPECIAL FORMS OF ECZEMA AND CONTACT REACTIONS: *PROTEIN CONTACT DERMATITIS*

In 1976, a group of Danish investigators described eczematous reactions to foods in food service workers, with irregular results on patch testing but positive immediate sensitivity. Not all of these individuals were atopic according to the report. These reactions appear as early as 30 min, which is much earlier than ordinary contact dermatitis. The first report found most reactions to food were to meats, but a few were to vegetables. The published antigens causing protein contact dermatitis have been divided into (1) fruits, vegetables, spices, plants; (2) animal proteins; (3) grains; and (4) enzymes. Atopic eczema patients commonly are sensitive to house dust and some health care workers are sensitive to latex or glove powder. Such sensitivity is picked up with testing for immediate sensitivity. Several methods have been reported, including prick testing, RAST testing, rubber testing, scratch testing and scratch chamber testing. Patch testing may or may not be positive. Persons with protein contact dermatitis may may or may not have contact urticaria.

Patch Testing

The most important confirmatory test in allergic contact dermatitis (and in establishing a diagnosis of irritant dermatitis) is the patch test. Here one attempts to prove the presence of allergy by reproducing the disease in a controlled situation. Usually standard commercial allergens (Table 3) are used for screening examinations. There are two commercially available sources of patch test materials in the United States. One set available from Chemotechnique or Trolab, as the European Standard Series, contains 24 allergens (Table 3). The other series marketed as the TRUE test contains 24 ready-to-use allergens (Table 3). Both series contain single allergens as well as mixtures. The TRUE test can be applied by removing the cover on each set of 12. These are marked by number with the antigens loaded.

Patch testing is done on clear skin on the upper back. Otherwise aluminum (Finn) or polypropylene chambers on Scanpor tape are usually used to hold the antigens. These are packaged 10/strip with two rows of five. One should mark the first of these with numbers 1–5 and 6–10 along the left and right rows, and the second set of ten chambers is marked 11–15 and 16–20, prior to removing the cover to load the chambers. The reason for this is that when the cover is removed and the strip is placed on the table for loading, the chambers can easily be turned around. If chambers are not marked, one could easily load the strips backward or even apply them upside down.

The chambers in the TRUE test are already loaded. The European standard tests are loaded from syringes into the aluminum or polypropylene chambers. Chambers are filled about half to two-thirds full, with liquids loaded last. To hold liquids, one must use a cellulose pad inside the chamber. A dab of petrolatum applied to the chamber prior to adding the cellulose pad will prevent the pad's falling out. Strips are applied with a rolling motion, from below upward, to the upper back while the patient is in a slightly flexed position. The external (upper) arm is an acceptable alternate site, but the forearm is not. The site is marked with a fluorescent highlighter by outlining the paper tape strip and marking each chamber's position on both sides as well as top and bottom. Then the second strip is applied. Remember, the liquids are not loaded until everything else is ready. Chambers are left on for 48 h and read at 72 h, and once more 1–4 d later. Accurate records, including a diagram, are kept detailing the substances applied, the location of each, the date of application and the vehicle and concentration used. Since much of this is routine, printed forms can be made up in advance. It helps to include a drawing of the back or the site of application to help identify responses when marks are difficult to locate. It does little good to find a reaction without knowing what caused it.

An important step for those new to the procedure is learning the discipline of reading the tests. This often requires experience. Standard criteria for scoring reactions are as follows: +/– reactions show erythema only; 1+ reactions are erythematous, and sometimes raised slightly or with a few papules but not vesicular; 2+ reactions are vesicular; 3+ reactions are bullous and often irritant.

Table 3
Sources of Standard Contact Allergens

Compound	Tests available	Description
Benzocaine, (caine mix)	E, T	Local anesthetic, OTC preparations, crossreacts with procaine, PABA sunscreen, sulfa, etc.
2-MBT	E, T	Rubber accelerator
Colophony	E, T	Rosin in pine and other conifers. Solder flux, tape, mascara, topical and dental medications, varnishes, putty, paint, pine products, etc. May indicate allergy to fragrance, flavor, chrysanthemum
p-Phenylenediamine	T	Permanent hair dyes, may crossreact with black rubber (some), color film developer, sulfa, PABA sunscreens, the benzocaine group and some epoxy hardeners.
Imidazolidinyl urea		Preservative found in a variety of cosmetic products
Cinnamic aldehyde		Fragrance and flavor ingredient. Cinnamon
Wool alcohols	T	Sensitizing component in lanolin. Found in many cosmetic products and lotions. Found in other materials from veterinary products to furniture polish. Will not detect all lanolin reactors, so some add Amerchol 101.
Carba mix	T	Accelerator in rubber products. Also found in agricultural chemicals, slimicides, etc.
Neomycin sulfate	E, T	Topical antibiotic. Often crossreacts with other aminoglycosides. Coreacts with bacitracin.
Thiuram mix	E, T	Rubber accelerator, especially in latex gloves. Closely related to carba mix chemicals. Rubber products, agricultural chemicals, animal repellents.
Formaldehyde	E, T	In wrinkle-free fabric finishes, cosmetics, shampoo, biocides, paper, plywood and many other products. Released by many preservatives.
Ethylenediamine	T	In one topical steroid-nystatin generic. May crossreact with Merthiolate, aminophylline, hydroxyzine
Epoxy	E, T	Resin used in many epoxy adhesives, paints, electrical dielectrics (insulation).
Quaternium-15	E, T	Cosmetic preservative. Releases formaldehyde. In many liquid soaps, shampoos and other wet products.
p-tert-Butylphenol formaldehyde resin	E, T	Adhesive in shoes, fiberglass, wood, etc.
Mercapto mix	E, T	Rubber accelerator related to 2-MBT.
(IPPD) Black rubber mix	E, T	Antioxidant in (esp. outdoor) rubber.
Potassium dichromate	E, T	Cement, mortar, leather, inks, paints.
Balsam of Peru	E, T	Used in US to detect fragrance allergy. Crossreacts with citrus peel, vanilla, eugenol, colas, flavored beverages.
Nickel sulfate	E, T	In steel, jewelry, many metal objects. Said not to be available from stainless.
Methyl(chloro) isothiazolinone	E, T	Preservative in wet products, coolant, shampoo, creams, lotions, air conditioners, etc.
Fragrance mix	E, T	Mixture of eight perfume chemicals used as screen for fragrance and flavor sensitivity. Found as flavors in foods and medications, as perfumes in personal care products from cosmetics, shampoo and soap to toilet tissue, laundry and household products.
Cobalt	E. T	Ingredient in metal products, jewelry. Commonly coreacts with nickel.
Clioquinol	E	Less frequent reactor. Contains iodo chlorhydroxyquin or clioquinol (in Vioform) and chlorquinaldol. May also be in veterinary products
Paraben mix	E, T	Preservatives in cosmetics, medications, foods and industrial products
Primin	E	Active ingredient in *Primula obconica,* German primrose
Sesquiterpene lactone mix	E	Screen for Compositae dermatitis
Thimerosal	T	Preservative in contact lens solutions, eye drops, allergy injections, immunization reagents, tincture of Merthiolate; may predict piroxicam photoreaction. Many true positives not relevant.
Control	T	Negative control

E, European series; T, TRUE.

Table 4
Potential Causes of False Positive and False Negative Reactions
to Patch Testing for Contact Dermatitis

False-Positive Reactions	False Negative Reactions
Nonspecific (irritant) responses	Technical Failure
Inappropriate solvents, acids, alkalis, etc.	Separation of patch from skin (inadequate
Irritant interaction of aluminum	occlusion time)
chamber with metal antigens	Loss of occlusion
Nonspecific pustular responses to metals	Time of reading (too early or too late)
Concentration, evaporation of liquid,	Material not fresh
edge effect	Improper marking
Unknown materials	Only one reading done (*see* text, this page)
Contamination	Failure to employ light in photodermatitis
Concentration errors	reactions
An "angry" back (skin responds	Patient taking systemic corticosteroids
nonspecifically to multiple stimuli)	or applying topical corticosteroids at site
Mislabeling	of application
Misreading	Inadequate penetration
Allergy to test apparatus (tape, chambers, etc)	Wrong site used to apply patch
Color left by colored allergens	Test applied to hairy skin
Phototoxic reactions	Inadequate dose of allergen
	Time of application too brief

Potential causes of false-positive and false-negative readings are given in Table 4. Once significant (2+ or nonirritant 3+) reactions are found, the relevance must be assessed by comparing the reaction with the probabilities of exposure. The patient should be provided detailed instruction on how to identify sources of that antigen or those antigens. Printed handouts in the patient's language can be found in Guin, 1995.

HOW DOES ONE MANAGE A PATIENT WITH SUSPECTED CONTACT DERMATITIS?

The principal rules for complex cases of suspected contact dermatitis involve the following procedure:

1. Remove the patient from all possible contact sources in the involved area. Of course, in some situations, e.g., clothing dermatitis, one cannot go without clothing. However, all white, polyester textiles are seldom a problem, and such materials are a good substitute. Many women are reluctant to omit wearing makeup, but they are much more receptive when shown the potential for developing additional allergy (meaning they will have difficulty eventually finding products they will tolerate) if not removed from a source of allergic contact dermatitis.
2. Patch test the patient to lotions he or she has applied and to cosmetic materials used on the site, provided they are known to be nonirritant. One can usually test to a moisturizer lotion by placing it in an aluminum patch-test chamber using the cellulose pad. One should not test to mascara, cleansing cream, soap, shampoo, and so on, as these are irritant. A cavalier willingness to apply unknown and often irritant materials, especially from work, can result in deep ulcers and scarring and can even sensitize the patient.

3. Avoid all products giving a positive test and all products possibly containing a chemical giving a positive test.
4. Reinstitute products giving a negative test, one at a time.
5. Treat with a steroid in petrolatum (only) and test to this to be sure it is tolerated. Hydrocortisone has to be tested as an intradermal (Solu-Cortef 1 mg/0.05–0.1 ml) and read at 72 h. Any erythema at that time is suspect; most can be confirmed with a usage test to one area.

    Application to the face should be done without touching the area with the hands. A vinyl glove or a finger wrapped in Saran wrap can be used to apply the steroid ointment. This avoids hand transfer.
6. Finally, the solution to managing allergic contact dermatitis is to avoid contact with all offending agents. In addition, and especially for hand eczema, the patient must be taught how to perform normal daily functions without irritation, as the inflamed skin is *very* easily irritated, which will prolong the time to recovery.

Making It Work

The most important aspect of the management of chronic contact dermatitis is the identification of the causative agent. Subsequent to the identification, of course, the treatment is avoidance. Patients with chronic contact dermatitis obviously should not be treated with long-term systemic corticosteroids, and continuous use of potent topical glucocorticoids also can be followed by complications. Avoidance, however, makes treatment unnecessary, unless another cause is present.

For acute contact dermatitis, such as poison ivy dermatitis, patients who do not have a contraindication can be treated with short courses of oral corticosteroids. For example, prednisone given in an initial dose of 60 mg. daily, and tapered over a 10–14 d period, is sufficient to suppress symptoms in most cases. One should avoid potential sensitizers to prevent developing new allergies (the extended allergen syndrome). Calamine lotion (not Caladryl) and tap water compresses are relatively safe. Midpotency (or at least less than category 1) topical steroids are sometimes used under occlusion for a 24-h wrap, and this can be combined with systemic treatment in severe cases.

HAND ERUPTIONS IN HEALTH CARE WORKERS

Health care workers with hand eruptions may have irritant dermatitis, atopic hand eczema, dyshidrotic eczema, psoriasis, allergic contact dermatitis, contact urticaria (usually to natural rubber latex), contact urticaria or dermatitis to glove powder, protein contact dermatitis or many other conditions. Glove reactions have become so common, however, and the consequences so serious on occasion, that protocols for health care workers are appearing in many hospitals.

When health care workers develop hand eczema the reactions may or may not be related to gloves. Similar to any other hand eczema, management requires avoidance of irritants, and it requires a search for possible allergy to rubber chemicals in latex gloves (especially thiuram and carbamates), contact urticaria to latex proteins, and occasionally to rubber chemicals, or cornstarch in glove powder and rarely to other gloves. We generally test persons to the rubber chemicals with a patch test to rubber chemicals for both 20–30 min (for contact urticaria to rubber chemicals) and the standard 48-h application for contact dermatitis. We also test to gloves other than latex, as well as formaldehyde, glutaraldehyde and contents of soaps to which they are exposed, e.g., chlorhexidine, cocamidopropyl betaine, the standard patch test series and other preservatives used in soaps and shampoos, including parachlorometaxylenol, quaternium-15 and other preservatives. A RAST test can be ordered to corn and latex, and if negative, prick testing can be done by an experienced allergist or by a dermatologist set up to do these tests. One should understand the dangers of anaphylaxis and other severe reactions and be prepared for them if one does prick testing to latex in the office.

Nitrile gloves contain carbamates and 2-MBT sometimes. Neither vinyl (polyvinyl chloride) gloves nor nitrile gloves normally contain natural rubber latex protein (although one should read the label on the box carefully). Powder-free gloves are free of cornstarch. However, highly allergic persons may come into contact by handling objects (such as charts) that were also handled by physicians and nurses wearing powdered natural-rubber latex gloves, and glove powder in the air may transfer latex protein causing asthmatic symptoms in highly allergic persons. Persons with urticarial reactions to natural rubber latex proteins may also be allergic to certain foods, especially banana, avocado, chestnut and kiwi, but the list of reported foods is long.

HOSPITAL PROTOCOLS FOR SUSPECTED NATURAL RUBBER LATEX SENSITIVITY

Many hospitals are now beginning to incorporate into their routine, management of hospital employees with hand eruptions suspected of possibly being from natural rubber latex or other glove reactions. Such protocols often contain one or more of the following components:

1. New employees are questioned about latex allergy when hired, and if positive are instructed to use latex-free gloves and to so inform their supervisor to assure availability in the workplace.
2. Work areas where latex materials are used are to develop protocols to allow avoidance by the employee.
3. The hospital employee health service will usually evaluate each ostensibly sensitive employee on a case-by-case basis. The employee's chart is commonly marked, and some hospitals require a special identification bracelet.
4. Appropriate referrals for workup by a dermatologist or allergist are usually done by the employee health section.
5. Appropriate substitute materials should be available in the workplace. Therapeutic protocols usually include latex-free resuscitation equipment.

SUGGESTED READING

Adams RM. *Occupational Skin Disease*, ed 3. New York, Grune and Stratton, 1999.

Cronin E. *Contact Dermatitis*, Edinburgh, Churchill Livingstone, 1980.

Guin JD. *Practical Contact Dermatitis*. New York, McGraw-Hill, 1995.

Rycroft RJG, Menne' T, Frosch PJ, eds. *Textbook of Contact Dermatitis*, ed. 2. New York, Springer Verlag, 1994.

15 Food Allergy and Intolerance

John A. Anderson, MD

INTRODUCTION

Definitions and Classifications

Adverse reactions to foods can be divided into two major groups: food allergy, which depicts an immunological, usually involving IgE, reaction to a food, and food intolerance, which involves all other adverse reactions, some of which are the result of unknown mechanisms, but none of which involves immune reactions (Table 1). Food anaphylaxis is an IgE-mediated, generalized, clinical reaction to a food because of mast cell/basophil chemical mediator release after first sensitization and then re-exposure to the same food. Anaphylactoid reactions to a food or food additive clinically resemble food anaphylaxis, but do not involve IgE sensitization and are the result of direct chemical mediator release from the mast cell/basophil.

Other terms that are occasionally used to describe types of food intolerance include food toxicity or food poisoning, idiosyncratic reactions and pharmacological reactions to foods. *Food toxicity* may be the result of natural or acquired toxins in some foods or the result of microorganisms or parasitic contamination of natural or processed foods. Some of these clinical reactions are allergic-like and must be differentiated from food allergy. An idiosyncratic reaction to a food also resembles allergy, but does not involve immune mechanisms. Primary and secondary lactose sugar intolerance, because of the lack of bowel wall enzyme lactase to digest the sugar, is an example of such a reaction. Finally, a pharmacological reaction occurs to some foods containing chemicals (e.g., caffeine), and some food additives (e.g., food colors) have drug-like effects.

From: *Current Clinical Practice: Allergic Diseases: Diagnosis and Treatment, 2nd Edition*
Edited by: P. Lieberman and J. Anderson © Humana Press Inc., Totowa, NJ

Table 1
Classification of Adverse Reactions to Foods

Food allergy (immunologic reaction)	Food anaphylaxis and urticaria/angioedema (IgE-mediated)
	Other immunological reactions to foods
Food intolerance (nonimmunologic reaction)	Anaphylactoid reactions to foods or food additives
	Food toxicity or poisoning (usually owing to contamination)
	Idiosyncratic reaction to a food (e.g., enzyme deficiency)
	Pharmacological reaction to a food (drug-like effect)

Incidence and Prevalence

The incidence of food intolerance reactions greatly exceed food allergies in all age groups. Only some food intolerance reactions resemble allergic reactions. One well-documented study of 480 consecutively born infants found that the incidence of adverse reactions to foods confirmed by double-blind, placebo-controlled food challenge (DBPCFC) during the first 3 yr of life was 8%. In three well-done studies involving infants (United States, Sweden, Denmark), the incidence of allergic and intolerance reactions to cow's milk protein was found to be 2%. One study, based on the prevalence of documented food additive reactions among 4274 Danish schoolchildren, found the incidence of such reactions in children in general to be 1–2%.

In a study involving the prevalence of serious anaphylaxis and anaphylactoid reactions seen in 73 emergency departments in the state of Colorado over a 2-yr period (ages 2–71), it was estimated that the overall incidence of such reactions that occur yearly in the United States is 0.004% or 1:250,000 population. In a recent Midwest USA study, food allergy was found to be the most common cause of anaphylaxis. In a well-controlled study involving adults, the incidence of food allergy and food intolerance (allergic-like reactions) was estimated in the Netherlands to be 1.5% of the total population.

Natural History of Clinical Reactions to Food Allergy

Among children, in whom allergic and allergic-like food reactions have been documented by DBPCFC during infancy, 80–87% were able to tolerate that food upon rechallenge by 3 yr of age. The usual foods to which these children originally were clinically sensitive were cow's milk, eggs, peanuts, soy, or wheat proteins. In general, the more severe the original reaction to the food, the longer it takes for clinical tolerance to be achieved.

In studies among children and adults who have had documented anaphylaxis to peanuts, the susceptibility to anaphylaxis upon re-exposure lasted at least 14 yr. On the basis of this study and numerous case reports, peanut allergy as well as allergy to other foods commonly associated with systemic anaphylactic type of generalized reactions, such as crustacean sea food (shrimp, lobster, crab, crayfish), fish, tree nuts (walnut, pecan, almond, Brazil nut, filberts, cashews) and seeds, are lifelong sensitivities. (Tables 2 and 3)

Table 2
Clinical Reactions to Food and Food Additives

Anaphylaxis	General reactions
	Isolated reactions to the skin (e.g., urticaria with and without angioedema)
	Systemic reactions (laryngeal edema, rhinitis/conjunctivitis, asthma, shock, death)
	Oral allergy syndrome (OAS)
	Food-dependent exercise-induced anaphylaxis (F-EIA)
Atopic dermatitis exacerbated by food allergy	
Gastrointestional reaction (involving food)	Infant formula allergy or intolerance and enterocolitis/colitis
	Vomiting, diarrhea and blood loss
	Eosinophilic gastroenteritis
	Celiac disease
Pulmonary reaction (involving food)	Heiner's syndrome
	Rhinitis and asthma
Other food-intolerance reactions that may be confused with allergy	Food poisoning and toxicity (including anaphylactoid reactions to histamine-containing foods)
	Primary and secondary lactose intolerance
	Migraine and other headaches
	Vasoactive amines
	Specific food-induced mediator release
	Reactions to specific food additives
	Chinese restaurant syndrome due to MSG
	Asthma due to SO_2/sulfites
	Urticaria due to colors and possibly other agents (sodium benzoates, BHA, BHT, nitrates)
	Behavioral effects
	Sugar
	Color in ADD
	Pseudo food allergy

In individuals who are allergic to pollens, usually with allergic rhinitis and conjunctivitis, some are also allergic to fresh fruits and vegetables. This tendency is due to a crossreactivity (e.g., ragweed pollen and melons plus bananas) (Table 3). Although the natural history of this association is not entirely clear, it appears that this type of food sensitivity correlates with the degree of clinical reactivity to pollens.

MECHANISMS OF ALLERGIC AND ALLERGIC-LIKE INTOLERANCE REACTIONS TO FOODS AND FOOD ADDITIVES

Food Allergy

Almost all cases of allergic reactions to foods are due to type I immune reaction involving IgE antibody directed to that food. As with other allergic reactions, the susceptible person must be first exposed to the food protein, usually intermittently over a time, before sensitization occurs. This process involves the development of IgE antibody to that specific food protein.

Table 3
Usual Foods and Food Additives Associated with Adverse Reactions

Condition	Likely causative food or additive	
Anaphylaxis (generalized systemic and urticaria/angioedema)	Egg and cow's milk (children); peanuts; tree nuts (almond, Brazil nut, cashew, filbert, pecan, walnut), crustacean seafood (shrimp, lobster, crab, crayfish), fish, seeds	
Oral allergy syndrome	Pollen sensitivity	Raw food
	Ragweed	Melons (watermelon, cantaloupe), bananas
	Birch tree	Apple, pear, hazel nut, carrot, potato, celery, kiwi
	Grass	Peaches, celery
	Mugwort	Celery
Food-dependent exercise induced anaphylaxis (F-EIA)	(Within 2 h) any meal, or celery, shrimp, oyster, chicken, peach, wheat	
Infantile atopic dermatitis	Egg, cow's milk, peanut, wheat, soy	
Infantile formula intolerance	Conventional cow's milk- or soy protein-based infant formula	
Celiac disease	Gluten: wheat, oat, rye, barley	
Heiner's syndrome	Cow's milk protein	
Scromboid fish poisoning	Tuna, mackerel, bonita, mahi mahi, bluefish	
Urticaria from histamine-containing or -releasing foods	Histamine-containing foods	
	Parmesan and Roquefort cheese, spinach, eggplant, wines	
	Histamine-releasing foods	
	Chinese restaurant foods, alcoholic beverages (especially red wine), strawberries, seafood	
Lactose intolerance	Lactose sugar in cow's milk, cheese, yogurt	
Headaches (especially migraine)	Vasoactive amine	Food
	Caffeine	Coffee, cola
	Phenylethylamine	Cheeses (especially Gouda and Stilton)
	Serotonin	Banana, pineapple, plantain, avocado, plum, tomato
	Theobromine	Chocolate
	Tyramine	Camembert and Cheddar cheese, yeast, red wine, pickled herring, chicken livers
Chinese restaurant syndrome	MSG	
Asthma due to a preservative	SO_2, sulfites, yellow color (uncommon), MSG (rare, if any)	
Urticaria due to a food additive	Colors, especially yellow, red, blue (BHA, BHT, sodium benzoate, nitrites—rare, if any)	
Attention deficit syndrome	Colors, especially yellow	

Once the IgE antibodies are formed, they tend to stick to tissue mast cells on the surface of the body, and, in some cases, circulating basophils. The mast cells and the basophils are the effector cells of allergy and contain either preformed chemical mediators or are able to facilitate formation of other mediators in the immediate tissue around the cell once stimulated (*see* Chapter 5). Re-exposure to the same food protein results in chemical mediator release or formation in the tissue, which causes the clinical allergy signs and symptoms.

Purified major antigens have been identified for cow's milk (e.g., casein, β-lactoglobulin, α-lactalbumin), chicken egg, peanut, soy, fish and shrimp. These major

---

Proven Food Alergy in Infants

The most likely foods involved in allergic reactions in children below the age of 2 in the United States are

- Cow's milk
- Eggs
- Peanuts
- Wheat
- Soy

---

food allergens are heat stable. Thus, individuals who are allergic to foods such as milk, peanut, or fish can develop symptoms, once sensitized to re-exposure to very small amounts of these specific foods in a natural, cooked or processed form. There are also minor food allergens, such as those found in fresh fruits and vegetables, that crossreact with pollens, as is seen in the oral allergy syndrome. In this condition, reactions are due to homology between food and pollen to common plant proteins such as proflin. These latter allergens are heat labile. Individuals allergic to a fresh fruit, such as apple, can usually eat an apple pie. A recent study would seem to indicate that short microwave exposure to a fresh fruit is enough to denature the allergen to allow it to be tolerated to some degree by individuals who develop symptoms to these fresh fruits.

Although there is some immunological crossreactivity between different foods, especially those in the same food family, characteristically, individuals react clinically more often only to a few foods in a given food family. For example, in the legume family, most individuals are clinically sensitive only to peanut and can tolerate peas, beans and soy protein, even though IgE antibodies to these foods can be detected either in IgE immediate-reacting skin tests or in vitro IgE food protein-specific antibody assays.

Exposure to food protein usually occurs orally. Occasionally, individuals can become sensitized or, after developing a food allergy, have a reaction to re-exposure of food through either the aerosol or contact route. Examples include bakery workers who develop IgE-mediated wheat protein sensitivity (and subsequent asthma called baker's asthma) from exposure and then re-exposure to wheat flour dust. Another example is the fish-allergic individual who may develop urticaria or systemic anaphylaxis when exposed to odor/steam of cooked fish.

In food-dependent exercise-induced anaphylaxis (F-EIA) (*see* Table 2), increased histamine release is induced by exercise. IgE reactions to foods only become clinically evident within 2 h of a meal, following vigorous activity. Atopic dermatitis is a skin condition, primarily in children, whose pathogenesis involves both nonimmune and immune factors. IgE antibody formation in general is usually enhanced in this condition. However, in only one third of children with atopic dermatitis is food allergy clinically important.

It has been shown in studies with atopic dermatitis individuals who are proven to be allergic to a food by DBPCFC that, while eating that food, in vitro histamine release is increased nonspecifically owing to the presence of "IgE-dependent histamine-releasing factors" in the serum. This tendency has a definite connection with the broad-based chronic inflammation found in the skin of the atopic dermatitis patient who is allergic to specific food proteins. The IgE reaction that results in the eczema type of rash in atopic dermatitis may be an example of a late-phase IgE reaction.

Another type of immunological reaction to food is a rare syndrome called the Heiner's syndrome (Table 2). In this syndrome, infants develop high IgG antibody titers to cow's milk through aspiration and sequestration of the milk protein in the lung. Subsequently, on repeated oral milk exposure, pulmonary infiltrates result. This reaction is felt primarily to be due to a type III immune reaction resulting from IgG milk antigen-antibody complexes with activation of complement. There is some evidence for a type IV cell-mediated immune reaction due to this cow's milk protein.

In celiac syndrome, the pathogenesis points toward both a toxic reaction to wheat gluten and a type IV cell-mediated immune reaction to this wheat protein.

Allergic-like Food Intolerance Reactions

The mechanisms for most food intolerance reactions are not known. Most infants who develop isolated gastrointestinal symptoms (vomiting, diarrhea, blood in stool) resulting from formula intolerance do not demonstrate IgE antibody reactions. This condition can occur while the child is ingesting cow's milk-based conventional formula, breast milk from mothers eating a normal diet or soy protein-based infant formulas. Approximately one half of the individuals with documented eosinophilic gastroenteritis are allergic. The rest are not, yet the disease pathology between the allergic and nonallergic group is similar.

An example of an anaphylactoid reaction to food is a "scromboid fish poisoning" (*see* Tables 2 and 3). In this situation, certain fish that are spoiled or contaminated with either *Proteus* or Klebsiella species of bacteria such as tuna, mackerel, bonito (scromboid varieties) or mahi and bluefish. The bacteria decarboxylate histidine in fish tissue to create histamine. When the fish is cooked and eaten, the diner experiences a sharp peppery taste, burning of the mouth parts, followed by nausea, vomiting, diarrhea, facial flush and headache—all resulting from the high levels of histamine in the tissue. This is the same major chemical mediator released from the mast cell or basophil as the result of an allergic reaction.

Other common foods that may contain a significant amount of histamine include Parmesan and Roquefort cheeses, spinach, eggplant, red wines and some Chinese restaurant foods (Table 3). Other pharmacoactive agents in foods that may produce symptoms that could be confused with allergy include caffeine (in coffee and cola), tyramine (in cheese), phenylethylene (in cheese, red wine and chocolate), serotonin (in banana, pineapple, avocado, tomato) and theobromine (in chocolate) (Table 3).

The possible effects of these various natural vasoactive amines is variable, but there are reports of these chemicals aggravating migraine headaches. Patients taking monoamine oxidase (MAO) inhibitor drugs for the treatment of conditions such as depression need to be very careful about eating these types of foods, since MAO is important for the metabolism of vasoactive amines. Thus, eating these foods and taking these inhibitor drugs may result in increased blood levels of the vasoactive amines. Both severe blood pressure elevation and headache have been reported.

Lactose intolerance is an idiosyncratic reaction caused by the lack of bowel wall lactase, which is necessary to metabolize lactose sugar found in cow's milk. Individuals with lactose intolerance who ingest milk cannot digest it, and the sugar ferments in the bowel, causing gas, discomfort and perhaps diarrhea. Primary lactose intolerance is a

---

Food Additive Reactions

- In general, proven adverse reactions to food preservatives, colors or flavor enhancers are uncommon.
- Chewing foods containing sulfites may release SO_2, which, when inhaled, may exacerbate asthma.
- Very few patients have been proven to develop urticaria after ingesting food coloring agents.
- Behavioral abnormalities in children usually cannot be attributed to diet content (e.g., amount of sugar, presence of allergic protein, or type of food additive).

---

common inborn error of metabolism in certain population groups (e.g., approximately 80% of North American African-Americans, Arab and Asian populations). This condition is a less common problem in other ethnic groups (10% incidence in North European Caucasian populations).

The symptoms begin about age 7, but may occur earlier if the patient develops a severe viral or bacterial gastrointestinal infection. Lactose intolerance may occur after any gastrointestinal infection and is usually a temporary condition lasting about 2 wk. Secondary lactose intolerance of a more permanent nature, however, can occur with chronic gastrointestinal conditions, such as sprue or cow's milk allergy. Each patient with lactose intolerance is different, and many may tolerate some degree of lactose sugar in their diet.

Food Additive Intolerance Reactions

Allergic reactions have been reported to occur to the preservative sulfites (and SO_2), sodium benzoate, butylated hydroxyzole (BHA), and butylated hydroxytyluene (BHT), the sugar substitute aspartame, artificial colors (especially yellow, red and blue), and the flavor enhancer monosodium glutamate (MSG). The symptoms of principal concern are urticaria and asthma. In most cases, even if it is proven that the food additive is involved in the clinical symptoms, the exact mechanism of the reaction is unknown.

In sulfite-induced asthma, the principal mechanism is believed to be the inhalation of SO_2 as sulfite-containing foods are chewed in the mouth. In addition, a small number of individuals have been identified who have a sulfite oxidase enzyme deficiency, which prevents metabolism of this preservative and could result in high blood levels. In a few cases of documented urticarial reactions to color, histamine and prostaglandin increase has been found in the urine after specific food allergy additive challenge.

In the attention deficit disorder syndrome with hyperactivity (ADD), food colors, especially yellow, have been implicated in 3% or less of the cases in inducing a drug-like effect on the patient's ability to learn.

The evidence for IgE-mediated food immune reactions as being involved in the pathogenesis of migraine headaches is very poor. However, there are a small number of documented cases of migraineurs who, on DBPCFC, demonstrate increases in plasma histamine PGF_α and PGD_2 that correlate with specific food protein challenge and headache.

```
┌──────────────────────────────────────────────────────────────┐
│                        Food Anaphylaxis                        │
│                                                                │
│     Lifelong sensitivity may occur at any age to these commonly│
│   eaten foods:                                                 │
│   • Peanuts                                                    │
│   • Seafoods (especially shrimp, lobster and crab)             │
│   • Tree nuts (e.g., almonds, Brazil nuts, cashews, filberts,  │
│     walnuts and pecans)                                        │
│   • Fish                                                       │
│   • Seeds                                                      │
└──────────────────────────────────────────────────────────────┘
```

CLINICAL REACTIONS TO FOODS AND FOOD ADDITIVES (TABLE 2)

Food Anaphylaxis

The signs and symptoms of anaphylaxis resulting from food allergy are no different from those due to anaphylaxis as the result of allergy to β-lactam antibiotics, stinging insects or natural rubber latex (*see* Chapter 5). The symptoms and signs may be mild or severe. Milder symptoms/signs include contact urticaria, generalized pruritus, erythema and urticaria with or without angioedema. More severe symptom/signs occur with generalized systemic anaphylaxis due to a food and may be multiple or single in nature. These symptoms include laryngeal edema, rhinitis with or without conjunctivitis, asthma, blood pressure decrease or shock and possible cardiovascular collapse and death. Occasionally, additional symptoms include nausea, vomiting, abdominal cramps, diarrhea and uterine or bladder cramps.

Most generalized anaphylactic reactions to foods of any significance are biphasic in nature with an early and late phase separated by about 1–8 h. Some very serious reactions are protracted and last continuously for 5–32 h without remission.

Individuals tend to develop serious anaphylactic reactions to a relatively small group of foods, including cow's milk and eggs (usually infants and children), peanuts, tree nuts (walnut, pecan, almond, cashew, Brazil, filbert), crustacean seafood (shrimp, lobster, crayfish), fish and seeds. (Table 3).

Most individuals who die or nearly die with food anaphylaxis are very allergic in general and reactive to many things in their environment, including pollen, animals, house dust and mold allergens. Most of these patients have allergic rhinitis and asthma. Many of the children with food allergies have, or have had, atopic dermatitis. Individuals who have been reported either to have died from or nearly died from a systemic reaction from food are usually aware of their specific food allergy. Most deaths occur when the individual is away from home. The specific food to which the individual is allergic is usually eaten in a disguised form (e.g., in a pastry, candy, salad, sandwich, or hors d'oeuvre). Often the difference between life and death is whether or not adrenaline was given quickly (e.g., within 1 h after the start of a reaction) when the dangerous food is ingested or the exposure occurs.

There are two special anaphylaxis syndromes that are specific for food allergy. The first is called the oral allergy syndrome (OAS) or the fruit and vegetable syndrome (Table 2). In this syndrome, individuals with pollen sensitivity, usually manifested by allergic rhinitis/conjunctivitis or hay fever, develop specific food sensitivities to fresh fruits and vegetables upon contact of these raw foods with the mouth. The mechanism is due partly to crossreactivity between the pollen protein and the food protein (*see* Mechanisms). The food crossreactivities include melons and bananas among US ragweed–allergic individuals; apples, pears, potatoes, hazelnuts, carrots, celery and kiwi among birch pollen–allergic individuals; peach, tomato, celery among grass–allergic individuals; and celery allergy among European mugwort weed–sensitive individuals (Table 3).

These crossreactivities between foods and pollens may be further complicated by the fact that individuals with anaphylaxis to natural rubber latex may also be sensitive to certain foods, including bananas, chestnut, avocado and kiwi and that these sensitivities may be due to crossreactivity between pollens, such as ragweed and grass.

The symptoms of OAS are usually confined to exposure to raw foods to either the mouth or hand, and the type of symptoms include pruritus, swelling, tingling or fullness. In some cases, full-blown systemic anaphylaxis may result. In the majority of cases, however, symptoms begin within 5 min of raw food contact and may be ameliorated by discontinuing contact and washing the hands or rinsing the mouth, so that symptoms resolve within 30 min.

A second food–specific anaphylactic syndrome is the food-related exercise-induced anaphylaxis (F-EIA). EIA is a relatively newly described physical urticaria in which vigorous exercise is associated with urticaria or shock. In half the cases, this syndrome requires a cofactor, such as eating a meal (in general) or ingestion of a specific food, including celery, shrimp, oysters, chicken, peaches or wheat (Table 3). All symptoms begin within 2 h of a meal, and usually the individual can eat the specific food in spite of the presence of IgE antibodies to that food, as long as he or she does not exercise in this 2-h period.

Atopic Dermatitis

Although atopic dermatitis is a primary skin disorder of children, in approximately 80% of the cases children are allergic in general and have high total IgE and many positive skin test reactions or evidence of in vitro antiallergic antibodies. Some of these reactivities are directed to foods. It has been proven, using DBPCFC, that about one third of children with atopic dermatitis react with an exacerbation of their rash to specific food challenge, such as egg, cow's milk, peanut, wheat and soy (Table 3). Other clinical reactions to foods in this group of patients are less common.

It has been found in studies using DBPCFC involving food-allergic atopic-dermatitis children that the allergy skin test or in vitro test is usually positive to the offending food, but that in food skin-test–positive situations, the likelihood of that food being clinically significant in the rash is no more than 50%.

In these studies, if the food skin test was negative, the DBPCFC was almost always also negative. It was found in these studies that the skin test and in vitro IgE food-antibody tests results were more reliable as an index of possible food involvement than was the mother's history of such reactions. Individuals who were found allergic were usually sensitive only to a few foods, not multiple foods. A negative food skin test or in vitro IgE food-antibody test practically ruled out the possibility that the DBPCFC would be positive to that food.

Allergy and Gastrointestinal (GI) Food Reactions

- Most GI reactions to diet are *not* due to fool allergy.
- Milk protein allergy/intolerance usually occurs in infants.
- Lactose (milk sugar) intolerance usually is a problem in older children or adults and runs in families.
- Food protein anaphylaxis (allergy) occurs within minutes to 2 h after food ingestion and almost always includes urticaria—with or without GI symptoms.
- The findings of eosinophils on GI biopsy is suggestive but not diagnostic of food alergy.

It has also been shown that if the food to which the patient was found to be allergic on DBPCFC was strickly eliminated from the diet for a time, the dermatitis would improve (*see* Mechanisms).

Gastrointestinal Reactions Involving Food

A wide variety of signs and symptoms involving the gastrointestinal tract could be attributed to a food allergy. However, most are not specific, and the possible causes for most of these signs and symptoms are multiple. Itching and swelling of the mouth, however, are certainly suggestive of an allergic reaction as in the OAS. Infants who have formula intolerance can develop vomiting, have diarrhea or simply have blood loss in the stool. Some individuals simply fail to thrive.

In food-induced enterocolitis, both the small and large bowel are usually involved. The bowel wall of the small intestine, in particular, is infiltrated with lymphocytes, plasma cells and eosinophils. Formula (usually cow's milk protein)-induced colitis resembles ulcerative colitis and is characterized by friable mucosal surfaces, eosinophilic infiltrates and either occult or gross blood loss. In these infants, often the elimination of conventional cow's milk–based infant formula feeding and replacement with a casein hydrolysate infant formula, plus rechallenge to conventional formula, is the only way to prove the etiology, since IgE antibodies to the food protein may not be found on in-vitro studies.

In studies, 30–42% of infants with gastroesophageal reflux were found to have eosinophilic infiltrates in the esophagus wall and milk allergy/intolerance. Food-induced protolitic occurs in infants, most of whom are breast fed. This condtion occurs in both allergic and nonallergic children.

Eosinophilic gastroenteritis is a chronic problem of older children and adults that involves the entire gastrointestinal tract (especially stomach and small intestine). These tissues are infiltrated with eosinophils. The symptoms include cramping, abdominal pain, nausea, vomiting diarrhea, and blood loss in the stool. Only one half of the reported cases of eosinophilic gastroenteritis are highly allergic, including reactions to many foods. When these specific foods are eaten, the condition is exacerbated. When the patient switches to a diet devoid of offending foods, however, the condition does not completely clear.

Celiac syndrome is less commonly diagnosed now than previously. The primary cause is gluten, usually from wheat protein (Table 3). The classic, full-blown picture of the once-thriving infant who becomes wasted, has an obvious protracted abdomen and suffers from chronic diarrhea and rickets is not now generally seen. When this condition is diagnosed currently, it is usually in a child with growth retardation and anemia or in an adult with chronic weight loss and persistent diarrhea.

Infant colic is not due to food allergy. It occurs in 20% of children regardless of the diet, including maternal breast milk. Recurrent abdominal pain in older children usually has nothing to do with food allergy. Intermittent bouts of diarrhea, along with abdominal cramping, are again not likely to be due to food allergy. Probably the most common problem diagnosed under these circumstances is an irritable bowel syndrome. However, other conditions, such as ulcerative colitis and regional ileitis, polypoid disease and cancer must be ruled out.

Pulmonary Reactions Involving Food

In 1956, D. Heiner and his colleague J. Sears, identified a group of infants with recurrent anemia and pneumonia associated with in vitro cow's milk precipitins in the serum. Some of these children later developed pulmonary hemosiderosis. This syndrome is believed to be the result of pulmonary aspiration of milk formula just after birth and the development of IgG cow's milk antibody titers due to sequestration of milk in the lung (*see* Mechanisms). Later, upon repeated exposure to cow's milk in the diet, both a type III immune complex and a type IV cell-mediated reaction occur. Today, such reactions in infants are rare, but should be considered in infants with recurrent pneumonia and anemia of undetermined etiology.

Rhinitis and/or asthma-like symptoms (wheezing, respiratory distress) occur as part of systemic anaphylaxis to foods. It has been shown in studies of children with atopic dermatitis who are allergic to foods that after specific food avoidance, followed by DBPCFC 2 wk later, one thid are likely, upon challenge, to develop respiratory symptoms, such as rhinitis or asthma, along with exacerbation of their skin rash. Other than this situation, rhinitis and asthma are unlikely to be triggered by food. This is particularly true of adults or older children with these conditions.

Other Food Intolerance Reactions That May Be Confused With Allergy

Reactions, such as anaphylactoid events following ingestion of scromboid fish protein, are described under Mechanisms to the foods listed in Table 3. Urticaria may occasionally occur following ingestion of certain foods containing histamine or as histamine reactors as listed in Table 3. Examples include cheese, red wine or strawberries.

One of the most common gastrointestinal problems that is confused with milk allergy is primary (and secondary) lactose intolerance. The pathogenesis of this reaction is described under Mechanisms. As pointed out, the problem with milk usually begins around age 7 among North American African-Americans, but may start earlier in childhood if the child has had significant gastroenteritis. Then, for the rest of his or her life, ingestion of cow's milk is a problem. This sequence of events is different from that of the individual who is milk protein allergic in that the milk-allergic individual has trouble during early childhood and later is usually able to tolerate milk clinically.

In the lactose-intolerant patient, the degree of exposure to milk sugar is important. Certain foods are better tolerated than others: Cheese is better tolerated than whole milk and naturally fermented yogurt is better tolerated than cheese. Since the problem is common in certain ethnic groups, older family members may report the same problem with milk ingestion, and lactose intolerance is usually simple to diagnose. If it is important to document this syndrome, this can be done by a gastroenterologist using a breath hydrogen test after lactose ingestion.

The triggering of headaches by vasoactive amines naturally or by food additives may occur with the foods listed in Table 3 and described under Mechanisms. Although the issue of allergy being involved in migraine headache pathogenesis has been long debated, it is rarely proven. In a few cases of patients with migraine headaches, chemical mediator release while eating a specific food may be involved in the headache. Migraines are very common in the general population (e.g., 25% of all adult women and 15% of all adult men). In addition, allergies are also common (20% of the population in general). Therefore, it would be easy to find both conditions (migraine headache and atopic disease) present in the same individual.

Adverse reactions to food additives are not nearly as common as is generally believed. Reactions to BHA, BHT, benzoates and nitrates are very rarely substantiated by objective measurements. The most common FDA-reported food additive reactions are those due to aspartame, and the usual type of symptom is headache. Fifteen percent of reports of adverse effects due to aspartame, however, are "allergic-like," usually urticaria. Although there are two documented cases of aspartame-induced urticaria/angioedema reported in the world literature, a recent large nationwide, multicenter study using DBPCFC was unable to confirm a significant association between aspartame and urticaria. The types of adverse reactions to food additives that have been confirmed over the years include the Chinese restaurant syndrome resulting from MSG, asthma resulting from SO_2 or sulfites in food and occasional episodes of urticaria/angioedema resulting from food coloring (*see* Tables 2 and 3).

The first report of the Chinese restaurant syndrome was a self-report of a Chinese physician in 1968 who ate at a Chinese restaurant and experienced symptoms of nausea, headache, sweating, thirst, facial flushing, tightness and burning of the face and chest, abdominal pain, tearing of the eyes and a sensation of "crawling" in the skin. Typically, the symptoms begin 15–30 min after eating a meal containing a large amount of MSG, which is a salt of a glutamic acid. These symptoms usually subside without specific medical treatment once the individual discontinues ingestion of the MSG-containing food.

The second most likely food additives (after aspartame) to be reported to the FDA as being responsible for an adverse reaction are sulfites and SO_2. Although a few cases of anaphylactoid type of reactions, usually involving urticaria/angioedema, have been reported, most reactions are the result of asthma exacerbation in a known asthmatic. Some of the early cases were serious, and a few led to death. Although SO_2 and sulfites have been used for many years as food and beverage preservatives, it was not until the 1970s to 1980s that reports emerged about serious asthma attacks being precipitated directly upon opening a package containing SO_2-preserved foods or eating (and inhaling SO_2 indirectly) sulfite-containing foods (*see* Mechanisms). Of particular importance were fresh vegetables and fruits in salad bars in restaurants (especially lettuce) to which a sulfite solution had been applied to preserve that food. The FDA has estimated that approximately 5% of all asthmatics are at risk for a reaction to SO_2 or sulfite, and studies have shown that the more serious asthmatic is at greater risk of an exacerbation of the asthma than a mild asthmatic.

In the late 1980s, the FDA made significant changes in the regulations concerning the maximum level of sulfites that could be in foods in the United States, as well as restrictions on the use of sulfites in restaurants, especially in salad bars. Since that time, the number of reports of sulfite- induced asthma has dropped dramatically. Although there have been reports of MSG–induced asthma exacerbations (in Chinese restaurants in Australia) that were confirmed by challenge studies in the 1980s, there has not been a similar problem with MSG in the United States.

Although in Europe food additives of all types have been implicated as primary causes of chronic urticaria in about 15% of the cases, most studies in the United States have failed to confirm a significant relationship with any additive except for a few isolated cases of color (particularly yellow)-induced urticaria and angioedema (Table 3).

Tartrazine (FD&C yellow #5) was originally felt to "crossreact" in some way with aspirin and to be a factor among asthma exacerbation in aspirin-sensitive asthmatics. Careful DBPCFC with tartrazine in proven aspirin-sensitive asthmatics have failed to confirm this association with yellow #5. Independent of aspirin sensitivity, there are a few isolated asthmatic patients who are sensitive to yellow #5.

Food additives (particularly colors, especially yellows) have been implicated in causing or exacerbating behavioral problems in children. Probably the most widely known theory regarding this relationship was the Feingold theory about colors (and other food additives) causing hyperactivity in patients with attention deficit disorder (ADD) (see Tables 2 and 3). Most subsequent studies have shown that colors do have a drug-like effect, but that this effect occurs in no more than 5% of children with ADD, and the effect has to do with learning abilities. There are no studies that show that colors in the market today are not safe for the general population.

In the mid to late 1980s, diets high in sugar were believed to cause abnormal behavior, especially hyperactivity in normal children, those with ADD and juvenile delinquents. The misnomer *sugar allergy* was coined. DBPCFC studies have documented the fact that sugar in the diet does not have an adverse effect on behavior and, in some cases, may have a calming effect. In the 1960s, D. Pearson coined the term *pseudo food allergy* to describe a syndrome that usually occurs in adults who believe they have food allergy and restrict their diet to such a degree that they develop signs of malnutrition (see Table 2). Almost all the patients who have been reported with this condition, have been found to have psychological problems, especially depression. The symptoms they complain about include fatigue, headaches, "mental fuzziness," malaise, arthralgia and myalgias. When DBPCFC studies were done, none of the patients studied reacted to the foods to which they were supposedly sensitive. With psychological counseling, all resumed a normal diet without adverse effect.

DIAGNOSIS OF FOOD ALLERGY OR INTOLERANCE

History

As outlined in Table 4, a good history is the most important factor in diagnosing a food allergy or intolerance. The history should include:

1. The description of the problem
2. The timing of the onset in relationship to the specific food or additive in the diet and the duration of the event

Table 4
Diagnosis of Food Allergy and Intolerance

History	Description of problem
	Timing of onset and duration of event related to diet
	Frequency of symptoms
	Other important circumstances
IgE-reacting skin testing and in vitro IgE antibody testing	
Food diary and diets	
Confirmatory food challenges	Open
	Double-blind, placebo-controlled
Other tests	Mast cell tryptase
	Analysis of potential food allergen ingredient content in processed foods
	Breath hydrogen and lactose tolerance

3. The quantity of the suspected food ingested
4. Whether similar symptoms to this same food (or other foods) have occured before
5. The frequency of symptoms (continuous or intermittent in nature)
6. Additional circumstances

Most individuals who develop food allergies have other manifestations of allergy personally or have family members with allergic disease. This includes atopic dermatitis, urticaria, asthma, allergic rhinitis/conjunctivitis. A history of asthma in a food-allergic individual should be considered a risk factor for possible serious life-threatening reactions of an anaphylactic nature to that food.

Certain foods are associated with different types of allergic and intolerance reactions (Table 3). This should be kept in mind when taking a history of the presenting complaint. Most food anaphylactic reactions (e.g., urticaria or systemic anaphylaxis) occur within minutes (and almost always within 2 h) after exposure to the food. In these types of cases, it is often easier to pin down a likely food candidate because of the close association in time. More difficult are cases in which the problem is chronic (e.g., atopic dermatitis) and in which many nonallergic factors play a role. In studies involving children who were allergic to food and had atopic dermatitis, the patient's history of the likelihood of a specific food being involved was often not helpful. Food-allergy skin testing or in vitro IgE-specific food-antibody testing were more helpful in narrowing the field of likely foods responsible for the allergic reaction. Finally, being a "good detective" may take a great deal of time, especially when the culprit food responsible for the adverse reaction is not obvious and/or a part of a prepared food.

IgE Food-Allergy Skin Testing or In Vitro Food Allergen-Specific Antibody Testing

Only the epicutaneous (prick/scratch/puncture) type of immediate-reacting IgE (allergy)-skin testing is used to diagnose food allergy. Tests are done with a drop of food allergen concentrate (usually 1:10 weight by volume) on the forearm or back

---

Confirming the Diagnosis of an Adverse Food Reaction

- DBPCFC is the "gold-standard" for the diagnosis of an adverse reaction to food.
- A positive DBPCFC does not identify the mechanism of reaction.
- In most cases of systemic (life-threatening) anaphylaxis, a DBPCFC is not clinically necessary since it is risky; the presence of IgE allergen-specific antibody can help establish a "presumptive" diagnosis.
- Food diaries and short-term elimination diets at home may be helpful tools, but in themselves do not confirm the diagnosis.
- IgE food prick tests or in vitro assays may assist the clinician in narrowing down the field of likely foods in suspected food allergy.

---

and read in 15 min. Either commercial allergy extract or fresh material (e.g., juice from a fresh apple in the oral allergy syndrome) can be used. Reactions in which the wheal is measured at 3 mm or more than the negative saline control are considered to be positive.

In vitro IgE food-allergen-specific antibody testing, either the radioallergosorbent test or the enzyme-linked immune assay methods are used. The in vitro tests are less sensitive than the skin test for foods and do not give more information (if the skin test is negative). The in vitro assay is the diagnostic method of choice in cases of systemic anaphylaxis, since it is safer. In these situations, any individual who had a recent systemic anaphylactic reaction to a food (e.g., peanut), is likely to have enough IgE-specific antibody in the serum to have a positive in vitro test.

The food allergy skin test (or in vitro test) is helpful to screen for food allergies. If one of these two tests is positive in infants, there is up to a 50% chance (for commonly eaten food) that the individual, if challenged, would be actually found to be clinically sensitive to that food. If the in vitro test is positive, there is approx a 40% chance that the individual, if challenged, would actually be clinically sensitive to that food. If the skin test or the in vitro allergy food tests are negative, however, almost 100% of the time if one would challenge with that food the challenge would be negative.

If either the immediate food allergy skin test or the IgE food allergy-specific in vitro test is positive in adults (in whom the frequency of true food allergies is less than in infants and children), with any food there is only a 3% chance that if the adult were challenged with the food, it would be clinically relevant. Again, if either the food skin test or the in vitro test is negative in adults, there is close to 100% chance that a food challenge would be negative.

In the case of systemic anaphylactic reactions to food, usually the in vitro allergy skin test is positive. In this case, a presumptive diagnosis of food anaphylaxis is made, the necessity for, without confirmation challenge studies.

Food Diary and Diets

Food diaries may be helpful in the patient with a history of several, but intermittent, episodes of acute urticaria or other symptoms suspected of being related to diet. If

Table 5
Major Food Allergen-Free Diet Foods and Beverages Allowed[a]

Apricots	Chicken	Pineapple	Sugar (cane or beet)
Arrowroot	Ginger ale	Plums	Sweet potatoes
Artichokes	Ham (boiled)	Poi	Tapioca (whole or
Asparagus	Kidney beans	Potatoes	pearl, not minute)
Bacon	Lamb	Potato chips	Turkey
Beef, all-beef	Lentils	Prunes	Vanilla extract
wieners	Lettuce	Rice	Water
Beets	Maple syrup or	Salt	White soda
Blueberries	maple-flavored	Soybeans	White vinegar
Carrots	cane syrup	Soybean sprouts	Yams
Celery	Navy beans	Soy milk	
Cherries	Olive oil	Spinach	
Any vegetable shortening or oleomargarine that contains no milk			

[a]All fruits and vegetables, except lettuce, must be cooked.

there is no obvious cause, a diary of events, including a diet for subsequent episodes, may be helpful in pinning down the ultimate diagnosis.

Temporary use of diets composed of foods to which most individuals have no allergy or intolerance are sometimes helpful when the patient has a chronic problem suspected of being related to diet, but not involving anaphylaxis. Examples of these allergen-free diets can be found in numerous textbooks and in Table 5. Usually the patient is kept on such a diet for 2 wk, and then one new food is added to the diet every 3 d (and the previously added food is kept in the diet—providing no adverse symptoms occurred). This is continued until a normal diet has been resumed.

Food Challenges

It is usually advisable to refer patients potentially requiring food challenge to an allergist/immunologist for evaluation of the problem. The gold standard in substantiating an adverse reaction to food regardless of the etiology is the DBPCFC. Usually if a food challenge confirmation is necessary, an open sequential food challenge, beginning with a small dose first, is done first under controlled conditions, followed by at least a 2-h wait. In most clinical situations, no challenge is indicated if the situation involves systemic anaphylaxis. A good history backed up by the finding of IgE antibody to that food in in vitro testing is enough for presumptive diagnosis. If open challenge is positive, to make absolutely sure of the cause of the reaction the DBPCFC technique is advised (Table 6 for this procedure). Details on the use of this type of challenge can be found in standardized text books.

Other Tests

Serum mast cell tryptase is a helpful tool in diagnosing serious systemic anaphylaxis and anaphylactoid reactions (see Chapters 5 and 16). Usually this enzyme is present in the blood for up to 2 h after the event, about the time the patient is seen by a physician in an emergency situation. Unfortunately, in many cases of anaphylaxis due to food, blood mast cell tryptase increase cannot be detected. Therefore, if the enzyme is

Table 6
DBPCFC Guidelines

The challenge should be performed by personnel knowledgeable in the management of
    anaphylaxis
The procedure should be done under controlled conditions, in the hospital, clinic, or office
The suspected food should be eliminated from the diet 10–14 d prior to challenge
Antihistamines should be discontinued 12 h prior to challenge
The individual to be challenged should be in a stable cardiovascular, pulmonary and metabolic
    condition prior to challenge
The individual to be challenged should be in a fasting state (6–12 h) when challenged
The challenge should start with a low dose (e.g., 125–500 mg or lyophilized food) so as *not*
    to provoke symptoms
Gradual increases in dose (suspected food or placebo) should occur by doubling the amount
    every 15–20 min
The maximum dose of food used in challenge should approximate 10 g of lyophilized food
The minimum recommended observation period following completion of the DBPCFC
    procedure for:
    Suspected anaphylaxis is 2 h
    Isolated GI signs/symptoms is 4–8 h
    Food intolerance reactions is 4–8 h
In followup of negative specific food challenge, open feeding with this food is recommended
    for the subsequent 24–48 h

From Sampson HA, Metcalfe DD. Food allergies. *JAMA* 1992;268:2840–2844.

detected (test is positive), it is helpful information. If the test is negative, however, it
does not rule out a systemic food reaction.

In some situations, it is necessary to do a detailed analysis of a meal or processed
foods, using immunological techniques to pin down a particular type of food protein
suspected of being responsible for an allergy or an intolerance. Even trace amounts of
food protein may be important in precipitating anaphylaxis in very sensitive individuals.
The label on processed foods may not indicate a contaminant or an offensive food
protein that ended up in the final product through some misadventure during the food
processing.

The idiosyncratic reaction of lactose intolerance (commonly mistaken for cow's
milk allergy), can be confirmed by means of a breath-hydrogen analysis after lactose
ingestion.

MANAGEMENT OF FOOD ALLERGY OR INTOLERANCE

The management of proven or suspected food allergy consists of strict avoidance of
that food. In some food-intolerance reactions, such as lactose intolerance, the reaction
is quantitative, since small amounts of lactose sugar–containing foods can be tolerated.
This is in contrast to the case of systemic anaphylaxis, in which food allergens in trace
amounts can trigger a serious life-threatening event once the patient is sensitized and
preformed IgE antibodies exist to that food.

Long-term specific food avoidance may be a problem for patients, especially when
they are away from home, while at school eating in the cafeteria, at a restaurant, or
at a party. Some foods, like nuts and peanuts, are easily disguised in candies, bakery

Table 7
Management of Food Allergy or Intolerance

Strict avoidance of the offending food (anaphylaxis) or in small amounts (some food
   intolerance)
Food substitution (e.g., infant formula)
Future role of allergen immunotherapy
In case of systemic allergen immunotherapy:
   EpiPen autoinjector (0.3 mg aqueous epinephrine) or EpiPen Jr (0.15 mg epenephrine) use
   in <6 yr of age) (Dey Lab.; Napa, CA 94556)
Systemic anaphylaxis: Medic Alert jewelry (Medic Alert Foundation, Turlock, CA
   (800) 642-0045)
Patient support:
  Food Allergy Network
  4744 Holly Avenue
  Fairfax, VA 22030
  (800) 929-4040; (703) 691-3179; fax (703) 691-2713
  Asthma and Allergy Foundation of America (AAFA)
  1125 Fifteenth Street NW
  Washington, D.C. 20005
  (800) 727-8462

products, hors d'oeuvres, or in salads or salad dressings. The cooking steam from fish or seafood may precipitate a reaction for specifically sensitive individuals. Processed foods may not have detailed labeling to identify a dangerous food. Particular ingredients in a restaurant meal may be difficult to identify (it is usually not advisable to take the waiter's viewpoint—only the cook knows!).

In a situation in which a definite food allergy is known or a presumptive diagnosis has been made, it is best for the individual to carry an EpiPen (0.3 mg) or an EpiPen Jr. (0.15 mg) and to wear Medic Alert jewelry about that sensitivity or intolerance (Table 7). Patient information concerning food allergies and food intolerance can be obtained through the Food Allergy Network (Table 7).

Allergen immunotherapy has been used to treat other allergic diseases, such as allergic rhinitis. Although food allergen injection therapy using conventional methods has been employed experimentally, this treatment method is not currently clinically accepted. New methods of allergen immunotherapy using specific foods (e.g., peanut) are now under investigation. The alternative medicine practice of using food drops under the tongue to attempt to neutralize symptoms as a method to prevent food reaction symptoms is *unproven* and *unapproved* treatment.

Infant Formula Substitution

A particular problem exists for infants who are allergic or intolerant to conventional cow's milk-based formula. Although some individuals who are milk allergic and have urticaria can use a soy-based formula substitute, any child with a gastrointestinal problem should be given a casein protein hydrolysate infant formula. Table 8 lists the substitute infant formulas available commercially in the United States for milk allergy. Nutramigen™ or Alimentum™ is usually preferable to Pregestimil™ in the United States. An elemental amino acid formula should be tried in the few infants who are very

Table 8
Commercial Substitute Infant Formulas for Milk-Allergic and -Intolerant Children

Cow's milk-based
  Casein protein hydrolysate
    Nutramigen[a]
    Progestamil[a]
    Alimentum[b]
  Whey hydrolysate
    Carnation Good Start[c]
  Soy protein-based
    Numerous, such as Isomil,[a] ProSoyBee[b]
  Elemental amino acid-based
    Neocate[d]

[a]Mead Johnson, Evansville, IN 47721.
[b]Ross Lab., Columbus, OH 43216.
[c]Clintec Nutrition Co., Deerfield, IL 60015.
[d]Scientific Hospital Supplies, Inc., Gaithersburg, MD 20877.

sensitive to cow's milk protein and cannot tolerate a protein hydrolysate formula. The only one on the US market that is designed for infants is Neocate™.

Prevention of allergy has been attempted in infants born to allergic parents by the use of special diets. Studies have compared the use of

1. Dietary restriction in the mother in the last trimester (of a diet devoid of allergy-type foods);
2. breast feeding; or
3. casein hydrolysate formula feeding in the infant; and
4. avoidance of allergic-type solid food in the infant for 1 yr to conventional formula feeding.

The results of these investigations demonstrate that the specially fed infants had less food-related allergy symptoms for the first 2 yr of life than infants who were fed conventional diets. However, at 2 yr and later in children, there were no differences in the respiratory allergic symptoms between the two groups.

The whey hydrolysate formula, Carnation GoodStart™, instead of conventional cow's milk formula, is not a good substitute for individuals proven to be allergic to cow's milk, since serious reactions may occur. The use of this formula, however, has been shown to be less likely to result in clinical allergy than the use of conventional cow's milk infant formula. Therefore, this type of feeding as an alternative to prolonged breast feeding (9 mo) is a suitable preventive measure in an infant born to allergic parents to reduce possible food allergy symptoms in the first 2 yr of life (Table 8).

SUGGESTED READING

Anderson J. Milestones marking the knowledge of adverse reactions to foods in the decade of the 1980s. *Ann Allergy Asthma Immunol* 1994;72:143–154.

Anderson J. Tips when considering the diagnosis of food allergy. *Top Clin Nutr* 1994;9:11–21.

Anderson JA. Allergic reactions to food. In: Clydesdale, FM, ed. *Critical Reviews in Food Science and Nutrition*, Allergenicity of foods produced by genetic modification (suppl.) 1996;36:519–38.

Bock SA. Prospective appraisal of complaints of adverse reactions to foods in children during the first three years of life. *Pediatrics* 1987;79:683–688.

Bock SA, Adkins FM. The natural history of peanut allergy. *J Allergy Clin Immunol* 1989;83:900–904.

Bock SA, Sampson HA, Adkins FM, et al. Double-blind, placebo-controlled food challenge (DBPCFC) as an office procedure. A. Manual. *J Allergy Clin Immunol* 1988;82:986–997.

Metcalfe D, Sampson H, Simon R., eds. *Food Allergy—Adverse Reactions to Foods and Food Additives.* Oxford, England, Blackwell Scientific, 1991; pp. 1–418.

Perkin J, ed. Food Allergies and Adverse Reactions, Gaithersburg, MD; Aspen, 1990, pp. 1–288.

Sampson HA, Albergo R. Comparison of results of skin test, RAST, and double-blind, placebo-controlled food challenge in children with atopic dermatitis. *J Allergy Clin Immunol* 1984;74:23–26.

Sampson HA, Metcalfe DD. Food Allergies. *JAMA* 1992;268:2840–2844.

Sampson HA, Mendelson L, Rosen J. Fatal and near-fatal anaphylactic reactions to foods in children and adolescents. *N Engl J Med* 1992;327:380–384.

Sampson HA. Food allergy. *JAMA* 1997;278:1888–1894.

Sampson HA, Anderson JA, eds. Workshop proceedings: Classification of gastrointestinal disease of infants and children due to adverse immunologic reactions. *J of Ped Gastroenterol and Nutrition*; 200:30(suppl 1):S1–S96.

Sicherer SH, Sampson HA. Cow's milk protein-specific IgE concentrations in two age groups of milk-allergic children and in children achieving clinical tolerance. *Clin Exp Allergy* 1999;29:507–512.

Yocum MW, Khan DA. Assessment of patients who have experienced anaphylaxis: A 3-year survey. *Mayo Clin Proc* 1994;69:16–23.

16 Allergic and Allergic-Like Reactions to Drugs and Other Therapeutic Agents

John A. Anderson, MD

CONTENTS

INTRODUCTION

Definition

Drug allergy is a common term often used to depict any unexpected and unwanted event or effect that occurs when an individual is taking a specific drug or therapeutic agent. A better, overall term to describe these circumstances would be an adverse reaction to a drug (Table 1).

These reactions can be further classified into either drug allergy (reactions due to an immunological mechanism) or drug intolerance (reactions due to nonimmunological or unknown mechanisms). Some reactions closely resemble allergic reactions and are termed allergic-like or pseudo-allergic. This includes anaphylactoid reactions that clinically resemble anaphylaxis, since in both situations, chemical mediator release or activation is responsible for these symptoms. Some idiosyncratic reactions to drugs can be confused with drug allergy.

From: *Current Clinical Practice: Allergic Diseases: Diagnosis and Treatment, 2nd Edition*
Edited by: P. Lieberman and J. Anderson © Humana Press Inc., Totowa, NJ

Table 1
Definition of Terms Used to Describe Adverse Reactions to Drugs and Therapeutics

Drug allergy: drug reactions resulting from an immunological mechanism
Drug intolerance: adverse reaction to drugs resulting from nonimmunological or unknown
  mechanisms
  Drug overdose: toxic reaction owing to excess drug dose or impaired excretion
  Side effect to a drug: unavoidable secondary pharmacological action of a drug
  Drug interactions: actions of two or more drugs on the toxicity or effects of each
    individual agent
  Idiosyncratic drug reaction: a measurable, abnormal response to a drug that differs
    from its pharmaceutical effect
Other terms used to describe allergic/intolerant reactions
  Allergic-like or pseudo-allergic reactions to drugs: drug reactions that clinically
    resemble those of drug allergy; the mechanism usually involves clinical mediators
    or activators, enzyme inhibition, or may be unknown
  Anaphylaxis and anaphylactoid reactions to drugs: generalized drug reactions owing to
    chemical mediator release/activation either involving IgE (anaphylaxis) or direct action
    of the drug on the mast cell (anaphylactoid)

Classification

Because of the different mechanisms involved in adverse reactions, it is impossible to classify all reactions to drugs and therapeutic agents under one heading. Table 2 classifies adverse reactions to these agents under four categories: generalized, immunological, organ specific and allergic-like reactions. A specific drug reaction may be classified under more than one category.

Incidence

The exact incidence of all types of adverse reactions to drugs and therapeutic agents is unknown. However, it is estimated that 1–2 million individuals in the United States experience a drug reaction each year. The most frequent manifestation of a drug reaction is a skin rash. Reports indicate that 2% of adult medical admissions each year to a community hospital are the result of drug reactions. Studies involving adults admitted to either medical or surgical wards in tertiary care hospitals demonstrate a yearly serious adverse reaction rate of 6.7%. The overall proportion of both serious and nonserious adverse resctions was 23.8% . Most drug reactions involve nonimmune or unknown mechanisms and are thus defined broadly as drug intolerances, not drug allergies (*see* Table 1).

In the case of two types of drug reactions, penicillin and other β-lactams as well as conventional radiocontrast media (RCM), the incidence of allergic and allergic-like reactions has been calculated. The risk of developing an allergic reaction, usually a rash, to a single course of penicillin is 2%, and to cephalosporin it is 2–3%. The risk of developing anaphylaxis to penicillin is no more than 0.04% (1/2500 courses of the drug), but it is rare to have such a reaction with a third-generation cephalosporin. Fatalities to penicillin are unusual. The risk ranges between 0.0015 and 0.002% (1 death/50,000–75,000 courses of the drug).

The overall reaction rate to conventional RCM (hypermolarity) has been reported in a review of 10,000 consecutive intravenous pyelogram (IVP) procedures to be 1.7%.

Table 2
Classification of Different Manifestations of Adverse Reactions to Drugs or Therapeutics[a]

Generalized reactions
    Mast cell–derived mediator reactions
        Systemic anaphylaxis and anaphylactoid reactions
        Generalized urticaria and angioedema
    Serum sickness-like reactions
    Drug fever
    Drug-induced vasculitis
    Drug related lupus
    Stevens-Johnson/toxic epidermal necrolyis
    Anticonvulsant drug hypersensitivity syndrome

Immunological reactions
    Type I: IgE-antibody–mediated (e.g., β-lactam antibiotics, insulin urticaria or anaphylaxis)
    Type II: antitissue cytotoxic antibodies (e.g., drug-induced hemolytic anemia
        or thromocytopenia)
    Type III: antigen-antibody immune complex involving complement reactions (e.g., serum
        sickness-like drug reactions)
    Type IV: cell-mediated hypersensitivity (e.g., neomycin contact dermatitis)

Organ-specific drug reactions
    Skin (e.g., pruritus, maculopapular, morbilliform and erythemic rashes, urticaria/
        angioedema, erthema multiforme, fixed drug eruptions, phototoxic and photoallergic
        reactions)
    Blood (e.g., drug-induced hemolytic anemia, thrombocytopenia)
    Liver (e.g., hepatitis)
    Lung (e.g., fibrosis)
    Kidney (e.g., nephritis)

Pseudo-allergic (allergic-like) reactions
    Ampicillin/amoxicillin rash
    RCM reactions
    Reactions to aspirin and nonsteroidal anti-inflammatory agents
    Reactions to enzyme inhibitors (e.g., ACE inhibitor–induced angioedema)
    Reactions involving histamine release (e.g. vancomycin red man syndrome)

[a]A specific drug reaction may be classified under more than one category.

The frequency of fatalities has been reported to be 1/50,000 IVP procedures. Overall reaction rates to lower-molarity RCM have been less than conventional high-molarity material and have been reported to be approx 2%. Serious reactions to RCM that require subsequent hospitalizations are estimated to be 1/2900 conventional RCM infusions and 1/8400 infusions with the low-molarity RCM. Death from conventional RCM is reported to be 1/10,900, but rare with low-molarity RCM use (1/165,00–500,000 procedures).

Factors that Influence Incidence

Table 3 lists important factors that may influence the likelihood of an adverse reaction during the use of a drug or therapeutic agent. Some drugs are more likely to be involved

Table 3
Factors Influencing the Frequency of Adverse Reactions
to Drugs and Therapeutic Agents

Drug type	Familial history of reactions
Degree of drug exposure	Atopy
Routes of administration	Viral infections
Age and sex	Concomitant drug use

in reactions than others. Antibiotics, especially β-lactams and sulfonamides, followed by aspirin and nonsteroidal anti-inflammatory drugs (NSAIDs) and central nervous system (CNS) depressants, are most commonly involved in these serious reactions. The β-lactam antibiotics, trimethoprim sulfamethoxazole (TMP-SMX) and whole blood are most likely to be involved in skin rashes, the most common manifestation of adverse reactions. Minor drug reactions (e.g., nausea) are more often involved with narcotic use, antibiotics and cardiovascular drugs.

Allergic sensitization to drugs is more likely to occur after multiple, intermittent courses of a drug than with continuous administration of that drug. All types of reactions to medicine occur more often when patients are treated with multiple agents than with single agents. Allergic drug sensitization is least likely to occur with oral administration. Topical application of drugs/chemicals favors contact sensitization. Once sensitization has occurred, however, elicitation of a drug reaction upon re-exposure to that drug may occur by any route, but the oral route is the safest, and the intramuscular route (im) is more risky than the intravenous (iv) route.

There are probably less adverse drug reactions in children and the elderly. Drug-induced skin rashes are reported to be one-third higher in females. Individuals who have a severe reaction to one drug (e.g., β-lactam antibiotics) may be at increased risk for reactions to other antibiotics. Children of parents with a confirmed reaction to a β-lactam antibiotic have more risk than the general population to develop an allergic reaction to β-lactam antibiotics. Although being "allergic" or atopic does not increase the risk of development of an allergy to β-lactam antibiotics, it may increase the risk of having an anaphylactoid reaction to RCM exposure.

A maculopapular (toxic) rash due to amoxicillin/ampicillin is more likely to occur when the patient treated with this drug has an Epstein-Barr virus infection (acute infectious mononucleosis). Both drug allergies (e.g., to β-lactam antibiotics) and drug intolerance reactions (e.g., systemic or skin reactions to many types of therapeutic agents) are more likely to occur in patients afflicted with the human immunodeficiency virus (HIV) than HIV-seronegative individuals. The risk of drug reactions increases with the degree of immunosuppression. The presence of other viral infections and altered drug metabolism because of chronic disease may also be an important factor effect in risk. Concomitant administration of β-lactam adrenergic agents with other drugs increases the risk of anaphylaxis in the case of β-lactam antibiotic use, and of serious anaphylactoid reactions in the case of RCM use. Concomitant use of ACE-inhibitor agents with other drugs may also increase the risk of a serious anaphylactic or anaphylactoid reaction.

Overview of Adverse Drug Reactions

- Most reactions do not involve immune events.
- A skin rash is the most common type of drug reaction.
- Most drug reactions occur in adult females and those individuals who are frequently intermittently exposed to multiple medications.
- More allergic drug reactions occur to β-lactam antibiotics than to other antibiotics.
- Reactions to RCM and aspirin/nonsteroidal anti-inflammatory agents are frequent causes of allergic-like or nonimmunological reactions.

MECHANISMS OF ALLERGIC AND ALLERGIC-LIKE REACTIONS DRUGS AND THERAPEUTICS

The exact mechanism involved in most reactions to drugs and therapeutic agents is unknown. Fully 90% of adverse reactions fall into the drug intolerance group. Of those reactions that are classified as a drug allergy, the best-studied reactions are those to β-lactam antibiotics, particularly penicillin and insulin.

β-*Lactam Antibiotics*

β-lactam antibiotics include the penicillins, cephalosporins, carbapenems and monobactams. These drugs have a common β-lactam ring chemical structure (Fig. 1). In the human body, penicillin is metabolized to form various products (Fig. 2). Most of the parent drug is broken down into penicilloyl, which readily combines with a carrier protein to become a complete antigen. This is called the major determinant (most common metabolic by-product). The remainder of penicillin stays either in its native state or is metabolized to other chemical structures. such as penicilloate. These agents, coupled with a protein, are referred to as minor determinants (less common metabolic by-products).

The ease by which these penicillin metabolites and the parent penicillin couple to tissue proteins is believed to be important regarding why these drugs are so often involved in allergic reactions and other drugs are not.

In individuals who have become allergic to penicillin, most develop type I (*see* Table 2) IgE-specific reactions to the major determinants alone or in combination with sensitization with the minor determinant—not sensitization to the minor determinants alone. In individuals sensitized to the major determinant, urticarial rash is the usual manifestation. In individuals sensitized to the minor determinant, specific systemic anaphylaxis is more of a risk.

Penicillin and other β-lactam antibiotics may also be responsible for a type II or type III immune reaction (Table 2). Immune hemolytic anemia can result from the binding of the drug or its metabolites to the surface of a red cell, followed by a specific antibody-mediated cytotoxic reaction that is directed against the drug antigen

BETA LACTAM CHEMICAL STRUCTURES

```
  -    CH – CH–
         |    |
        CO – N –
```

Beta Lactam Ring

```
                      S
                    /   \
R₁ – CO – NH –   CH – CH     C (CH₃)₂
                 |    |       |
                CO – N  —  C COOH
```

Basic Penicillin

```
                      S
                    /   \
R₁ – CO – NH –   CH – CH     CH₂
                 |    |       |
                CO – N       C – CH₂ – R₂
                      \     /
                        C
                      COOH
```

Basic Cephalosporin   Fig. 1. β-Lactam chemical structures.

or at the cell membrane component altered by the drug. This reaction and immune thrombocytopenia may occur with other drugs as well.

In type III immune reactions, soluble immune complexes are responsible for the syndrome of serum sickness. Although originally this term depicted reactions to "horse serum," penicillin and other β-lactams as well as other drugs can react in a serum sickness-like fashion. Clinically, events are characterized by fever and a rash that includes a papular urticaria and/or urticaria, lymphadenopathy and arthralgia, which occur 2–4 wk after the beginning of the drug therapy. At this point, drug and drug antibody immune complexes are in slight antigen excess, and the complement system is activated. Clinical symptoms of serum sickness begin to subside when the drug/metabolites are eliminated from the body by the reticuloendothelial system.

Insulin

Human insulin has a mol wt of approximately 6000, and its amino acid sequence differs from pork insulin by only one amino acid and beef insulin by three amino acids. Animal-derived insulins make up the majority of replacement insulins used today in the United States. Insulin is a potent antigen. Approximately 40% of patients receiving bovine/porcine insulin therapy develop IgE antibodies. These antibodies are almost always directed against the insulin molecule itself, even though animal-derived insulin

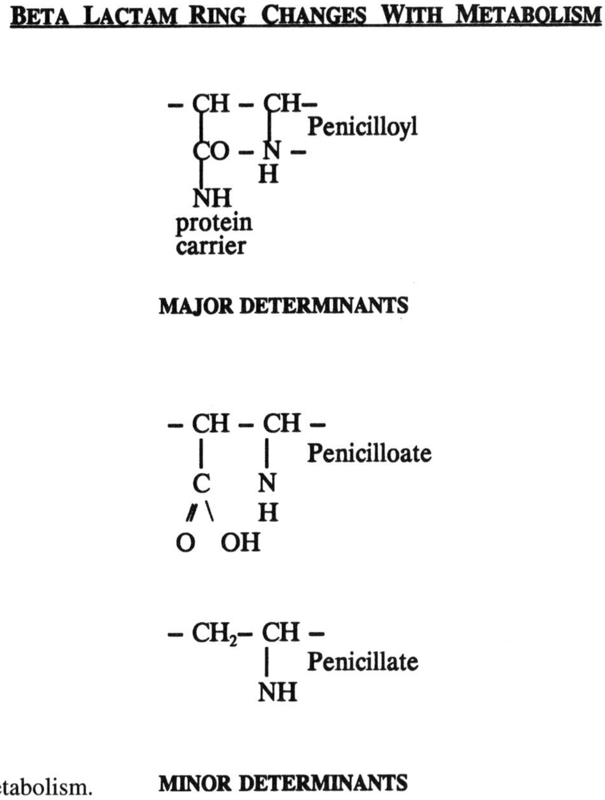

BETA LACTAM RING CHANGES WITH METABOLISM

$$- \text{CH} - \text{CH}-$$
$$\quad | \qquad | \quad \text{Penicilloyl}$$
$$\text{CO} - \text{N} -$$
$$\qquad \quad \text{H}$$
$$\text{NH}$$
protein
carrier

MAJOR DETERMINANTS

$$- \text{CH} - \text{CH} -$$
$$\quad | \qquad | \quad \text{Penicilloate}$$
$$\quad \text{C} \qquad \text{N}$$
$$\quad \text{// \textbackslash} \quad \text{H}$$
$$\text{O} \quad \text{OH}$$

$$- \text{CH}_2 - \text{CH} -$$
$$\qquad \quad | \quad \text{Penicillate}$$
$$\qquad \text{NH}$$

Fig. 2. β-Lactam ring changes with metabolism.   **MINOR DETERMINANTS**

contains other proteins that may stimulate an immune reaction. These individuals will have positive IgE allergy skin tests to insulin. Only 5%, however, will have severe enough local reactions at the injection site to be clinically relevant, and very few (0.1–0.2%) will be expected to develop systemic anaphylaxis to insulin.

Radiocontrast Media

The imaging efficacy of RCM depends upon the iodine concentration that can be delivered to a space within the body. Since RCM was first discovered in 1923, the character of the iodinated compound has progressed from a monoiodinated to a tri-iodinated benzoic acid compound. The conventional RCM is hypertonic, having osmolarity up to six times that of plasma. A newer, nonionic RCM has been developed that has an osmolarity <50% of the conventional material and retains the same iodine concentration. This change in osmolarity of the newer RCM material has reduced the vascular wall toxicity and allergic-like reactions with the use of these agents, presumably by reducing the capacity of the newer agent to form bonds with body proteins.

The exact mechanism by which RCM elicits an anaphylactoid reaction is unknown. However, in vitro histamine release does occur, probably through direct interaction between RCM and a cell membrane receptor. Unfortunately, there is no consistent documented relationship between histamine release by these agents and clinical adverse events.

RCM can activate the complement system. Conventional RCM has been shown to have a direct effect on C3 and C4 to produce C3b and C4b anaphylatoxins (which in turn can cause histamine release). The newer low-osmolarity RCM has been shown to activate complement through the alternate pathway by inhibition of factors H and I. The exact role activation of complement by either conventional or the newer RCM agents plays in the production of an anaphylactoid reaction is still speculative.

Mechanisms of Other Drugs Involved in Allergic-like Reactions

Aspirin and NSAIDs may both cause or excerbate urticaria/angioedema and anaphylactoid reactions. These drugs are responsible for a syndrome consisting of perennial rhinitis, sinusitis, nasal polyps and severe asthma. Current studies indicate an important role for increased leukotriene production (especially LTC_4, LTD_4 and LTE_4), kininogens and histamine release in these allergic-like reactions.

Vancomycin antibiotic iv infusion has been responsible for generalized flushing, the so-called red-man syndrome. The mechanism of reaction in this case is thought to be related to direct toxic release of histamine from mast cells/ basophils. Rare cases of vancomycin-IgE–antibody-induced anaphylaxis have been reported. Angiotensin-converting enzyme (ACE) inhibitors are now commonly used antihypertensive agents. These agents have been associated with both a cough and angioedema (anaphylactoid reactions) in different groups of patients. Although the mechanism of these reactionss is not entirely clear, increased histamine release, inhibition of bradykinin degradation, and abnormal prostaglandin and substance P metabolism are suspected.

Blood products and protamine sulfate (fish-derived protein), which is a component of some insulin preparations and is an anticoagulant, may result in anaphylactoid reactions through activation of the complement system and release of anaphylatoxins (C3a and C4a). Drug-induced vasculitis is often associated with c-ANCA* or p-ANCA† positive reactions. Cell-mediated immune reactions similar to graft vs host are suspected, but not proven, in drug-associated febrile mucocutantious reactions Stevens-Johnson Syndrome/toxic epidermal necrolysis (SJS/TEN)

SIGNS AND SYMPTOMS

Generalized Reaction

Anaphylaxis and anaphylactoid reactions to drugs and other therapeutic agents have the same signs and symptoms of reactions as other agents that frequently cause allergic reactions (e.g., insect stings, foods, natural rubber latex). Reactions range in severity from mild pruritus, skin erythema and urticaria/angioedema to more generalized and systemic reactions of laryngeal edema, rhinitis/conjunctivitis, asthma, shock and possibly death. IgE sensitization is involved with the following drug reactions: β-lactam antibiotics, insulins, protamine, blood products, chymopapain, vaccines, natural rubber latex used in drug delivery systems, ethylene oxide used to clean dialysis agents or neuromuscular agents used in anesthesia induction. Anaphylactoid reactions may occur to RCM, ASA, NSAIDs, ACE inhibitors, vancomycin, protamine and blood products.

---

*Antineutrophil cytoplasmic antibodies with a granular cytoplasmic pattern.

†Antineutrophil cytoplasmic antibodies with a perinuclear pattern.

Urticaria and Drug Reactions

- Severe urticaria may be a manifestation of cutaneous (mild) anaphylaxis/or anaphylactoid reactions.
- Urticaria is suggestive, but not diagnostic, or an allergic etiology.
- Urticaria may be caused by other factors, such as viral infections.
- A drug-induced skin rash that does not include urticaria does not rule out immunological involvement.

Other generalized allergic-like drug reactions (Table 2) include serum sickness, in which the symptoms begin 7–21 d into drug therapy. These drug-induced serum sickness-like reactions are characterized by fever, malaise, urticaria, arthralgia and lymphadenopathy. Reactions occur not only to blood products, but to β-lactam antibiotics, sulfonamides, thiouracil, cholecystographic dyes, hydantoin, aspirin and streptomycin as well as to other agents.

Isolated drug fever typically occurs between day 7 and 10 of therapy and may occur with many drugs, especially antibiotics and blood products. Drug-induced lupus erythematosus (DLE) is usually characterized by mild fever, malaise and arthralgias. Butterfly rashes on the face, renal and CNS involvement and Raynaud's phenomenon are less common in the drug form than in the idiopathic systemic form of the disease (SLE). The drugs usually involved with this condition include procainamide, hydralazine, isoniazid, chlorpromazine and hydantoin. The signs and symptoms usually improve or decrease with discontinuation of the specific drug involved. Drug-induced vasculitis may occur with hydralazine, antithyroid medications or penicillamine. The anticovulsant drug hypersensitivity syndrome is characterized by fever, facial edema, maculopapular rash and generlized lymphadenopathy. This syndrome may be induced by phenytoin, carbamazepine and phenobarbitol.

Skin Reactions

Isolated skin lesions due to drugs are the most common adverse symptoms of drug reactions. Almost any type of manifestation can occur (see Table 2). However, a maculopapular/morbilliform rash is the most frequent, followed by urticaria in allergic or allergic-like reactions. Usually, drug reactions are symmetrical and begin in the extremities in the ambulatory patient or on the back in bedridden patients. The ampicillin/amoxicillin rash typically occurs on the knees and elbows first, before spreading over the body. Urticaria/angioedema occurs with all types of reactions, including drug allergy, drug intolerance and infections. A fixed drug eruption is a rare localized patch of eczema that reappears at the same site with repetitive drug treatment. Many drugs can be involved, but the reaction is more commonly associated with phenobarbital or antibiotic treatments.

Phototoxic (sunburn-like) rash may occur with short-term sun exposure while patients are taking drugs such as doxycycline or chlorpromazine. Prolonged sun exposure may produce a photoallergic (urticarial or eczema) rash in individuals taking drugs such as griseofulvin, psoralens and sulfonamides.

Erythema multiforme (EM minor) "target" skin lesions as well as the combination of EM (major) fever, toxicity and ulceration of the mucous membrane (SJS) or sloughing

---

Febrile Mucocutaneous Reactions

- Includes Stevens-Johnson syndrome (SJS) and toxic epidermal necrolysis (TEN)
- Syndrome consists of fever, erythema multiforme rash and ulceration of two or more mucous membranes, plus with TEN, skin sloughing
- SJS and TEN are frequently drug associated; however, these reactions may be precipitated by viral infections and other unknown events
- If drug-associated, repeat exposure to the same drug is contraindicated

---

of the skin (TEN) may be both drug- and viral-infection associated. Cell–mediated immune events have been suspected but not proven in these febrile mucocutaneous reactions. EM minor is a mild condition, and the mortality in SJS is low. The mortality in TEN, however, may be as high as 30%, especially in the elderly. Drugs that have been repeatedly involved include the sulfonamides (especially TMP-SMX), seizure medications and β-lactams antibiotics. Drugs that have been associated with EM minor or systemic reactions (e.g., SJS or TEN) should be strictly avoided, since re-exposure may be associated with a more serious reaction.

Signs and Symptoms of Other Organ-Specific Reactions

Type II immune reactions (*see* Table 2) to drugs such as β-lactam antibiotics may result in a hemolytic anemia, usually 7 d after beginning therapy. Quinine, quinidine and heparin have been involved in immune thrombocytopenic-type reactions. Hepatitis has been shown to occur with several drugs, including sulfonamides, phenytoin and halothane. Methicillin as well as sulfonamides have been involved in producing interstitial nephritis in rare patients. Phenytoin and gold have been involved in reactions characterized by systemic eosinophilia and pneumonitis. Recently, the Churg-Strauss syndrome, a systemic, eosinophilc-granulomatosis and vasculitic process involving asthmatics, has been reported in increasing numbers of patients receiving leukotriene antagonists, glucocorticosteroids, and macrolide antibiotics.

GENERAL APPROACH TO THE DIAGNOSIS AND MANAGEMENT OF ALLERGIC AND ALLERGIC-LIKE REACTIONS TO DRUGS AND THERAPEUTICS

Initial Measures

Initially, when an adverse drug reaction is suspected, especially when associated with significant symptoms, the drug should be discontinued (Table 4). Any treatable signs and symptoms should then be promptly attended to. Simple pruritus and urticaria with or without angioedema will usually improve with an antihistamine (e.g., 10–25 mg of hydroxyzine (Atarax) or 25–50 mg of diphenhydramine (Benadryl) 2–4 times daily). Initially, aqueous Adrenalin 1:1000, 0.1–0.3 mL subcutaneously followed by Sus-

Table 4
General Approach to Diagnosis and Management of Allergic Drug Reactions

Initial measures
1. Discontinue suspected medication
2. Treat reaction
3. Draw blood for possible confirmation of etiology in select situations (e.g., tryptase in anaphylaxis/anaphylactoid reactions; complement assay (C) levels in serum sickness, Coombs' test in hemolytic anemia)
4. Substitute appropriate medication whenever possible
5. In very select cases and when appropriate, desensitize with original medication if no substitute is available (e.g., β-lactam, insulin, TMP-SMX, ASA)

Follow-up measures
Skin test in case of drug allergy (e.g., β-lactam antibiotics,[a] insulin, papain[a], and latex)
Skin test/subcutaneous drug challenge (local anesthetics)
Oral sequential challenge under controlled conditions (nonanaphylactic conditions)
Strict avoidance based on presumptive diagnosis
Preventive measures for inadvertent exposure in serious situations (e.g., Medic Alert, EpiPen auto-injector)

[a]In vitro tests available to some degree.

Phrine 1:200 0.05–0.15 mL subcutaneously will help the pruritus and the acute rash in an office or emergency room situation. Treatment of acute systemic anaphylaxis or anaphylactoid reactions from any cause is outlined in Chapter 5.

There are few (if any) absolute confirmatory tests available initially when an adverse reaction involves mediator release, is to a drug is suspected.. Diagnosis is usually, therefore, presumptive. Management is important in spite of this fact (e.g., drug discontinuation, treatment of signs and symptoms of the reaction, substitution of another drug if necessary).

One test (if positive) that can help confirm the fact that the reaction involves mediator release is an in vitro mast cell tryptase blood test. In severe cases of systemic anaphylaxis/anaphylactoid reactions, tryptase is released along with other mast cell chemical mediators. This enzyme remains increased in the bloodstream for several hours after the event, thus allowing the possibility of confirming a mast cell degranulation (and histamine and other mediator involvement) in the reaction at the time that the patient is seen in the office or emergency room for the acute symptoms.

When serum sickness is suspected, the complement system is usually activated and low serum levels of C3, C4, and possibly CH100 (total hemolytic complement assay at 100%), may, in retrospect, help confirm the suspicion of this condition. In cases of hemolytic anemia, a positive Coombs' test will help confirm the immune nature of this condition.

In almost all cases, the drug or therapeutic agent presumed to be responsible for the adverse reaction can be avoided, and a substitute medication should be available to treat the primary condition. Occasionally, this is not possible if the primary condition is serious and the offending drug is important to therapy. In some of these cases, medication pretreatment (RCM), graded oral drug challenge or drug desensitization may be necessary.

Follow-up Measures

Elective immediate reacting allergy skin testing is usually available only in the case of β-lactam antibiotic sensitivity and insulin sensitivity and with reactions to natural rubber latex. It is available experimentally for papain sensitivity and suspected sensitivity to neuromuscular blocking agents. In vitro blood/serum assays are available only for latex, β-lactam antibiotics (penicillin major determinant only) and papain (experimental). These in vitro assays are helpful only if positive. A negative test does not rule out sensitivity. At one time, in vitro cell–mediated drug lymphocyte transformation testing was available in some experimental laboratories. There is little or no current evidence regarding the value of this type of drug reaction testing.

In cases of suspected local anesthetic reactions, a well-studied protocol consisting of skin testing followed by a graded sc injection challenge helps confirm the safety of local anesthetics for subsequent use.

In some cases, when adverse symptoms are minor (maculopapular rash to an antibiotic that is usually not associated with systemic anaphylaxis or anaphylactoid reactions), a graded oral challenge may be done on an outpatient basis. When done, however, it should be done under controlled conditions in which the physician is prepared to manage the possibility of a serious reaction (e.g., systemic anaphylaxis). Usually the total amount challenged under these conditions is approximately the amount of a usual single dose (e.g., 250 mg of an antibiotic). The patient should wait for 2 h following challenge before going home. Usually, it is advisable to avoid starting therapeutic doses of the antibiotic until the next day (12–24 h) after challenge, providing no adverse reaction occurs during the interval. Table 5 is an example of a graded oral drug challenge protocol that can serve as a guide for specialists managing drug reactions.

In most cases, after a presumptive diagnosis of drug allergy or intolerance has been made, the individual is advised to avoid these medications. In some cases of reactions to drugs, drug desensitization is possible and necessary. In the case of anaphylaxis/anaphylactoid reactions and other serious systemic events (e.g., SJS or TEN), re-exposure to the medication is not advised.

In situations in which there is documented life-threatening drug reactions (e.g., systemic anaphylaxis) and inadvertent re-exposure is a risk, the patient should be advised to carry an EpiPen (0.3 mg epinephrine) auto-injector (Center Lab, Port Washington, NY). If the patient is below 6 yr of age, an EpiPen Jr (0.15 mg epinephrine) autoinjector is advised. In these cases, Medic Alert jewelry (Turlock, CA (800) 642-0045) is also advised (*see* Chapter 5).

DIAGNOSIS AND MANAGEMENT OF SELECTED ALLERGIC AND ALLERGIC-LIKE DRUG REACTIONS

β-*Lactam Antibiotics*

In patients with a history of an allergic reaction to penicillin or other β-lactam antibiotics, penicillin skin testing should be done electively. Only 20% of adults and 10% of children with this diagnosis turn out to be actually allergic based on allergy skin testing (the positive penicillin allergy skin test rate is higher in the first year after a reaction). There are three reasons why the true allergy rates are low in individuals labeled allergic to penicillin.

Table 5
Graded Oral Drug Challenge Protocol

Time (MIN)[a]	Challenge dose (mg/mL) [b]	
	Child	Adult
Initial[c]	1.25/0.005	2.5/0.1
20–30	5/0.2	10/0.4
40–60	25/1.0	50/2.0
60–90	50/2.0	100/4.0
80–120	75/3.0	150/6.0
Total Dose	156.25 mg	312.5 mg

[a] Time inteval should be increased in a clinically sensitive patient
[b] Stock drug conc.: 125 mg/5 mL.
[c] Initial dose should be no more than 1/100 of the anticipated therapeutic dose or no more than 0.1 mg in a clinically sensitive patient.

1. In many cases, the original reaction, usually a rash, is a result of an infection (usually viral) rather than the antibiotic used to treat that infection.
2. In cases of true penicillin allergy, the reaction rate dissipates about 10%/yr.
3. In children, toxic (nonallergic) maculopapular rash to ampicillin/amoxicillin and to some cephalosporins like Ceclor, are common (5% of antibiotic therapies).

In most cases, it is advisable to refer the suspected penicillin-allergic patient to an allergist/immunologist specialist for evaluation of the condition. Table 6 lists the penicillin skin tests based on commonly available agents. Penicilloyl polylysine is an example of the major breakdown product of penicillin drug metabolism coupled to a carrier protein. This test reagent is responsible for positive skin tests in patients with an isolated skin rash (especially urticaria, or urticaria and angioedema). Penicillin G is the parent drug. A positive skin test to penicillin G correlates with all types of allergic reactions. A positive minor determinant mixture skin test (minor or secondary penicillin metabolites) (*see* Fig. 2) correlates best with more serious life-threatening, systemic anaphylaxis, penicillin reactions. Unfortunately, this latter skin test reagent is not available commercially, but is available in many allergist/immunologist offices. The positive predictive value of skin testing to assess the future risk for allergic reactions to β-lactam antibiotics using only Pre-Pen and PenG is unclear. Skin test reactions to the Pen-minor determinant mix in studies range from 7–20%. The overall reliability of testing with these basic agents plus the minor determinant mixture is estimated to be between 92 and 99%. In the latter situation, if the skin test is negative, therefore, there is a 1–8% chance of a minor skin rash if the drug is given.

Penicillin skin testing also tests for other penicillin and cephalosporin antibiotics, since the penicillin skin test measures reactions to the β-lactam ring that is common to all of these agents (*see* Fig. 1). The overall crossreactivity rate between penicillin allergy and cephalosporin allergy is estimated tp be 3% (3rd generation) to 10% (1st generation). However, if the penicillin skin tests are positive, β-lactam antibiotics should be avoided, since any one individual is 100% at risk.

In cases in which the skin test results are equivocal, or the history of the prior reaction is severe but the skin tests are negative, a graded challenge with a single usual oral dose of the β-lactam antibiotic in question under controlled conditions followed

---

Penicillin Allergy Skin Tests

- β-lactams are the only type of antimicrobial agents in which a suspected reaction (allergic) can be verified by skin tests (reliability up to 96–99%).
- Of those patients with a history of a prior reaction, only 20% of adults and 10% of children have been found to be skin-test-positive.
- Positive skin test to penicilloyl-polylysine (Pre-Pen) correlates best with urticarial reactions; positive skin test to penicillin "minor determinant mix" correlates with anaphylaxis.
- Skin testing with penicillin G metabolites, alone, is usually a measure of potential clinical reactions to the β-lactam ring in amoxicillin and cephalosporins.

---

by a 2+ h wait is advisable (*see* General Approach to Diagnosis and Management and Table 4).

In cases in which the individual is found to be allergic (history of reaction positive, confirmed by skin test and/or challenge), all β-lactam antibiotics should be avoided. Usually substitute medications are used to treat subsequent infections, particularly the sulfonamides, erythromycin and clarithromycin (Biaxin, Abbott Laboratories, North Chicago, IL).

In select cases in which individuals who are proven β-lactam-antibiotic-allergic and need a β-lactam antibiotic (life-threatening or other serious infections without suitable substitutes available), then penicillin or the appropriate β-lactam antibiotic desensitization may be indicated. In these cases, it is advisable to consult an allergist/immunologist specialist.

Table 7 is an example of an oral penicillin desensitization protocol that can be used as a protocol for desensitization with penicillin and other β-lactam antibiotics. This procedure should be done only in the hospital under controlled conditions, such as an intensive care unit with a doctor present during the entire procedure. Each individual case is different, and published protocols are only guides to the procedure.

The oral route is felt to be safest, but the iv route may be preferable in some cases. Studies have shown that reactions during the procedure should be expected approximately 30% of the time. When these occur, the patient should be treated appropriately and stabilized before restarting the desensitization procedure. The next desensitizing dose should be less than the one producing the reaction.

Once the procedure is complete, the patient is usually maintained at a full treatment dose of the medication until the therapy is complete. Once the drug has been stopped for 12–24 h, the patient should be considered to have reverted to his previous sensitized (allergic) state.

Sulfonamides and Other Antibiotics

Reactions to sulfonamides (particularly rashes) are common in the general US population. There is marked accentuation of these rates in the patient with HIV infection. In particular, with TMP-SMX, which is frequently used for the treatment

Table 6
Penicillin Skin Testing

Reagent	Type of test	Dose
Penicilloyl-polylsine (Pre-Pen) [a] test strength	Prick/scratch/puncture (intradermal)	1 drop 0.02 mL
Penicillin G, 10,000 U/mL[b]	Prick/scratch/puncture (intradermal)	1 drop 0.02 mL
Penicillin—minor determinant mixture	Not commercially available in the US	

[a]Schwartz Pharma, Kremers Urban Co., Milwaukee, WI.
[b]Serial dilutions (10, 100, 1000 U/mL) advisable in very sensitive individuals.

Table 7
Oral Penicillin Desensitization Protocol

Desensitization dose[a]	Stock drug, 250 mg/5 mL concentration	Oral dose[a]	
		mL	mg
1	0.5 mg/mL	0.05	0.0025
2		0.10	0.05
3		0.20	0.10
4		0.40	0.20
5		0.80	0.40
6	5.0 mg/mL	0.15	0.75
7		0.30	1.50
8		0.60	3.
9		1.20	6.
10		2.40	12.
11	50 mg/mL	0.50	25
12		1.20	60
13		2.50	125
14		5.0	250

[a]Dose increased approximately every 20 min unless reaction occurs; then adjust accordingly.

and prophylaxis of Pneumocystis carinii pneumonitis, the reaction rates are as follows: general population 3%; immunodeficient patients (HIV seronegative) 12%; AIDS patients (HIV seropositive) 29–70%. Sulfa drugs are also likely to be associated with EM minor, SJS and TEN types of reactions.

The allergic-like reaction to sulfonamides is not felt to be IgE mediated or, for that matter, an immune event. Unfortunately, there is no skin test or no in vitro blood test to confirm a suspected reaction. In almost all cases, strict avoidance of the drug is recommended once a presumptive diagnosis has been made.

The exception is life-threatening situations, such as in patients with AIDS with *P. carinii* infection. In some cases, the infection can be successfully treated with antimicrobial agents other than the TMP-SMX, such as inhaled pentamidine. In other cases, this is not possible, and TMP-SMX is the optimal drug for treatment of active infection and/or use in P. carinii prophylaxis.

In some cases, adults with a documented history of a prior rash to TMP-SMX have later been given full doses of TMP-SMX without subsequent reaction. In other cases, serious reactions have resulted from this "full-dose" challenge.

Extended oral TMP-SMX desensitization procedures have proved successful in a limited series of patients: 10–23 d (19/21 patients); 10 d (23/28 patients); 2 d (6/7 patients). Use of full-dose challenge or desensitization is not advised for any patient who has a prior history of drug–associated erythema multiforme, SJS or TEN. The management of these situations is best left to the allergist/immunologist specialist.

Documented allergic-like reactions to other antibiotics are uncommon. Usually, they are not life-threatening in nature. Most reactions to iv vancomycin result in a red flush ("red man syndrome") resulting from direct histamine release and can be controlled symptomatically and with adjustment of the iv drug administration rate.

In the case of reactions to other antibiotics, in almost all situations long-term avoidance is usually recommended, and the event is documented in the patient's records. Since there are usually substitute antibiotics available, it is not a problem for most individuals.

In a few individuals, however, multiple antibiotic sensitivities of different types occur. This type of patient presents a problem when the primary care physician tries to treat common infections. In most cases, the β-lactam antibiotics are involved, so penicillin skin testing can be done. (Often, the tests are negative.) There are no convenient tests for reactions involving other antibiotics. Reproducible reactions of any kind, especially those that are systemic in nature, are unusual. If the history of reaction is minor, and the drug is necessary for therapy, a graded oral challenge followed by a 2-h wait in the office can usually be done without difficulty to prove the safety of this alternative antibiotic. (*see* General Approach to Diagnosis and Management and Table 5).

Insulin

Approximately 50% of humans given insulin regularly as a replacement therapy, especially the animal-derived forms, develop some IgE antibody to the insulin molecule that can be validated by a positive immediate–reacting IgE skin test. Most of these individuals do not have clinical reactions to insulin. A few, however, do have bothersome local swelling at the insulin injection site.

Management of this local reaction problem consists of the following:

1. Division of the insulin dose in half and administering these doses at different sites
2. Trial of an added oral antihistamine
3. If steps 1 and 2 fail, switching to another commercial type of insulin

Generalized urticaria or systemic anaphylaxis to insulin is very uncommon (0.1–0.2% of diabetics). Usually the systemic reaction is the direct result of a diabetic discontinuing insulin replacement therapy regularly, for a time, and then resuming regular therapy. About 12 d after restarting of the insulin, systemic anaphylaxis occurs.

Patients who have a systemic reaction to insulin should be hospitalized after treatment first of the acute symptoms. If the reaction is mild and the patient is seen within 24–48 h, the total insulin daily replacement can be decreased by one third

> **Drug Challenge and Desensitization**
>
> - Graded drug challenges, or drug desensitization, should be done only when necessary, with informed consent, and under controlled conditions by specialists familiar with these techniques
> - Any serious (anaphylaxis or anaphylactoid) reactions following drug challenge usually start within 2 h of drug exposure
> - Reactions during drug desensitization procedures, such as with β-lactam antibiotics, should be expected to occur in one third of patients.

and subsequently the dose can usually be safely increased 5 U/dose until therapeutic levels have been achieved.

In the situation in which the reaction is more severe or the interval between reaction time and examination is more than 48 h, the patient will require specific insulin allergy skin testing by an allergist/immunologist specialist to identify the least reactive insulin type (usually human insulin). The patient then requires desensitization over the course of a week with this new insulin.

Anesthetic Agents

Some patients given local anesthetics complain of allergic-like symptoms. Few, if any, of these reactions have been shown to be Ig mediated. When a patient is confronted with such a problem, the goal is to find one local anesthetic the patient can tolerate. The allergist/immunologist will usually skin test the individual complaining of symptoms with more than one type of local anesthetic, including the one that the surgeon/dentist wants to use.

The specialist will select one of the nonreacting agents and then administer a graded sc injection challenge using dilutions of the local anesthetic at 1:100 (dose: 0.1 mL), 1:10 (dose: 0.1 mL), and full-strength local anesthetic (dose; 0.1, 0.5 , 1.0 and 2.0 mL) at 20-min intervals, under controlled conditions.

Most patients successfully complete the local anesthetic challenge without difficulty. The referring physician is then informed regarding the safety of the drug used in the challenge.

It is common for an allergic-like reaction to occur during the induction of general anesthesia (1:5,000 to 1:15,000 inductions). The symptoms include urticaria, wheezing, rapid heart rate, low blood pressure and shock. Two types of allergic reactions should be considered should these symptoms occur: (1) reactions to natural rubber latex and (2) allergic reactions to one of the neuromuscular blocking agents used in the induction period (e.g., tubocurarine chloride, alcuronium, gallamine triethiodide, pancuronium bromide, succinylcholine chloride, fluphenazine hydrochloride, thiopental, amytal sodium and methohexital).

Certain individuals (e.g., health care workers, children with spina bifida or multiple operations, highly allergic individuals and individuals with atopic dermatitis) are at increased risk for systemic reactions to natural rubber latex. Usually there is a history of prior contact dermatitis or contact urticaria to latex products, before the patient has

---

Adverse Effects of ASA/NSAID

- GI bleeding
- Exacerbation of urticaria/angioedema from any cause
- Asthma; especially in nonatopic adults with chronic rhinitis and nasal polyps
- Anaphylaxis/urticaria-angioedema

---

a systemic reaction. Latex proteins can be transferred via aerosol coupled to glove powder, so that severe reactions may occur in very sensitized individuals just by being in a room where latex is being used.

In situations in which systemic anaphylaxis has occurred in an operating room, it is advisable to draw blood from the patient as soon as possible after the event so that in vitro testing can be subsequently performed for mast cell tryptase (as a sign of mast cell release, *see* General Approaches to Diagnosis and Management) and IgE latex–specific antibodies. If the latex in vitro test is positive, it is diagnostic of this type of allergy. If the test is negative, the patient can be skin tested by most allergists/immunologists using a common latex rubber source (no commercial allergen for testing is available).

Although the allergist/immunologist specialist may attempt direct skin testing with various neuromuscular blocking agents, such a type of testing procedure is not standardized. Positive allergy skin testing to neuromuscular agents would provide helpful information, but a negative skin test result to these agents does not rule out an association between these agents and clinical reactions.

Aspirin (ASA) and NSAID

There is no skin test or in vitro test available to confirm the presumptive diagnosis of ASA/ NSAID intolerance in patients who have a history of allergic-like reactions (e.g., urticaria or asthma). The only management is to advise the individual to avoid these drugs strictly. Although a graded drug challenge (beginning with no more than 3 or 30 mg of ASA, depending upon the history of sensitivity, and advancing to 60, 100, 150 and 300 mg at 3-h intervals) has been studied experimentally, such a challenge is usually not advocated in most clinical situations. Also experimental is ASA desensitization. ASA desensitization has proven successful in some patients with ASA-sensitive asthma, but not with most individuals with ASA/NSAID-induced urticaria, angioedema or anaphylactoid reactions. This procedure is not recommended for the usual ASA-sensitive patient.

RCM

RCM is used in imaging diagnostic procedures, and adverse reactions to RCM are fairly common. Therefore, one allergic-like problem that a primary care physician is likely to face is the patient with a prior history of RCM reaction who needs another diagnostic imaging procedure.

There is no skin test or in vitro diagnostic test that can be done to predict whether or not the patient with a history of prior reaction to RCM will have another reaction. Studies have shown that the chances a patient with a previous reaction to conventional

Table 8
Pre-RCM Treatment Protocol for Prevention of Repeat RCM Anaphylactoid Reactions

Time	Agent/Dose
18, 12 and 6 h before procedure	Prednisone 50 mg every 6 h for 3 doses (total 150 mg)
Immediately before procedure	Diphenhydrammine hydrochloride (Benadryl) 50 mg po, im, 1 h or iv 5 min before RCM Cimetidine (Tagamet) 300 mg or ranitidine (Zantac) 300 mg po, 1–3 h before, or 5 min before RCM
During procedure	Low-ionic RCM

RCM will have another reaction to the same material is approx 30%. This risk can be reduced to 10% by using a preprocedure treatment of prednisone and diphenhydramine (Benadryl). It may be reduced to a risk of 0.5% by using a low-molarity RCM material plus a preprocedure treatment of medications as outline in Table 8.

In spite of these preprocedure treatments and the use of a low-ionic RCM during the procedure, the individual with a prior RCM reaction is at some risk, and the radiologist should be prepared to treat anaphylaxis should it occur (*see* Chapter 4). In addition to the usual treatments, the radiologist should be prepared to treat an unusual but occasionally severe RCM reaction that mimics excess vagal stimulation, inducing bradycardia and resistant shock. Under these special circumstances, the addition of atropine to the anaphylactoid treatment regimen may be lifesaving.

Angiotensin-Converting Enzyme Inhibitors (ACE-I)

The incidence of cough with the use of ACE-I ranges up to 25%—usually starting within 2 wk of therapy. In approximately one half of the cases, the problem is severe enough to discontinue the drug. Switching types of ACE-I is not advisable. Potentially life-threatening angioedema is estimated to occur in 0.1–0.2% of patients receiving ACE-I (usually not those with cough). In 25% of these cases, serious laryngeal edema has been reported. Although swelling usually occurs within a few weeks or months of initial ACE-I therapy, late-onset reactions, over 2 yr, have been reported—often intermittently. When such a reaction is suspected, all ACE-I should be discontinued.

SUGGESTED READING

Anderson JA. Allergic reactions to drugs and biological agents. *JAMA* 1992;268:2845–2857.

Anderson JA. Antibiotic drug allergy in children. *Curr Opin Pediatr* 1994;6:656–660.

Anderson JA. Drug desensitization. In: Spector SL, ed. *Provocation Testing in Clinical Practice*. New York, Marcel Dekker, 1995, pp. 761–783.

Anderson JA. Drug allergy. In: Kaliner M, ed. *Current Review of Allergic Diseases*. Philadelphia, Current Medicine, 1999, pp. 191–202.

Bates DW, et al. eds. Incidence of adverse drug events and potential adverse drug events. *JAMA* 1995;274:29–34.

DeShazo RD. Allergic reactions to drugs and biologic agents. *JAMA* 1997;278:1895–1906.

DeSwarte RD. Drug allergy. In: Patterson R, Grammar LC, Greenberger PA, Zeiss CR, eds. *Allergic Diseases—Diagnosis and Management*, ed.. 4, Philadelphia: JB Lippincott, 1993, pp. 395–552.

Lieberman P. Difficult allergic drug reaction. *Immunol Allergy Clin North Am* 1991;11:213–231.

Macy E, Richter PK, Falkoff R, Zeiger R. Skin testing with penicillote and penilloate prepared by an improved method: Amoxicillin oral challenge in patients with negative skin test responses to penicillin reagents. *J Allergy Clin Immunol* 1997;100:586–591.

Patterson R, DeSwarte RD, Greenberger PA, Grammar LC. Drug allergy and protocols for management of drug allergies. *N Engl Reg Allergy Proc* 1986;7:325–342.

Sogn D, Evans R, Shepard SM, et al. Results of the NIAID collaborative clinical trial to test the predictive value of skin testing with major and minor penicillin derivatives in hospitalized adults. *Arch Int Med* 1992;151:1025–1031.

VanArsdel PP, ed. Drug allergy. *Immunol Allergy Clin North Am* 1991;11:461–700.

17 Antihistamines

Phil Lieberman, MD

CONTENTS

HISTAMINE

To prescribe antihistamines rationally it is important to be familiar with the role of histamine in the production of allergic disease. Histamine is widely distributed through the body with the highest concentrations in the lung, skin and gastrointestinal tract. Mast cells and basophils contain the majority of histamine, but it is also found in gastric mucosa, epidermal cells, rapidly growing tissue, enterochromaffin cells and the central nervous system.

Histamine exerts its action through three receptors (H_1, H_2, H_3). The activities of these three receptors are seen in Table 1. H_1 receptors are most important in the production of allergic symptoms. H_1-receptor stimulation produces contraction of bronchial smooth muscle, reflex bronchoconstriction through stimulation of the vagus nerve, stimulation of peripheral nerve endings to produce pruritus and pain, and increased vascular permeability.

The most important actions mediated through the H_2 receptor are an increase in gastric acid production, a down-regulation of a number of immunological and inflammatory responses and a direct inotropic/chronotropic effect on the heart. The combination of H_1- and H_2-receptor stimulation is necessary for the maximal expression of effects such as peripheral vasodilatation (producing flush, headaches, hypotension) and the induction of mucous secretion.

Histamine has specific effects on target organs. In the vascular tree the overall effect of histamine produces vasodilatation. This results in flushing, lowering of peripheral resistance and hypotension. In addition, there is increased vascular permeability resulting in fluid shifts into the extravascular space. The vasodilatation, as noted, is mediated through H_1 and H_2 receptors with maximal vasodilatation achieved by stimulation of both. However, the majority of the effects on the vascular bed are

From: *Current Clinical Practice: Allergic Diseases: Diagnosis and Treatment, 2nd Edition*
Edited by: P. Lieberman and J. Anderson © Humana Press Inc., Totowa, NJ

Table 1

Biological Effects of Histamine Mediated Through Various Histamine Receptors

H_1	H_2	$H_1 + H_2$	H_3
Elevates cyclic GMP (cGMP)	Increases cyclic AMP (cAMP)	Produces vasodilatation	Inhibits histamine synthesis in central nervous system, lung and skin
Induces smooth muscle contraction	Increases gastric acid and pepsin secretion	Produces flush	Reduces peptide release from airway nonadrenergic, non-cholinergic nerves
Increases vascular permeability	Produces positive inotropic and chronotropic effect on heart	Produces headache	Modulates cholinergic neuro-transmission in human airways
Stimulates nerve endings	Decreases fibrillation threshold of cardiac muscle	Produces hypotension	Affects CNS functioning
Pruritus	Immune down-regulation	Modulates eosinophil chemotaxis	
Vagal irritant receptors (cough and bronchospasm)	Decreases basophil histamine release	Alters mucus glycoprotein secretion from goblet cells and bronchial glands (H_1 increases viscosity and H_2 increases amount)	
Induces vasodilatation	Inhibits basophil chemotaxis		
Direct	Inhibits lymphokine and lysosome release		
Stimulation of endothelial cell production of relaxing factors	Decreases lymphocyte proliferation		
Discharges neuropeptides during axon reflex	Inhibits T-cell-mediated cytotoxicity		
Increases histidine uptake in basophils	Activates suppressor T-cell		
Induces epinephrine secretion from adrenal medulla	Causes lymphocyte production of histamine-induced suppressor factor		
Increases rate of depolarization of SA node	Decreases monocyte secretion of complement components		
Slows rate of atrioventricular (AV) conduction	Inhibits neutrophil superoxide and peroxide generation		
	Modulates neutrophil chemotaxis		

324

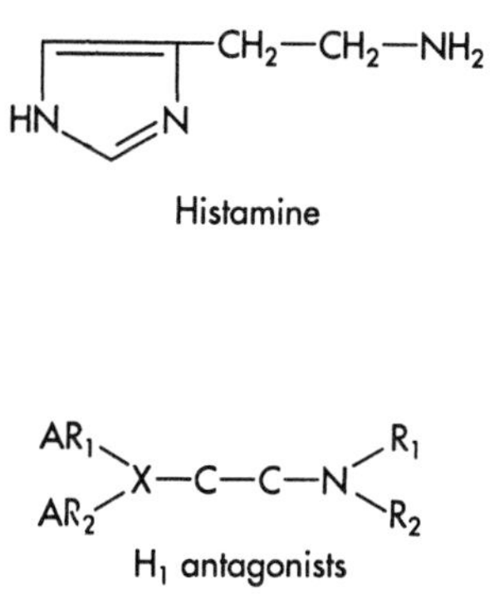

Histamine

H₁ antagonists

Fig. 1. Structure of histamine compared to prototype structure of first-generation antihistamines.

mediated through the H_1 receptor, which has a higher affinity for histamine and is stimulated by a lower concentration of the amine.

The effects of histamine on the heart are mainly mediated through the H_2 receptor, but the H_1 receptor also plays a role. Vasodilatation is responsible for reflex tachycardia. In addition, histamine exerts a direct effect on the heart that is both inotropic and chronotropic with the H_2 receptor increasing the rate and force of both atrial and ventricular contraction. The H_1 receptor speeds the heart rate by hastening diastolic depolarization at the SA node. In addition, H_1-receptor stimulation contracts coronary arteries.

Smooth muscle contraction in the bronchial tree is mediated solely by the H_1 receptor. The H_1 receptor also produces modest contraction of the smooth muscle of the uterus. Histamine effects on gastrointestinal smooth muscle vary from species to species, but the predominant effect is contraction, mediated through the H_1 receptor.

Glandular secretion is mediated through both H_1 and H_2 receptors. The H_2 receptor increases the amount of mucous glycoprotein secretion from goblet cells in bronchial glands, whereas the H_1 receptor increases the viscosity of mucus.

CLASSIC, FIRST-GENERATION ANTIHISTAMINES

Structure/Function Relationships

All H_1 antagonists are competitive or noncompetitive inhibitors of histamine at the target organ. Their activity depends on the prevention of histamine binding to tissue receptors. Most, but not all, first-generation antihistamines have a structural resemblance to histamine (Fig. 1) in that they contain a substituted ethylamine moiety. It was previously felt that this structural similarity was necessary for competitive inhibition. However, with the development of newer agents it has been shown that antihistamine activity can occur without an obvious shared structural relationship between histamine and its antagonist. The proposed difference between the mechanisms of action of antihistamines with an ethylamine moiety (thus exhibiting a structural resemblance to histamine) and those without this entity is that the former group actually binds to the same site on the histamine receptor as histamine, whereas the latter group binds to the seven-chain G-protein–coupled histamine receptor at other sites to sterically hinder the binding of histamine.

> All antihistamines are rapidly absorbed from the gastrointestinal
> tract and usually begin to work within an hour. It is important to
> note that tissue activity extends beyond serum half-lives.

First-generation antihistamines have classically been separated into categories based on the atom linking the ethylamine grouping to aromatic substituents (Fig. 1). For example, if the link is via oxygen, the drugs are classified as ethanolamines; if via carbon, they are called alkylamines; and if via nitrogen, they are called ethylenediamines (Fig. 2). Certain biological activities have been attributed to these differences; however, clinically it is unclear whether or not these are significant. For example, it is said that alkylamines cause less drowsiness in general than do ethanolamines. Examples of first-generation antihistamines classified according to their structural differences are seen in Table 2.

Pharmacokinetics

The pharmacokinetic and pharmacodynamic properties of selected first-generation antihistamines are presented in Table 3.

All first-generation H_1 receptor antagonists are rapidly absorbed and reach peak serum concentration within 3 hours when given in liquid form. All are extensively metabolized in the liver, and little, if any, of these drugs is excreted unchanged in the urine. All of these agents are metabolized through the hepatic cytochrome P-450 system. Rates vary from patient to patient and are age dependent with children having shorter and the elderly having longer elimination half-lives. Severe hepatic dysfunction can prolong the half-life and require dosing adjustments.

Pharmacodynamics

An important principle of the pharmacodynamic activity of these drugs is that their tissue effect is delayed relative to peak serum levels and can extend far beyond the life of the drug in the serum. For example, hydroxyzine can suppress histamine-induced wheal and flare for as long as 60 h despite maintaining a negligible serum concentration at this time.

The tissue effect however is delayed compared to peak serum concentrations. For example, with hydroxyzine, maximal suppression of wheal and flare does not occur until 7 h after peak serum concentrations have been achieved. Based upon these pharmacodynamic observations, it can be concluded that it is best to administer H_1 antagonists before allergen exposure.

Other Pharmacological Actions

First-generation antihistamines have a number of pharmacological activities unrelated to their antihistaminic properties. They can exert antimuscarinic, anti-α-adrenergic, antidopaminergic, antiserotonergic, local anesthetic, antiemetic and antimotion sickness activity.

Side Effects

By far the most common significant side effect of first-generation antihistamines is drowsiness. All first-generation antihistamines cross the blood-brain barrier. The exact

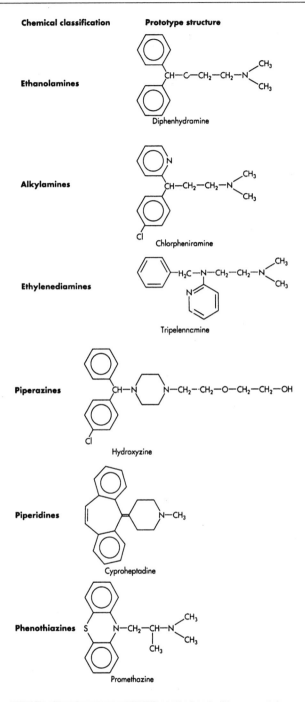

Fig. 2. Structural classification of classic H_1 antagonists.

mechanism of production of drowsiness by these drugs is unknown, but may include antihistaminic, anticholinergic, antiserotonergic, and antiadrenergic activities. It should be noted that the antihistaminic activity does not necessarily correlate with the sedative potential, suggesting that this is not the sole cause of this side effect. The degree of

Table 2
Characteristics of Representative First-Generation H_1 Antagonists
Based Upon Chemical Classification

Chemical class	Examples	Comments
Ethanolamines	Diphenhydramine Clemastine Carbinoxamine	Significant antimuscarinic effects. Can be potent sedatives, but sedative potential varies, with clemastine producing the least amount. Low incidence of gastrointestinal side effects. Can have some antimotion sickness activity. Diphenhydramine and clemastine both available over the counter
Alkylamines	Chlorpheniramine Brompheniramine Dexchlorpheniramine Tripolidine	Relatively moderate incidence of drowsiness. Moderate anti-cholinergic effect. No antiemetic or antimotion sickness activity. Little gastrointestinal side effect. All available over the counter. Occasional paradoxical central nervous system stimulation, especially in children.
Ethylenediamines	Tripelennamine Pyrilamine Antazoline	Mild to moderate sedation. Slight anticholinergic effect. Some local anesthetic effect. Pyrilamine is sold over the counter and is oldest antihistamine preparation available today. As a group, may have more frequent gastrointestinal side effects.
Piperazines	Hydroxyzine Meclizine Cyclizine	Hydroxyzine has highest sedative activity in group. Meclizine and cyclizine relatively low sedative activity with main use being for vertigo, antimotion sickness, and antiemetic activity. Hydroxyzine has significant anti-cholinergic activity.
Piperadines	Cyproheptadine Phenindamine Azatadine	Mild to moderate sedation. Little anticholinergic activity, antiemetic activity and anti-motion sickness activity. Cyproheptadine has potent antiserotonin effect. As a class, has relatively high incidence of paradoxical central nervous system stimulatory activity.
Phenothiazines	Promethazine Methdilazine Trimeprazine	Usually highly sedating. Strong antiemetic, anticholinergic activity. Main clinical use is as antiemetics.

sedation depends on many factors, including age, the pattern and quality of nocturnal sleep and concurrent medication. First-generation antihistamines clearly potentiate the activity of other sedative drugs such as alcohol.

Of importance is the fact that the subjective degree of drowsiness does not necessarily correlate with the objective measurement of central nervous system impairment. For example, drowsiness can occur without impairment and impairment without drowsiness. Although drowsiness can be overcome by the exertion of will, impairment

Table 3
Pharmacokinetic and Pharmacodynamic Characteristics
of Selected First-Generation H_1 Antagonists

Drug	Peak serum concentration reached after oral dose (h approx)	Half-life (h approx)	Duration of biological activity (suppression wheal and flare; h approx)	Route of metabolism
Diphenhydramine	0.75–2.5	8–9	6–10	Liver
Chlorpheniramine	1.5–2.5	20–24	24	Liver
Hydroxyzine	1–2.5	20	36	Liver
Brompheniramine	2–3	24	9	Liver
Tripolidine	1–2	2.1	—	Liver

of cognitive functions and psychomotor performance cannot, and will persist until the effect of the drug abates.

Paradoxical central nervous system stimulation can occur in some individuals, especially children. Other central nervous system side effects include dizziness, tinnitus, blurred vision and tremors.

The next most common group of side effects produced by first-generation antihistaminics relate to their antimuscarinic activity. These include dryness of the mouth, urinary retention, blurring of vision, difficulty in urination and constipation.

Other side effects are uncommon and include loss of appetite, nausea, abdominal pain and diarrhea. Drug allergy to first-generation antihistamines is extremely rare, but has been reported. Leukopenia, agranulocytosis and hemolytic anemia have all been seen. Teratogenic effects have been noted in animals, but there has been no documentation of this in human beings.

SECOND-GENERATION ANTIHISTAMINES

Second-generation antihistamines available for oral administration in the United States at this time include loratadine (Claritin), cetirizine (Zyrtec) and fexofenadine (Allegra). Azelastine (Astelin) is available as a nasal spray, and levocarbastine (Livostin) and olopatadine (Patanol) are available as eye drops. The term *second-generation antihistamine* is used loosely in this chapter to refer to antihistamines available since 1981. In general, these drugs are distinguished from classic sedating antihistamines by the fact that they are considered either nonsedating or lesser sedating drugs. Loratadine and fexofenadine are the currently available nonsedating antihistamines.

Second-generation antihistamines differ from first-generation antihistamines as well by the fact that it is more difficult to classify them by structure (Fig. 3). They do not always contain a readily accessible ethylamine side chain as do first-generation drugs. Thus their structure-function relationships are less well defined. Nonsedating antihistamines are diverse in chemical structure, and many can be considered as drugs with multiple pharmacological effects in addition to their antihistaminic activity. For example, azelastine was originally produced as an anti-asthma drug. These multiple

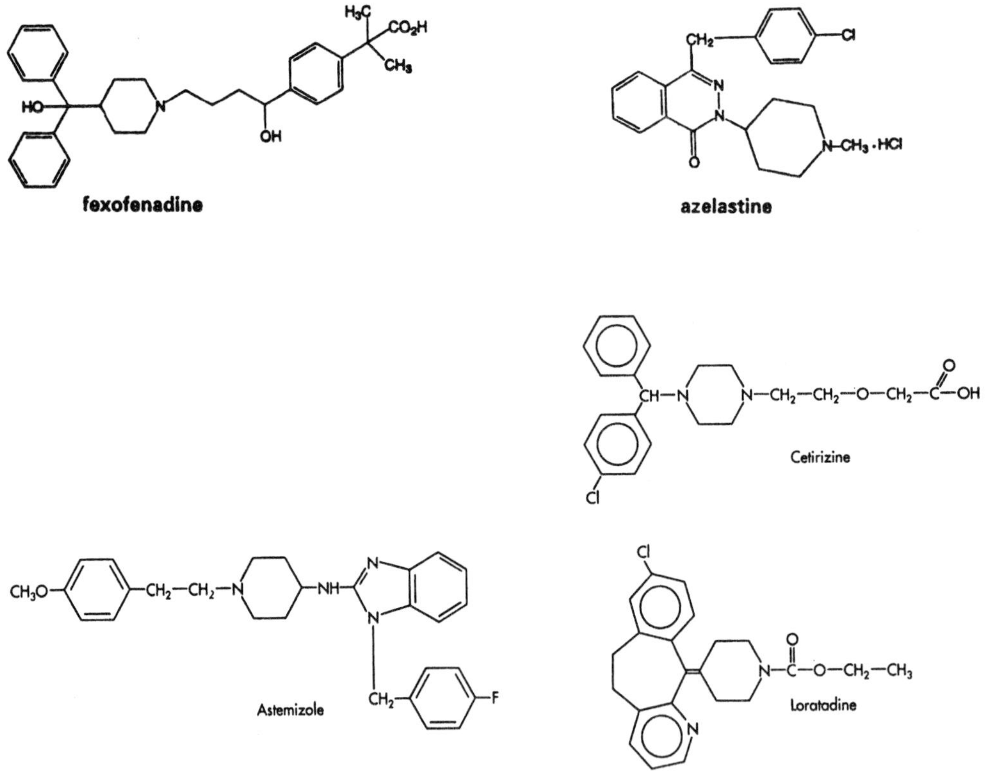

Fig. 3. Structures of representative second-generation H_1 antagonists.

pharmacological effects, however, differ from those noted for the first-generation antihistamines. First-generation antihistamines, as noted, have antimuscarinic, antiserotonergic and anti-α-adrenergic effects. These activities are probably related to the fact that all of these mediators act through a G-protein–coupled receptor that is analogous in structure to the receptor for histamine. Thus the receptor, for example, for α-adrenergic agents differs from that for histamine only by several amino acids. Therefore, these activities of second-generation antihistamines are presumably due to their nonspecific ability to hinder the effect of other mediators at the receptor site in a manner less efficient than their ability to hinder the activity of histamine. However, the other pharmacological activities of nonsedating antihistamines are termed antiallergic effects and are probably related to more diverse pharmacological activities as described later.

The most clinically important factor that distinguishes second-generation from first-generation antihistamines is their lack of sedative activity. The most likely explanation for this lack of sedation is the fact that they do not readily pass the blood-brain barrier. The basis for the failure to cross the blood-brain barrier likely includes several properties of these agents: (1) a relative lack of lipid solubility compared to first-generation antihistamines; (2) an increased tendency to bind to serum proteins; (3) a relatively large molecular size with larger side chains; (4) their electrostatic charge; (5) and the presence of chemical groups that ionize at physiological PH. In addition, their relative specificity for the H_1 receptor negates the antimuscarinic, antiserotonergic

> Central nervous system impairment as detected by objective testing can exist in the absence of drowsiness, and patients can feel drowsy without showing detectable signs of impairment on objective tests.

and anti-α-adrenergic soporific effects of first-generation antihistamines. Finally, these second-generation antihistamines have a greater affinity for peripheral vs central H_1 receptors. Thus, the lack of sedative activity of these agents is probably related to a multiplicity of pharmacological properties—the major one of which is their failure to pass the blood-brain barrier.

Pharmacokinetics

The pharmacokinetic properties of second-generation antihistamines (Table 4) allow for once- or twice-daily therapy. As with first-generation antihistamines, all second-generation drugs are rapidly absorbed after oral administration. Peak plasma levels occur 1–2 h after administration. Loratadine and azelastine are all extensively metabolized in the liver, through varying cytochrome activities. Cetirizine is partially metabolized in the liver, but is renally excreted for the most part. Fexofenadine differs in that it is, for the most part, excreted unchanged in the feces.

The elimination half-life of cetirizine and loratadine are between 7 and 10 h and 12 and 15 h, respectively. Fexofenadine has an elimination half-life of approximately 14½ h. Loratadine, astemizole and azelastine have active metabolites. Fexofenadine and cetirizine have no active metabolite. All of these drugs have strong serum protein–binding activity (Table 4).

Pharmacodynamics

As with first-generation antihistamines, the pharmacodynamic activity of these drugs is relatively unrelated to their serum levels. The peak pharmacodynamic activity is delayed relative to the peak serum levels and can extend far beyond the life of the drug in the serum. The ultimate duration of their antihistaminic activity, therefore, is not predictable solely on the basis of their metabolic half-life because of the degree of reversibility of receptor binding. Therefore, clinical activity cannot be assessed by measuring serum concentrations. Astemizole is perhaps the most obvious example of this. Although the drug appears in significant amounts in the serum 1 h after administration, it has a delayed effect at the tissue level. This effect does not occur until approximately 4 h after ingestion, thus making astemizole unsuitable for "prn" administration. In addition, its inhibitory activity can persist for 18 d after administration, long after there are detectable plasma concentrations.

Antiallergic Effects of H_2 Antagonists

Second-generation antihistamines have been shown to have diverse antiallergic or anti-inflammatory pharmacological activities. The clinical significance of these activities has not been well documented, but based upon their nature, it can be presumed that part of the therapeutic effect of these agents may indeed be related to these

> Second-generation antihistamines differ from first-generation drugs in that they are selective for the H_1 receptor and do not readily cross the blood–brain barrier.

properties. The antiallergic activities of second-generation antihistamines include the following: (1) prevention of histamine release from mast cells and basophils; (2) down-regulation of intracellular adhesion molecules such as ICAM-1 on epithelial membranes; (3) decreased eosinophil influx into tissues; (4) prevention of the generation of superoxide; (5) prevention of the generation of leukotrienes; and (6) prevention of the production of interleukins. For example, fexofenadine has been shown to decrease the expression of ICAM-1 on epithelial cells and prevent the release of interleukin-I and granulocyte-macrophage–colony stimulating factor (GM-CSF).

Sedation and Psychomotor and Cognitive Impairment

It is important to distinguish sedation from cognitive and psychomotor impairment. Sedation refers to the subjective sensation of sleepiness, fatigue, drowsiness, decreased ability to concentrate and loss of alertness. Of note is the fact that these subjective sensations can occur independent of objective detection of psychomotor and cognitive impairment. For example, patients can feel sedated without being impaired and can show impairment without being sedated. It has been shown that, in general, all second-generation antihistamines are less sedating and produce less impairment that do first-generation antihistamines. Loratadine and fexofenadine are the only two that are nonsedating. Thus, these drugs are the only second-generation antihistamines approved by the US Federal Aviation Administration (FAA) to be taken before or during a flight. Again, it is important to make the distinction between sedation and impairment. Sedation, being subjective, can be overcome by the exertion of will in many circumstances. However, impairment will still persist, and cannot be overcome through conscious effort. Patients therefore may not be aware of impairment when they are not subjectively sedated. The growing recognition of this is reflected in the increased number of states that have enacted laws prohibiting the operation of a motor vehicle by someone taking sedating medications, including sedating antihistamines. At the time of this writing a majority of states have enacted such laws.

Perhaps of singular importance regarding the distinction between subjective drowsiness and the objective ability to perform occurs in children. It has been shown that the learning capacity of allergic children may suffer during the allergy season and that a first-generation sedating antihistamine (although improving allergy symptoms) may actually worsen performance. On the other hand, the use of a nonsedating antihistamine will, presumably by controlling symptoms without affecting performance, enhance learning ability in children.

Based upon the above observations, it is quite clear that nonsedating second-generation antihistamines such as loratadine and fexofenadine have a clear advantage over first-generation antihistamines in terms of their ability to relieve symptoms without affecting performance. However, because of their increased cost, health care providers under managed care have attempted to reduce their usage by recommending a second-generation antihistamine during the day and a first-generation antihistamine at night.

Table 4
Comparison of Second-Generation Antihistamines

Drug	Route of administration	Adult dose (mg)	Effect of food on absorption (AUC)	Plasma protein bound (%)	Elimination T 1/2 (Hours)[a] parent	Elimination T 1/2 (Hours)[a] metabolite	Onset of action (H)	FDA cautionary label	Metabolized in liver	Pregnancy category	Possible cardiac side effects
Loratadine (Claritin)	Oral	10 q.d.	↓40%	97–99	12–15	17	1	No	Yes	B	No
Cetirizine (Zyrtec)	Oral	10 q.d.	0	93	7–10	—	1	Yes	Minimally[b]	B	No
Fexofenadine (Allegra)	Oral	60 b.i.d.	NR	60–70	14.4	—	1	No	Minimally[c]	C	No
		180 q.d.	NR	60–70	14.4	—	1	No	Minimally[c]	C	No
Azelastine (Astelin)	Intranasal	0.137/spray 2 sprays each nostril b.i.d.	0	78–88	22–36	42–54	1	Yes	Yes	C	No

[a] Loratadine and azelastine have active metabolites; cetirizine and fexofenadine do not.
[b] Mainly excreted in urine.
[c] Majority excreted in feces.
NR = Not reported; AUC = Area under the curve; NAM = No active metabolite.

333

> Antihistamines are usually more effective for the rhinitis symptoms of sneeze, itch and rhinorrhea than for those of congestion and postnasal drainage.

Unfortunately it has been shown, as noted above, that tissue effects of first-generation antihistamines persist beyond their serum level, and thus it can be expected that the performance-impairing activity of a first-generation antihistamine given at bedtime can persist during the following day. Therefore, this strategy may be ineffective in preventing impairment due to the administration of first-generation antihistamines.

Uses of Antihistamines

RHINITIS

It is quite clear that nonsedating second-generation antihistamines are the recommended first line of therapy for patients with allergic rhinitis. They are usually sufficient to treat symptoms of sneezing, rhinorrhea and itching associated with mild to moderate allergic rhinitis. They are also helpful for ocular symptoms. However, they have little effect on nasal congestion. There is no distinct difference in the efficacy between first- and second-generation antihistamines for the therapy of allergic rhinitis. However, the lack of effect on performance makes second-generation antihistamines the drugs of choice.

For rhinitis induced by the common cold, second-generation antihistamines are not effective. However, first-generation antihistamines, presumably because of their anticholinergic effects, are somewhat beneficial for the therapy of rhinorrhea and sneezing.

URTICARIA

As with allergic rhinitis, antihistamines are the drug of choice in patients with urticaria. The primary symptom in urticaria is pruritus. Antihistamines exert their major suppressive activities on this symptom. They are usually less effective in reducing wheal size.

ATOPIC DERMATITIS

There are very few studies examining the use of second-generation H_1 receptor antagonists in atopic dermatitis. Because of the inflammatory nature of this disease it is expected that they would be less effective than they are in urticaria. Nonetheless, it is customary to use antihistamines in the therapy of atopic dermatitis, and, since at least a portion of the symptoms appears to be related to the release of histamine, there is strong rationale for their use. However, in the treatment of atopic dermatitis, the use of antihistamines is considered adjunctive rather than first-line therapy.

ASTHMA

It has long been thought that antihistamines might be contraindicated in the therapy of asthma because of their "drying effect." This is of course untrue. Antihistamines are certainly not contraindicated and have been shown to have a beneficial effect to some extent in the therapy of this condition. Second-generation H_1 antagonists have been studied extensively in the therapy of asthma. A number of these drugs have been reported to be effective. Thus there is certainly no reason to withhold these drugs in asthmatics, and in fact, their administration may be helpful.

SUGGESTED READING

Casale TB, et al. Safety and efficacy of once daily fexofenadine, HCL hydrochloride ACL, in the treatment of autumn seasonal allergic rhinitis. *Allergy Asthma Proc* 1999;20:193–198.

D'Agostino RB, et al. The effectiveness of antihistamines in reducing the severity of runny nose and sneezing: A meta-analysis. *Clin Pharmacol Ther* 1998;64:579–596.

Dykewicz MS, Fineman S. Diagnosis and management of rhinitis: Parameter documents of the joint task force on practice parameters in allergy, asthma, and immunology. *Ann Allergy, Asthma Immunol* 1998;81:501–505.

Horak F, Stubner UP. Comparative tolerability of second generation antihistamines. *Drug Saf* 1999; 20:365–401.

Lieberman P. Antihistamines. In: Rich RR, Mosby, eds. *Clinical Immunology Principles and Practice*, vol. 2. St. Louis, Mosby, 1996, pp 1968–1979.

Nathan RA. The new antihistamines. In: Kaliner, M, ed. *Allergic Diseases* Philadelphia, Current Medicine, 1999, pp 87–100.

Simons FER. Antihistamines. In: Middleton E, et al, eds. *Allergy Principles and Practice*, vol. 2. 1998; pp 612–637.

Slater JW, Zechnich AD, Haxby DG. Second generation antihistamines, a comparative review. *Drugs* 1999; 57:31–47.

18   β-Adrenergic Agonists

Clifton T. Furukawa, MD

CONTENTS

INTRODUCTION
β-ADRENERGIC RECEPTORS
β₂-ADRENERGIC AGONISTS FOR THERAPY
METHODS OF ADMINISTRATION
ADVERSE EFFECTS
UNITED STATES OLYMPIC COMMITTEE DRUG RULES
SUGGESTED READING

INTRODUCTION

β-adrenergic agonists, and especially β₂-adrenergic agonists, are generally prescribed for all asthmatics as backup medication to anti-inflammatory therapy or, in the case of exercise-induced asthma, as the primary drug. Technological advances have led to the development of increased β₂-specific adrenergic agonists of longer duration of action. The effectiveness of β-adrenergic agonists in treating asthma is indisputable. However, the very effectiveness of these drugs causes problems of overuse, and consequent side effects, raising issues such as whether other drugs or other parameters should be preferentially utilized.

β-ADRENERGIC RECEPTORS

Initially, adrenergic receptors were classified as either α or β, based upon the tissue response to various sympathomimetic amines. The receptor population that mediated excitatory responses was called α, and the potency ranking was epinephrine > norepinephrine > α-methyl norepinephrine >α-methyl epinephrine > isoproterenol. The receptor population that mediated inhibitory responses was designated as β, and had an agonist order of potency of isoproterenol > epinephrine > α-methyl epinephrine >α-ethyl norepinephrine > norepinephrine. It later became recognized that although generally correct, this classification was overly simplified, and the α- and β-receptors were further subclassified. For β-adrenergics it is now recognized that there are three receptor groups, β₁, β₂, and β₃. The β₁-adrenergic receptors are primarily located in

From: *Current Clinical Practice: Allergic Diseases: Diagnosis and Treatment, 2nd Edition*
Edited by: P. Lieberman and J. Anderson © Humana Press Inc., Totowa, NJ

the brain, the heart and the pineal gland, the β_2-adrenergic receptors are primarily in the lung and prostate, and the β_3-adrenergic receptors are found in brown and white adipose tissue. Improved techniques to identify receptors have led to the discovery that although these receptors have preferential primary locations, they may also be present in other tissues. The β_2-adrenergic receptor is the predominant β-receptor in the lung, but is also found in adipose tissue, the brain, heart and placenta. This is of particular importance in understanding the side effects of the β_2-specific adrenergic drugs.

β_2-ADRENERGIC AGONISTS FOR THERAPY

Advances in therapeutic β-adrenergic agonists has been accomplished by modification of chemical structures of adrenergic agents (Fig. 1). Although the specific chemical structure determines the specific class of drugs (e.g., catecholamines, noncatecholamines, saligenins), it may be more convenient to consider the available therapeutic agents as first, second, third and fourth generation, dependent upon the newness of the drug, the β_2 specificity and the duration of action.

First Generation Agents (α and β)

Probably the oldest adrenergic drug is ephedrine, used in China as ma huang for centuries before the use of epinephrine. Although ephedrine is rarely used for treatment today, it was commonly combined with theophylline and sometimes a sedative as treatment for asthma until more effective and more specific bronchodilators were developed. The major problem with ephedrine was that it easily crossed the blood-brain barrier and even modest doses had significant side effects, particularly headache. The amount of bronchodilation was also relatively weak.

Epinephrine has both α- and β-adrenergic actions, which make it the drug of choice for the treatment of anaphylaxis. It is effective as an injection, but not orally, because epinephrine and other catecholamines are rapidly inactivated by the action of catechol-o-methyltransferase (COMT), an enzyme present in the gastrointestinal wall. Epinephrine can also be aerosolized, but this particular treatment is more popular for acute laryngobronchitis (croup).

Second-Generation Agents (Relatively β)

Two other catecholamines are of note: isoproterenol and isoetharine. Isoproterenol is available for aerosol administration for asthma, but also is available for sublingual and injectable routes. As an inhaled bronchodilator, isoproterenol has good immediate potency, usually accomplishing peak bronchodilation within 5 min. However, the effectiveness rapidly declines and usually is lost completely by 2 h. This makes isoproterenol useful acutely, but not useful for any maintenance bronchodilator therapy, or even for prophylactic use before exercise. If high doses are used, cardiac stimulation becomes an unacceptable side effect.

Isoetharine is the first β-agonist that clearly had increased β_2 activity. Because it also is a catecholamine it cannot be used orally because of deactivation by COMT. It is, however, resistant to monoamine oxidase and so has a slightly longer duration of bronchodilation than the other catecholamines. Its clinical usefulness, however, has been greatly overshadowed by the more specific and longer-acting β_2 drugs.

Metaproterenol is a resorcinol, not a catecholamine. The resorcinol group has a modification in the 3,4 hydroxyl groups of the benzene ring. The hydroxyl groups

Adrenergic Bronchodilators

Classification	Molecular Structure	Formulations in the USA	Duration of effect (h)
First Generation Ephedrine	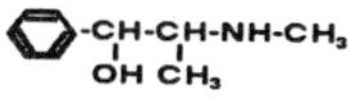	Liquid, tablet	2-3
Epinephrine	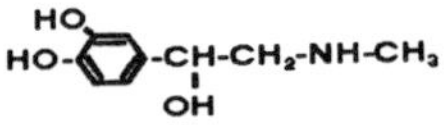	Injection, MDI	<1
Second Generation Isoetharine	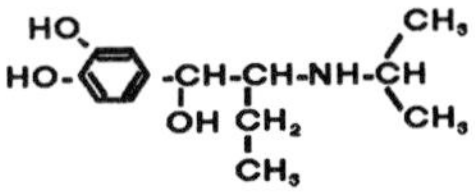	MDI, nebulizer solution	3
Isoproterenol	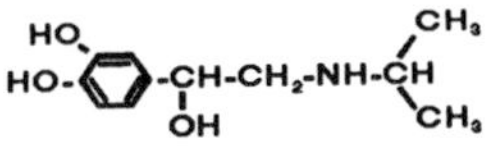	Injection, liquid, MDI, nebulizer solution, tablet	1-2
Metaproterenol	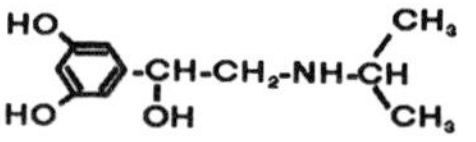	Liquid, MDI, nebulizer solution, tablet	3-5
Third Generation Albuterol	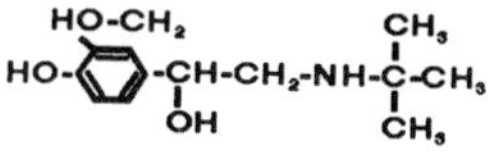	Dry powder inhaler, liquid, MDI, nebulizer solution, tablet	4-6
Bitolterol	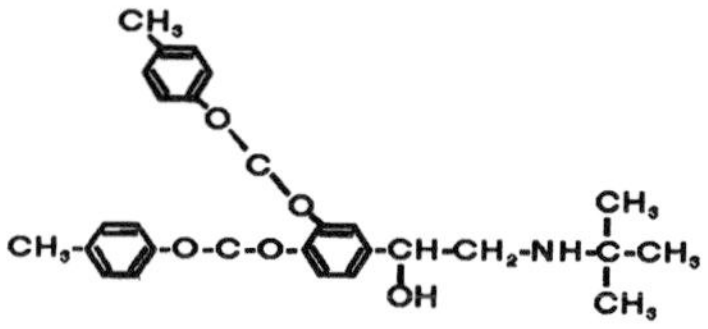	MDI, nebulizer solution	6-8
Fenoterol	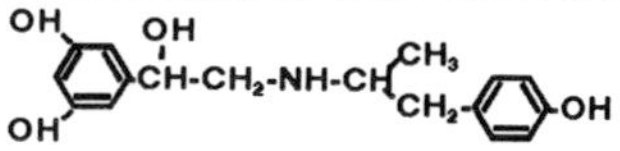	Not available	6-8
Pirbuterol	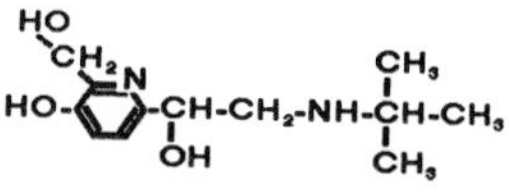	MDI	4-6
Terbutaline	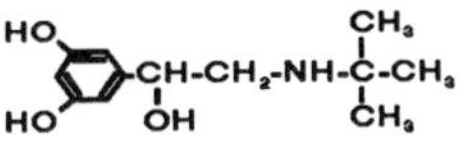	Injection, MDI, tablet	4-6
Fourth Generation Formoterol	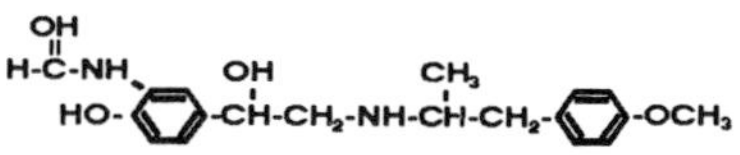	Not available	8-12
Salmeterol	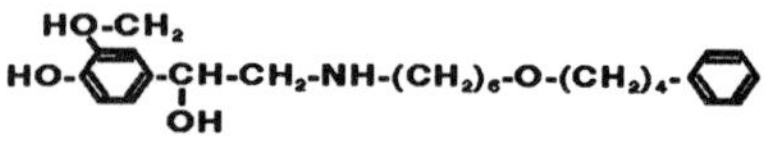	MDI	12

MDI = metered dose inhaler

Modified from Kemp JP. Making best use of today's bronchodilators. J Respir Dis 1994;15 (4 suppl):S21-S27.

Fig. 1.

Inhaled Albuterol: Use and Overuse in Asthma

- Most asthma patients are advised to use Albuterol on an "as needed" basis.
- If use is > 2 × weekly, asthma controller medications are advised.
- Daily use of Albuterol (with controller medications) itself is generally not harmful—but usually indicates that the asthma is not under control.
- Prolonged daily use of more than one Albuterol MDI canister per month has been linked to an increased risk for asthma death.

---

repositioning from the 3,4 to the 3,5 positions makes metaproterenol resistant to inactivation by COMT, and this leads to the advantage of prolonged duration of action. The side chain of metaproterenol is essentially the same as isoproterenol, so, as would be expected, both drugs are similar in their effects relative to heart and lung. Since the relative cardiac effect is similar for both isoproterenol and metaproterenol, metaproterenol is less suited for maintenance bronchodilator treatment or for higher dose treatment than are the third-generation of β-adrenergic agonists.

Third-Generation Agents (Highly β, Longer Acting)

The third-generation group are those drugs that are highly β_2-specific with a longer duration of action. These characteristics make these the ideal choice for acute asthma treatment and prevention of exercise-induced asthma.

Albuterol, a saligenin, is resistant to the action of COMT because of the substitution of the 3 hydroxyl group with a hydroxymethyl group, In addition, albuterol has a tertiary butyl group that replaces the isopropyl group seen in isoproterenol and metaproterenol. This increased bulkiness of the side chain has resulted in substantially more selectivity for the β_2 receptor. Albuterol is resistant to degradation by COMT, making it effective orally as well as by aerosol and parenterally. With its high β_2 specificity, and its longer duration of activity, albuterol became the standard against which other bronchodilators are compared.

Bitolterol is resistant to COMT because the 3,4 hydroxyl groups are esterified to form a di-p-toluate ester. This modification substantially prolongs the bronchodilator activity; in addition, a tertiary butyl group replaces the isopropyl group, resulting in increased β_2 specificity and protection of the drug against degradation by monoamine oxidase (which then further increases the duration of activity). Bitolterol is also an interesting bronchodilator because when administered by inhalation, it acts as a pro-drug, which is slowly degraded to the active drug colterol. This gives bitolterol the potential of being much longer acting than the other bronchodilators in this group.

Pirbuterol is resistant to COMT because of the substitution of a hydroxyl methyl group for the 3 hydroxyl group. This plus the increased size of the terminal amino group increases the duration of the bronchodilator action. The side chain is also adequately bulky to account for more selectivity for the β_2 receptor.

Terbutaline is resistant to COMT because of the repositioning of the hydroxyl groups to the 3,5 positions. This modification increases the duration of the bronchodilator action and makes the drug potentially capable of oral administration. The side chain of

> ### Safety of β-Adrenergic Drugs when Used Appropriately
>
> - Intermediate Action
>   Albuterol, terbutaline, pirbuterol, bitoeterol—yes
>   Fenoterol[a]—No
> - Long activity
>   Salmeterol—yes
>   Formoterol[a]—yes
>
> [a]Not available in the United States.

terbutaline had a tertiary butyl group that increases the β_2 specificity and also protects against degradation by monoamine oxidase, increasing the duration of bronchodilation. As with the other drugs in this third-generation group, terbutaline is of current usefulness, but it also has unique advantages as the potentially most safe drug for use in pregnancy. It also is used by obstetricians to control premature labor.

Fenoterol is a drug that is not used in the United States, but has been part of substantial controversies about the safety of β-agonists. Fenoterol, as other members of this group, is resistant to the action of COMT because hydroxyl groups are located at the 3,5 positions. The side chain in fenoterol is much larger than the other members of this group with the use of a 4-hydroxybenzyl moiety. Nonetheless, in the case of fenoterol, the β_2 specificity is less than those drugs that use a tertiary butyl group substitution. It is this relative decreased β_2 specificity that makes fenoterol a drug that potentially could have more side effects than the other drugs in this group.

Fourth-Generation Agents (Highly β, Extremely Long Acting)

Salmeterol and formoterol induce a long duration of bronchodilation, in some studies reported to be more than 12 h. These two drugs resemble the noncatecholamine selective β_2-agents, but also posses bulky lipophilic side chains. It is thought that these side chains anchor the molecule next to the β-receptor site. The action of both of these drugs can be reversed by introducing a β-adrenergic blocking agent, but if the β-blocker is removed the receptor is restimulated. Because of their long duration of action, these drugs are particularly useful for long-term bronchodilator treatment, but are potentially less useful acutely and may pose problems of toxicity with overuse or increased dosage. Concerns about tolerance to the bronchoprotective properties are raised by studies showing rapid reduction of protection to methacholine or exercise with regular use of salmeterol.

There are some interesting differences between salmeterol and formoterol. Formoterol, when given by inhalation, has rapid onset of action, whereas salmeterol has delayed onset of action even when given by inhalation. Formoterol, if given orally, has a duration of activity about equal to albuterol. When given by inhalation, it and salmeterol both have bronchodilation which persists at least 12 h. However, if the subgroup studied are older nonsmoking asthmatics with some degree of fixed obstruction, formoterol activity can only be measured up to 8 h. At present, formoterol is not available in the United States, and salmeterol is recommended for use under very specific guidelines.

These include no more frequent use than two puffs 2 times a day, and warnings that it should not be initiated in patients with worsening or deteriorating asthma, should not be used for acute symptoms and should not be considered a substitute for oral or inhaled corticosteroids. Thus, most experts recommend use of salmeterol concomitantly with inhaled anti-inflammatory therapy, and availability of a shorter-acting inhaled bronchodilator for acute symptoms.

METHODS OF ADMINISTRATION

Oral

In general, oral dosing of β-adrenergic agonists requires larger administered doses than in other routes. Consequently, increased likelihood of side effects results. Of course, the only drugs useful orally are those that are resistant to COMT. However, variable absorption is also a concern because of conjugation of the drug in the gut wall or the presence of food in the stomach. Decreased bioavailability may result from rapid metabolism on first passage through the liver. In the case of terbutaline, this results in the bioavailability being only 7–26% when given by the oral route.

Sustained-release formulations have been particularly useful in nighttime asthma, but compared to sustained-release theophylline may cause more side effects. Overall the oral route of administration may be useful only for persons who are unable to use other routes of administration, such as very young children or elderly patients. However, nebulizer solutions can effectively be used by these patients.

Parenteral

Both terbutaline and albuterol have been used subcutaneously, by continuous iv infusion and by bolus iv infusion. Such use has been primarily limited to hospitalized severe asthmatics, but continuing therapy has been reported used up to several years. It is interesting that the principal side effect has been problems in sleeping and that tolerance did not occur.

Inhalation

Administration by inhalation is highly recommended, since drug effect is usually rapid and the dose required for adequate bronchodilation is usually accompanied by few side effects. It is interesting that when side effects do occur, these side effects usually are of less duration than the duration of bronchodilation. Overall, the major reasons to primarily recommend inhalation rather than the oral or injectable route of this class of drugs is that the effective dose is less and the side effects are less. In fact, many centers have as part of their protocol for dealing with severe hospitalized asthmatics the use of a continually nebulized selective β_2 bronchodilator as treatment prior to consideration of any more aggressive measures. This is particularly important in view of evidence that isoproterenol iv infusions have been shown to create myocardial injury.

There are, however, substantial problems in the use of the inhalation route if patients are not adequately trained in inhalation techniques. It is absolutely essential that all patients be taught how to use their inhaler or nebulizer and are given opportunity to demonstrate their competence at each follow-up evaluation. The use of spacers can also improve the efficiency of a metered-dose inhaler, but with the increasing concern of fluorocarbon use, it is expected that self-actuated inhalers will be the standard. Devices such as rotohalers, diskhalers and turbohalers will make the use of spacers unnecessary.

ADVERSE EFFECTS

Tremor is a specific β_2 effect upon skeletal muscles and thus is not separable from the bronchodilator action. However, tremor does decrease with continual use of β-adrenergic drugs. Side effects such as increased heart rate and palpitations are decreased with the more selective β_2 drugs. However, since there are β_2 receptors in the myocardium, and since there is reflex sympathetic stimulation of the heart as a consequence of β_2 relaxation of the vasculature that supports skeletal muscles, there is always some degree of increased heart rate and cardiac output if the dosage of the β_2 drug is high enough. With long-term use, hyperglycemia and hypokalemia may result. Hypokalemia does occur from direct stimulation of the sodium-potassium pump in the cell membrane, and so can occur acutely. Further hypokalemia occurs with steroid or diuretic treatment so that a hypoxemic patient could experience arrhythmias.

Since the 1960s this class of drugs has been implicated as contributory to asthma deaths. In the 1960s asthma mortality was increased in the United Kingdom at the same time that high-dose isoproterenol metered-dose inhaler sales increased. When these devices were made prescription and subsequent sales were decreased, there was a decline in the number of asthma deaths. In the mid 1970s New Zealand noted a sharp increase in asthma deaths at the same time that fenoterol as a metered-dose inhaler went into increased use in this population. In the last few years, studies of pharmacy use and morbidity and mortality in Canada implicated fenoterol and albuterol overuse in death and near-deaths from asthma. However, other studies and a meta-analysis of case-control studies noted that a relationship between β-agonist use and death from asthma is a weak relationship. More important may be overuse of medication in patients who are not adequately managing their disease. Consequently, comprehensive overall management of the patient's disease has been emphasized as the most effective way of minimizing potential adverse effects from the medications. Thus the emphasis on treatment being primarily directed toward the prevention and treatment of inflammation is appropriate. Except for use in preventing exercise-induced asthma, any use of this class of bronchodilators beyond three times per 24 h should be considered reason for re-evaluation of the asthmatic's management program.

UNITED STATES OLYMPIC COMMITTEE DRUG RULES

At present, this class of drugs falls under stimulants, so that the US Olympic Committee has banned certain forms of β_2-agonists. Thus, the only β_2-agonists that are permitted are albuterol, terbutaline, and Salmeterol. These are permitted by inhalation only, and only with written notification from the prescribing physician sent prior to competition indicating its appropriateness of use because of exercise-induced asthma or for asthma. All adrenergic medications by any oral or injectable route are banned, and β_2 agents other than albuterol, terbutaline, and Salmeterol are banned even if given by inhalation. The basic reason for this is that some of the β_2 agents possess anabolic properties, particularly if they are taken orally or by injection. The allowable list of medications is constantly being reviewed by the Committee and constantly revised and changed so that this information should be checked as to currency on a regular basis (US Olympic Committee Drug hotline phone number is 1-800-233-0393).

SUGGESTED READING

Blauw GJ, Westendorp RGJ. Asthma deaths in New Zealand: Whodunnit? Commentary. *Lancet* 1995;345:2–3.

Drotar DE, Davis EE, Cockcroft DW. Tolerance to the bronchoprotective effect of salmeterol 12 hours after starting twice-daily treatment. *Ann Allergy Asthma Immunol* 1997;79:31–34.

Drugs for asthma. *Medical Letter* 1995;37:1–4.

Furukawa CT, Kemp JP, Simons FER, Tinkelman DG. The proper role of β2-adrenergic agonists in the treatment of children with asthma. *Pediatrics* 1992;90:639–640.

Gibson P, Henry D, Francis L, Chuickshank D, Dupen F, Higginbotham N, et al. Association between availability of non-prescription beta 2 antagonist inhalers and undertreatment of asthma. *BMJ* 1993; 306:1514–1518.

McFadden ER. Perspectives in β2-agonist therapy: Vox clamantis in deserto vel lux tenebris? *J Allergy Clin Immunol* 1995;95:641–651.

Mullen M, Mullen B, Carey M. The association between β-agonist use and death from asthma. *JAMA* 1993;270:1842–1845.

Simons FER, Gerstner TV, Cheang MS. Tolerance to the bronchoprotective effect of salmeterol in adolescents with exercise-induced asthma using concurrent inhaled glucocorticosteroid treatment. *Pediatrics* 1997;99:655–659.

Suissa S, Ernst P, Boivin JF, Horwitz RI, Habbick B, Cockroft D, et al. A cohort analysis of excess mortality in asthma and the use of inhaled β-agonists. *Am J Respir Crit Care Med* 1994;149:604–610.

Taylor DR, Sears MR, Herbison GP, Flannery EM, Print CG, Lake DC, et al. Regular inhaled β agonist in asthma: Effects on exacerbations and lung function. *Thorax* 1993;48:134–138.

Taylor DR, Sears MR. Regular beta-adrenergic agonists. Evidence, not reassurance, is what is needed. *Chest* 1994;106:552–559.

Wahedna I, Wong CS, Wisniewski AFZ, Pavord AD, Tattersfield AE. Asthma control during and after cessation of regular beta-2 agonist treatment. *Am Rev Respir Dis* 1993;148:707–712.

19 Theophylline

Elliot F. Ellis, MD

CONTENTS

INTRODUCTION

Theophylline was introduced into clinical medicine almost 50 yr ago for the treatment of asthma. The drug was widely used for 20 yr after its introduction; however, following reports of adverse reactions, including death, there was a pronounced decline of theophylline prescribing, particularly for children. In the mid 1960s and the early 1970s when the pharmacokinetics of the drug began to be elucidated, an increase in the use of theophylline occurred, and it became the most commonly prescribed drug for the treatment of asthma. During the past decade, because of the introduction and widespread use of new potent anti-inflammatory inhaled steroids, doubts about theophylline's bronchodilatory activity in acute asthma and renewed concern about theophylline toxicity (well characterized in the 1950s and 1960s), prescription of theophylline substantially decreased. Very recently, however, evidence, first based on in vitro and subsequently on clinical studies, has strongly suggested an immunomodulatory role for theophylline even at low (5–10 µg/mL) serum concentrations.

Theophylline is a methylated xanthine, closely related to naturally occurring caffeine and theobromine. A theophylline derivative, dihydroxypropyl theophyline (dyphylline) marketed as Lufyllin® and Dilor®, is promoted as being safer than theophylline because it is eliminated principally through the kidneys, and its disposition is unaffected by the multiple factors that influence the biotransformation of theophylline in the liver. Unfortunately, dyphylline has substantially less bronchodilator activity than

From: *Current Clinical Practice: Allergic Diseases: Diagnosis and Treatment, 2nd Edition*
Edited by: P. Lieberman and J. Anderson © Humana Press Inc., Totowa, NJ

**Evidence for Anti-inflammatory/Immunomodulatory
Effects in Vitro**

- Reduces histamine release from human mast cells and basophils
- Inhibits T-cell proliferation after antigenic and mitogenic stimulation
- Inhibits production and release of IL-2
- Inhibits generation of eosinophil chemoattractants, e.g., LTB_4 and PAF, from human monocytes and release of eosinophil basic proteins

---

theophylline, and because of its water solubility, dyphylline is rapidly excreted from the body with an elimination half-life of approximately 2 h.

MECHANISM OF ACTION

Sixty years after the introduction of theophylline into clinical medicine its mechanism of action is still unclear. There are four theories, which have received the most attention, and it is possible that combinations of mechanisms maybe involved.

Phosphodiesterase (PDE) inhibition. Theophylline has been long known to be an inhibitor of the phosphodiesterase enzymes that are responsible for breakdown of cyclic 3,5-adenosine monophosphate (cAMP) and cyclic guanine monophosphate (cGMP), the intracellular concentrations of which regulate smooth muscle relaxation/contraction. It is now known that the cyclic nucleotide PDEs are a family of five isoenzymes (PDE I–PDE V). In the context of asthma, selective types III and IV and mixed III and IV PDE inhibitors relax smooth muscle in vitro. Theophylline causes smooth muscle relaxation by nonselective PDE inhibition of both PDE III and PDE IV. PDE III and IV inhibitors also play very important roles in affecting the activity of inflammatory cells involved in asthma. For example, infiltration and activation of inflammatory cells is attenuated by PDE IV inhibitors. The latter also inhibit cytokine activation of proinflammatory cells and attenuate cytokine release from these cells. Theophylline has been shown to have a number of important actions on eosinophil and lymphocyte function and as a modulator of cytokine production. It is of interest that many of these effects are observed at lower concentrations (5–10 µg/mL) than are thought to be necessary for optimal bronchodilator activity.

Adenosine receptor antagonism. Adenosine, a purine nucleoside that occurs naturally, causes contraction of smooth muscle from asthmatics in vitro and bronchoconstriction of asthmatics by inhalation by an indirect mechanism (release of histamine and leukotrienes from airway mast cells). Theophylline is a potent competitive antagonist of the three known types of adenosine receptors, A_1, A_{2a} and A_{2b}. However, theophylline-induced bronchodilation does not appear to be related to adenosine antagonism, since enprofylline (3-propyl xanthine), which has little inhibitory effect on adenosine receptors, is a potent bronchodilator. The absence of CNS stimulatory effect with enprofylline suggests that adenosine receptor antagonism is responsible for this (and possibly) other adverse effects of theophylline.

> **Evidence for Anti-inflammatory/Immunomodulatory**
> **Effects of Theophylline In Vivo**
>
> - Reduces allergen-induced eosinophil tissue infiltration
> - Inhibits airway hyperresponsiveness
> - Inhibits the late asthmatic reaction (LAR)
> - Reduces nasal plasma exudate secretion

Catecholamine release. Theophylline, particularly when given intravenously, causes catecholamine (principally epinephrine) release. Whether this effect is of sufficient magnitude to be clinically significant is doubtful.

Improvement in diaphragmatic contractility. There are reports that theophylline increases diaphragmatic and other respiratory muscle contractility and delays onset of fatigue. Since this effect is inhibited by calcium channel blockers and does not occur in the absence of extracellular calcium, it has been suggested that theophylline alters transmembrane calcium flux.

PHARMACOKINETICS

Absorption

RAPID-RELEASE FORMULATIONS

Theophylline is rapidly absorbed from orally administered liquid and uncoated tablets and from rectally administered (as an aminophylline)solutions. The absorption profile of rectally administered theophylline looks very much like that seen after iv administration. Theophylline suppositories (erratically absorbed) are no longer manufactured in the United States. The speed, but not the extent, of absorption is affected to a clinically insignificant degree by concurrent ingestion of food or antacid. For iv use, aminophylline continues to be the preferred product. The dose administered needs to be corrected for the fact that aminophylline is 80–85% theophylline.

SLOW-RELEASE FORMULATIONS

Slow-release theophylline formulations are indicated for patients in whom elimination half-lives are <6 h and for enhancing compliance, because less frequent dosing is required. Various products differ in terms of rate and extent of absorption. The ideal product releases the drug at a constant rate over the dosing interval. Slow-release formulations vary in rate of the drug released (from slow to slower to ultraslow). With the ultraslow products, the rate of the drug released is typically so slow that the drug may be out of the gut before it is completely absorbed. There is diurnal variation in theophylline absorption with slower absorption during the night, resulting in higher morning trough concentrations. It has been proposed that host factors, in addition to the drug itself, are responsible for some of the erratic absorption patterns. To minimize fluctuation in serum concentration over a dosing interval, the patient's theophylline elimination characteristics (slow or fast) should ideally be matched to the product's release characteristics (slow, slower or ultraslow). Most children over the age of 6–8 yr can be treated successfully with 12-h dosing intervals with some slow-release preparations (e.g., Slo-bid Gyrocaps, Uniphyl, Theo-Dur or Uni-Dur tablets). Patients

---

Theophylline Pharmacokinetics

- There is a linear relationship between the log of serum theophylline concentrations and improvements in FEV$_1$ between theophylliine concentrations of 5–20 µg/mL.
- Anti-inflammatory/immunomodulatory effects occur at serum concentrations in the 5–10 µg/mL range.
- The therapeutic window is relatively small, and toxic symptoms occur when this therapeutic window is exceeded; therefore, monitoring is often necessary.
- Multiple factors affect theophylline metabolism and, consequently, serum theophylline levels. These include age, smoking habits, other drugs and disease states.
- Each theophylline preparation has its own absorption characteristics, and the physician must be familiar with the preparation utilized.

---

with exceptionally rapid theophylline clearance require 8-h dosing intervals to prevent serum concentration fluctuation >100%. On the other hand, individuals, e.g., the elderly, who eliminate theophylline very slowly will maintain therapeutic levels of theophylline with once-a-day dosing of most extended-release products. Food taken concurrently with theophylline has an important effect on the rate of the drug release with some products and minimal or no effect with others. Once-a-day products are more vulnerable to variations in intestinal pH and mobility. The best example of the food effect on slow-release theophylline absorption has been reported with Theo-24. When given with a high-fat-content meal (50% carbohydrate, 20% protein and 30% fat), about half of the dose of Theo-24 is absorbed in a 4-h period (usually beginning 6–8 h after ingestion), and peak concentrations average two to three times higher than those observed when this drug was given during fasting. This phenomenon of "dose dumping" (defined as more than 50% of the total dose being absorbed in <2h) is a particular hazard with once-a-day products, in which the total dose is given at one time. Antacids may affect the rate of drug absorption from products with pH-dependent dissolution, in contrast to absorption of formulations whose dissolution is not pH dependent (e.g., Slo-bid Gyrocaps, Theo-Dur tablets).

Distribution

The pharmacokinetics of theophylline can be characterized by the use of a linear, two-compartment open model, because the multicompartment characteristics of theophylline are not very pronounced. After iv administration, theophylline distributes rapidly from the plasma to its site of action in the tissues; this distributive phase is virtually complete within 30 min. The volume of distribution averages about 0.45 L/kg in children and adults (within reasonable parameters of ideal body weight). Protein binding at physiological pH (approximately 40%) is not of sufficient magnitude to result in toxicity due to competitive drug interaction. Theophylline passes through the placenta and into breast milk and crosses the blood-brain barrier. Concentrations in the central nervous system (CNS) in children are about 50% of the serum concentration

(90% in premature infants). Salivary concentrations are approximately 60% of serum levels.

Metabolism/Elimination

Theophylline is eliminated from the body principally by biotransformation in the liver to inactive (with the exception of 3-methylxanthine) metabolites. The enzymes responsible for the metabolism of theophylline (and many other drugs) belong to the cytochrome P-450 family of oxidases located in the smooth endoplasmic reticulum of the liver. The isoenzymes involved are designated CYP3A3, CYP2E1 (cause hydroxylation to 1, 3-dimethyluric acid) and CYP1A2 (causes *N*-dimethylation to 1-methylxanthine and 3-methylxanthine). Initial pharmacokinetic studies of theophylline elimination reported that elimination occurred by a first-order process, i.e., the rate of elimination was proportional to the drug concentration remaining—a log linear decay. However, more recent investigation has shown that, particularly at high serum concentrations, dose-dependent nonlinear elimination comes into play. This means that there is a disproportionate increase in serum theophylline concentration for a given percent increase in dose. How many patients being treated with theophylline manifest this dose-dependent kinetics is not known, but in children a 15% incidence has been proposed. Theophylline metabolism is age dependent. In infants, drug biotransformation is slow as a result of immaturity of hepatic microsomal enzymes and slowly increases during the first year of life. By 8–12 mo of age, clearance rates approach those seen in early childhood. From 1–9 yr of age, the rate of theophylline metabolism accelerates. There is a gradual decline in the rate of theophylline biotransformation during the adolescent and early adult years. At about 16 yr of age, the metabolic rate approximates that seen in young adults. After 1 yr of age, approx 10% of the drug is excreted unchanged in the urine. In premature infants and normal newborns during the first month of life, 45–50% of an administered dose of theophylline is cleared by the kidney unaltered. At all ages, a small amount (approx 6%) of theophylline is *N*-methylated to caffeine. This minor conversion becomes clinically relevant only in premature infants, in whom caffeine has an extremely long half-life (mean, 96 h), which results in its accumulation and pharmacological effect.

Because liver microsomal enzyme activity is dependent not only on age but is also subject to the inducing and inhibiting action of a large variety of unrelated environmental conditions and disease factors, it is not surprising that there is intra-individual variation over time in the rate of metabolism of theophylline and resultant serum concentration. Individual variations in theophylline metabolism, however, are small, unless there are changes in disease factors (e.g., fluctuating cardiac function) or changes in concurrent drug therapy. Cigaret smoking causes a dose-related increase in theophylline clearance. Heavy smokers metabolize theophylline twice as fast as nonsmokers. A similar effect is seen with marijuana but to a lesser extent. Ingestion of a high-protein, low-carbohydrate diet accelerates theophylline metabolism, presumably by increasing liver enzyme activity. Dietary intake of methylxanthines, caffeine in particular, affects theophylline metabolism by acting as a competitive substrate for theophylline-metabolizing enzymes. The ingestion of charcoal-broiled meat, presumably because of a stimulating effect on liver enzyme function of polycyclic hydrocarbons produced during the charcoaling process, has been reported to increase metabolism of theophylline. Although of theoretical interest, dietary factors are seldom

Table 1
Factors Other Than Drugs That Influence Theophylline Clearance

Factors	Decreased clearance	Increased clearance
Age	Premature infants; neonates and up to 6 mo; adults over 60 yr	Ages 1–16 yr
Diet	Dietary methylxanthines	—
Habits	—	Cigaret smoking (tobacco or marijuana
Disease	Liver disease, hypothyroidism, congestive heart failure, acute pulmonary edema, chronic obstructive pulmonary disease, sustained fever usually with viral illness	Cystic fibrosis, hyperthyroidism, diabetes mellitus (poorly controlled)

a clinically significant problem. Although the data are conflicting, the effect of obesity on theophylline clearance appears to be negligible. Because theophylline distributes poorly into fat, dosage should be based on ideal body weight rather than actual weight.

Theophylline metabolism is affected by various disease states, including hepatic disease, cardiac disease and viral illnesses. Hepatic dysfunction is a major cause of altered theophylline biotransformation. Patients with decompensated cirrhosis, acute hepatitis and possibly cholestasis have reduced theophylline clearance. A correlation between slow hepatic metabolism and serum albumin and bilirubin concentration has been made in patients with cirrhosis. Cardiac disease, presumably causing decreased liver microsomal enzyme function by passive congestion of the liver secondary to congestive heart failure, may have a profound effect on theophylline metabolism. When heart failure is treated, theophylline clearance increases. Acute viral illnesses, especially influenza, associated with fever have been reported to prolong theophylline half-life. Symptoms of nausea, vomiting and headache are commonly observed in children during many viral infections; however, when these symptoms develop in a child receiving theophylline, the physician must consider the possibility of theophylline intoxication. If fever is high and sustained (e.g., temperature higher than 102°F for more than 24 h), the dosage should be reduced in a patient whose theophylline serum concentration was previously maintained within the therapeutic range (Table 1).

Drug interactions are another factor in altering theophylline elimination. All of the drugs listed in Table 2 caused a change (increase or decrease) of 20% or more (some more than 100%) in theophylline serum concentration. Drugs most likely to be encountered by allergists include cimetidine, macrolide antibiotics (particularly the estolate salt of erythromycin) troleandomycin and clarithromycin, estrogen-containing oral contraceptives, phenytoin, rifampin, and certain quinolone antibiotics (ciprofloxacin, enoxacin, and perfloxacin). Influenza vaccine immunization was originally reported to slow theophylline elimination with a consequent increase in serum levels and the potential for toxicity. More recently, studies have shown no significant effect, and hence, there is no reason to reduce theophylline dose coincident with influenza immunization.

Table 2
Clinically Important Drug Interactions with Theophylline

Decreases theophylline metabolism resulting in increase in serum concentration	*Increases theophylline metabolism resulting in decrease in serum concentration*
Alcohol	Aminoglutethimide
Allopurinol	Carbamazepine
Cimetidine	Moricizine
Ciprofloxacin	Phenobarbital (PB)
Disulfiram	Phenytoin
Mexiletine	Rifampin
Propafenone	Sulfinpyrazone
Pentoxifylline	
Propanolol	
Enoxacin	
Erythromycin	
Estrogen-containing oral contraceptives	
Fluvoxamine	
Methotrexate	
Interferon, human recombinant alpha-2a	
Tacrine	
Ticlopidine	
Thiabendazole	
Troleandomycin	
Verapamil	
Zileuton	

THERAPEUTIC DRUG MONITORING

The rationale for therapeutic monitoring of theophylline serum concentration is that it is a major determinant of both efficacy and toxicity. Theophylline has a narrow therapeutic index, which makes it imperative for the physician to understand that serum concentration may be affected by many factors that affect liver microsomal enzyme function and alter elimination kinetics.

During the treatment of an acute exacerbation of asthma, a serum theophylline level should be determined before administration of an iv loading dose of aminophylline if the patient has been receiving theophylline. In this circumstance, the initial bolus may need to be reduced by 25–50%, depending on the result. For a patient who is admitted to the hospital and receives a constant infusion ot theophylline after the bolus, it is important to obtain a 1-h level and adjust the serum concentration to the therapeutic range. Thereafter, serum theophylline levels should be monitored every 12–24 h.

The indications for monitoring theophylline serum concentrations in the management of chronic asthma are subject to some controversy. Some authors believe that all patients with chronic asthma should be monitored at regular intervals during the initial phase of theophylline adjustment. These intervals vary, and it is assumed that theophylline clearance is stable. Other clinicians reserve monitoring for patients who do not obtain optimal symptom control after an appropriate dose is given and for patients in whom adverse effects develop. In the event of symptoms associated with theophylline toxicity, immediate determination of serum theophylline concentration is mandatory. To interpret serum theophylline concentration properly in clinical situations, a significant amount of information must be provided with a sample, such as characteristics of the patient (age, weight) , formulation of the drug (rapid release or slow release), dosage , duration of therapy (to ensure steady state for maintenance-dose adjustment), dosing interval, exact timing of previous adjustment, exact timing of blood collection, concurrent drug therapy and presence of fever or other disease states, such as congestive heart failure or liver dysfunction. With a rapid-release theophylline product (liquid or tablet), a sample obtained 2 h after the dose approximates the peak concentration. The determination of the trough concentration (the sample obtained immediately before the next dose) does not provide much additional information except to show the magnitude of the peak-trough difference. Because of a circadian effect on theophylline absorption, specimens should be drawn during the same dosing interval when more than one measurement is being compared. Various slow-release products differ in their release characteristics (e.g., Theo-Dur tablets or Slo-bid Gyrocaps reach peak serum concentration approx 3–7 h after the morning dose). Slow-release products that have pH-dependent dissolution characteristics (e.g., Theolair and Theo-24) release drugs at variable rates, depending on whether they are given during fasting or with a meal. Intersubject and intrasubject variability in absorption of slow-release products may be the reason for a theophylline serum level to be inconsistent or lower than the expected level for a particular dose. An important reason for inconsistent levels of theophylline is poor patient compliance.

PHARMACODYNAMICS

It is well recognized that there is a linear relationship between the logarithm of serum theophylline concentration and improvement in forced expiratory volume in l s (FEV_1). This relationship was first noted in children by Maselli and colleagues, who showed a strong correlation between the intensity of bronchodilator effect (improvement in FEV_1) and the logarithm of the amount of drug in the tissue compartment. It was evident from this study that the effect on pulmonary function was not seen until 30 min after the bolus injection of iv aminophylline; this lag represented the time for the drug to be distributed from the plasma to the site of action in the tissues. Because the bronchodilator effect increases and then falls rapidly after a bolus, it is logical to give iv aminophylline by constant infusion rather than by repeated bolus injection after the initial bolus dose. Mitenko and Ogilvie also studied the log serum concentration–bronchodilator relationship in a group of hospitalized adult asthmatic patients and showed a proportionality between the log of the serum concentration and the bronchodilator effect over the 5–20 μg/mL range. Subjects with severe asthma (status asthmaticus) have a rather flat serum concentration–bronchodilator effect curve over the range of 5–20 μg/mL. In patients with mild asthma who may have an FEV_1 of 50–60% of the predicted level, the serum concentration–response curve is steep.

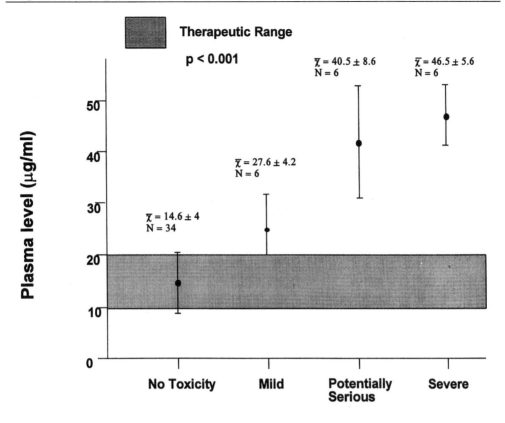

Fig. 1. Frequent toxicity from iv aminophylline infusions in critically ill patients. Modified from Hendeles L, Bighley L, Richardson RH, et al. *Ann of Pharmacotherapy* 1977;11:12–18.

THEOPHYLLINE TOXICITY

Like its bronchodilator activity, adverse effects are related to the logarithm of the serum concentration. Hendeles and associates demonstrated a relationship between serum concentration and symptoms of theophylline toxicity. Few toxic symptoms were noted when the steady-state serum concentration was <14.6 µg/mL. Adverse effects appeared as the serum concentration rose beyond 20 µg/mL. These included gastrointestinal, CNS, and cardiovascular effects (Fig.1). Of all adverse effects, those involving the gastrointestinal tract are most common. Vomiting, particularly if persistent, is very suggestive of theophylline toxicity. Hematemesis has been reported primarily in children; its exact pathogenesis is not clear. Gastrointestinal symptoms occur most often as a result of a central effect of an excessive serum theophylline concentration on the medulla rather than because of a local irritative effect on the stomach. Relaxation of cardioesophageal smooth muscle may lead to reflux and worsening of asthma by reflex stimulation of neural receptors in the distal esophagus or by aspiration of stomach contents into the upper airway and lung.

Theophylline stimulates the nervous system at various levels: the medulla (increased respiratory rate and sensitivity to carbon dioxide, nausea and vomiting), vagal effect (causing bradycardia), the cerebral cortex (restlessness, agitation, tremor, irritability, headache, seizures, difficulty in concentration), the hypothalamus (hyperthermia) and even the spinal cord (hyperreflexia). The mechanism of theophylline's effect on the nervous system is not known. Although seizures are a prominent manifestation of theophylline toxicity and are often difficult to control, they by themselves do not necessarily lead to death or to irreversible brain damage. Serum concentration associated with seizure activity varies substantially. The combination of seizures and cardiorespiratory arrest leads to the most disastrous consequences of theophylline intoxication. Individuals who are resuscitated and survive show signs of severe anoxic brain injury, much like those who have been resuscitated after drowning or strangulation. A recent meta-analysis of 12 studies with theophylline and 9 with caffeine showed no effect of either drug on behavior or cognition in children and adolescents. Concern about the effects of theophylline on the behavior, particularly learning, was raised by Rachelefsky and coworkers; however, there were many commentaries and critiques of this study. Furukawa and associates, in two studies of theophylline in asthmatic children, also interpreted their results to suggest that theophylline may impair learning and behavior. It is of interest that one important abnormal finding in their initial report was not substantiated in their second study. Creer and McLoughlin, after a critical review of the subject, commented that there is no definitive evidence that theophylline produces any type of learning disability. A similar conclusion was reached by the US Food and Drug Administration Pulmonary/Allergy Drug Advisory Committee in 1987 after a review of studies published until that time.

Theophylline has both inotropic and chronotropic effects on the heart. Although a number of opposing factors (direct effect on pacemaker tissue, effect on catecholamine release, peripheral vagolytic action, stimulation of the medullary center) confound the effects of theophylline on heart rate, the net result is usually tachycardia. In the therapeutic range, the effect of theophylline on the heart rate is modest, in the range of 3–16 beats/min. On the other hand, tachycardia is an almost constant finding in cases of significant theophylline intoxication. The arrhythmogenic potential of theophylline has been shown in experimental animals, but data in humans are less clear. Metabolic effects, principally hypokalemia and hyperglycemia, are commonly observed in cases of severe theophylline toxicity.

The appropriate treatment of theophylline toxicity is based on history, clinical signs and symptoms and theophylline serum concentration determinations. For patients with acute overdose and serum concentrations in the 20–30 µg/mL range, administration of oral activated charcoal 1 µg/kg up to 30 g for adults and monitoring of serum theophylline concentration for 2–4 h after the dose are often all that is needed. In acute overdose situations with serum concentrations between 30 and 100 µg/mL, administration of multiple doses of oral activated charcoal, as indicated above, given every 2 h with serum theophylline concentration monitoring, is appropriate. Since patients with theophylline toxicity are almost invariably vomiting, administration of the charcoal must often be via a nasogastric tube. If the oral activated charcoal therapy is ineffective and serum theophylline continues to increase, serious consideration should be given to institution of charcoal hemoperfusion if the facilities are available. In an acute overdose situation with serum concentrations of >100 µg/mL, prophylactic anticonvulsive therapy should be considered in addition to multiple-dose administra-

---

Theophylline Toxicity

- Symptoms of theophylline toxicity generally do not appear until serum concentration exceeds 20 μg/mL.
- Gastrointestinal symptoms (nausea, vomiting) are the most common manifestation of theophylline toxicity.
- Tachycardia almost invariably occurs in instances of significant theophylline toxicity.
- Seizures, often difficult to control, may lead to brain damage if associated with cardiorespiratory arrest.

---

tion of activated charcoal. If signs and symptoms of CNS irritation are such that a seizure is anticipated, anticonvulsive therapy should be initiated with an iv dose of a benzodiazepine (e.g., diazepam in a dose of 0.1–0.2 mg/kg every 1–3 min until seizure is terminated). If seizure control is not obtained, then a loading dose of phenobarbital 20 mg/kg should be infused over 30–60 min. Of course, monitoring of vital signs and electrocardiogram (ECG) should be instituted in all cases of significant theophylline toxicity. Recommendations for treatment of theophylline toxicity occurring in patients as a result of chronic overdosage are similar to those for acute overdosage with the following caveat: Young patients tolerate acute overdosage much better than older patients, who most often are suffering from chronic overdosage. Serious adverse events are more likely to occur at lower serum concentrations in the chronic overdose situation, and therefore, more aggressive measures are indicated in this setting. In patients older than 60 yr, seizures may occur at levels lower than 30 μg/mL and therefore, prophylactic anticonvulsive therapy should be instituted earlier than in the young individual suffering from acute theophylline overdosage. Communication with a poison control center should be sought in cases of serious theophylline concentration.

CLINICAL USE OF THEOPHYLLINE IN ASTHMA

Although iv aminophylline has been standard treatment for status asthmaticus since the early 1940s, the value of aminophylline in the emergency-room setting for acute asthma has been questioned recently. Various authors have suggested that theophylline adds little in terms of bronchodilator activity while increasing adverse effects when optimal therapy with aerosolized β-agonists has been given. In an early study of the use of iv theophylline in the treatment of acute asthma, theophylline was compared with sc epinephrine in an emergency department. The bronchodilator effect of theophylline was inferior to that achieved by the epinephrine. Subsequent studies have generally confirmed the observation that in acute asthma, the bronchodilator effect of aminophylline is inferior to that of optimal administration of aerosolized β_2 agonists. However, published data support the addition of iv aminophylline in the treatment of patients who fail optimal aerosolized agonist and steroid therapy and who require hospital admission. For example, Pierson and associates showed clinical benefit and pulmonary function improvement in status asthmaticus in a double-blind study of iv aminophylline in children with status asthmaticus. An emergency department study of adults with acute airway obstructive disease showed a threefold decrease in hospital admission rates for subjects treated with aminophylline in comparison with placebo recipients. Sakamoto and colleagues reported on results of a study of iv aminophylline administration in 12 asthmatic patients with acute episodes varying from mild to moderate to severe. They found progressive improvement in FEV_1 over the range of 5–15 µg/mL; the greatest bronchodilator effect was observed in patients whose initial airway obstruction was of a milder degree. Extrapulmonary effects of theophylline both in improving diaphragmatic function and delaying the onset of muscle fatigue are a useful additional benefit of theophylline administration. For iv therapy with aminophylline, some simple calculations can be used to determine the correct loading and maintenance therapy doses. In the case of drugs, like theophylline, that are distributed rapidly from the plasma to the tissues, there is a relationship among plasma concentration (C_p), dose (D) and volume of distribution (V_d) so that

$$C_p = D/V_d \qquad (1)$$

If an average V_d of 0.5 L/kg is assumed, it is easy to determine that for each mg/kg (ideal body wt) infused, there will be an increase of approx 2 µg/mL in peak plasma concentration. The loading dose (aminophylline) needed to achieve a given theophylline plasma concentration is determined as follows (in the following equations 0.8 is used in the denominator to correct for the fact that aminophylline is 80% theophylline):

$$\text{Loading dose (D)} = (V_d) \text{ [desired plasma concentration } (C_p)]/0.8 \qquad (2)$$

In this equation, it is assumed that the patient has not previously been receiving theophylline. If theophylline has been taken on an outpatient basis, the loading dose should be reduced, unless an immediate serum theophylline determination is available. Once the observed level of theophylline is known, it can be subtracted from the desired level and multiplied by the volume of distribution:

$$D = V_d \, (C_p \text{ desired} - C_p \text{ initial})/0.8 \qquad (3)$$

The dose of aminophylline required to maintain a desired steady state of serum theophylline concentration (C_{pss}) may be calculated as follows:

$$\text{Constant infusion rate} = (Cl) \, (C_{pss})/0.8 \qquad (4)$$

where Cl is the clearance L/h/kg, and C_{pss} is the average plasma concentration at steady state. A theophylline level determined from a serum sample obtained 1 h after the loading dose is useful in determining the need for an additional bolus loading dose. Therefore, Eq. 1 can be used to calculate the subsequent loading dose if needed. A subsequent determination 4 h after the initiation of a constant infusion shows the trend of the serum concentration; the rate can be either increased or decreased as needed. Additional samples after 12 and 24 h guide further iv dosing.

To convert the iv dose to an equivalent oral dose, the hourly dose is multiplied by the dosing interval to be used for oral therapy. It is important to correct the aminophylline dose to obtain the theophylline equivalent by multiplying the aminophylline dose by 0.8. In this calculation, it is assumed that the oral product is completely absorbed.

The use of theophylline in chronic asthma is being redefined. Over the 4-yr period from 1989 to 1993, prescriptions for theophylline written by pediatricians decreased from 27 to 7% of all asthma medicines. According to the most recent Expert Panel

Report of the NHLBI National Asthma Education of Prevention Program, theophylline has been relegated to a second-line position for patients who fail to respond to optimal β_2-agonist and inhaled steroid treatment. However, there are abundant data accumulated over the past 20 yr that indicate that theophylline is as effective as cromolyn in young children and provides additional control of symptoms even in patients taking inhaled steroids. In several well-designed studies of patients with severe asthma, withdrawal of theophylline resulted in significant deterioration in their clinical condition. In addition, many physicians have noted deterioration of asthma in patients previously well controlled with theophylline therapy in whom the drug was withdrawn as a requirement for a drug study, especially those subjects with moderate to severe asthma. Extended-release theophylline is more effective than extended release oral β_2-agonists in nocturnal asthma, although β_2-agonists cause less disturbance of sleep architecture. A recent study of twice-daily salmeterol and extended-release theophylline in nocturnal asthma demonstrated no major clinical advantage of one drug over the other. However, there was a small benefit in sleep quality, quality of life and daytime cognitive functioning with salmeterol.

When theophylline is used for the management of chronic asthma, it is most effectively administered as one of the sustained-release formulations. Use of sustained-release products minimizes the peak-and-trough fluctuation of serum concentration. Depending on an individual's serum theophylline clearance, an 8- or 12-h, or even 24-h, dosing interval is appropriate. In general, the younger the child (under 9 yr of age), the more likely it is that an 8-h dosing interval will be required to minimize peak-and-trough fluctuations in theophylline concentration. Determination of theophylline serum concentration during the initial weeks of treatment is useful in adjusting the dose and dosing interval. Sustained-release theophylline products that are completely absorbed and whose bioavailability is insignificantly affected by concomitant food administration are preferred. Once-a-day dosing is inappropriate in most children, who, because of their relatively rapid theophylline clearance, show unacceptable peak-and-trough differences in theophylline concentration and may become symptomatic toward the end of the 24-h dosing interval. With pellet formulations, the beads should be added to moist food (e.g., applesauce) to ensure their dissolution. Sustained-release tablets should not be crushed because this destroys their slow-release properties. An algorithm for initial dosing and final dosage adjustment based on serum concentration measurement may be found in a recent review of safety and efficacy of theophylline in children with asthma (Hendeles et al.). Because adverse effects of theophylline become manifest as the serum concentration of 20 µg/mL is approached, it is best to aim for the 8–15 µg/mL range in the majority of patients. Also in in vitro, animal models and human studies, theophylline has anti-inflammatory/immunomodulatory effects at serum concentrations in the 5–10 µg/mL range. (See dosing recommendations in Table 3.)

SUMMARY

Theophylline was introduced into clinical medicine 60 yr ago for treatment of asthma. Its role as a bronchodilator is undisputed, but it is not as effective as β_2-agonists in this regard. Most recently it has been discovered, as a result of studies in vitro and in animal and human models, that theophylline has very significant anti-inflammatory

Table 3
Dosing Titration (as Anhydrous Theophylline)[a,b,c]

Infants < 1 yr old
  Initial dosage
    Premature neonates
      <24 do postnatal age; 1.0 mg/kg every 12 h
      ≥24 d postnatal age; 1.5 mg/kg every 12 h
    Full-term infants and infants up to 52 wk of age
      Total daily dose (mg) = [(0.2 × age in wk) + 5.0] × (kg body wt)
        Up to age 26 wk; divide dose into three equal amounts administered at 8-h intervals
        >26 wk of age; divide dose into four equal amounts administered at 6-h intervals
  Final dosage
    Adjusted to maintain a peak steady-state serum theophylline concentration of 5–10
    µg/mL in neonates and 10–15 µg/mL in older infants. Since the time required to
    reach steady state is a function of theophylline half-life, up to 5 d may be required
    to achieve steady state in a premature neonate, whereas only 2–3 d may be
    required in a 6-mo-old infant without other risk factors for impaired clearance in
    the absence of a loading dose. If a serum theophylline concentration is obtained
    before steady state is achieved, the maintenance dose should not be increased,
    even if the serum theophylline concentration is < 10 µg/mL

Children (1–15 yr) and adults (16–60 yr) without risk factors for impaired clearance

Titration step	Children < 45 kg	Children > 45 kg and adults
Starting dosage:	10 mg/kg/d up to a maximum of 300 mg/d divided every 8 h	300 mg/d divided every 8 h
After 3 d, if tolerated, increase dose to:	13 mg/kg/d up to a maximum of 400 mg/d divided every 8 h	400 mg/d divided every 8 h
After 3 more days, if tolerated, increase dose to:	16 mg/kg/d up to a maximum of 600 mg/d divided every 8 h	600 mg/d divided every 8 h

Patients with risk factors for impaired clearance, the elderly (>60 yr), and those in
  whom it is not feasible to monitor serum theophylline concentrations:
  In children 1–15 yr of age, the initial theophylline dose should not exceed 16 mg/kg/d up
    to a maximum of 400 mg/d in the presence of risk factors for reduced theophylline
    clearance or if it is not feasible to monitor serum theophylline concentrations. In
    adolescents ≥16 yr and adults, including the elderly, the initial theophylline dose
    should not exceed 400 mg/d in the presence of risk factors for reduced theophylline
    clearance or if it is not feasible to monitor serum theophylline concentrations.
Loading dose for acute bronchodilatation:
  An inhaled β_2-selective agonist, alone or in combination with a systemically
    administered corticosteroid, is the most effective treatment for acute exacerbations
    of reversible airways obstruction. Theophylline is a relatively weak bronchodilator,
    is less effective than an inhaled β_2-selective agonist and provides no added benefit
    in the treatment of acute bronchospasm. If an inhaled or parenteral β-agonist is not
    available, a loading dose of an oral immediate release theophylline can be used as a
    temporary measure. A single 5 mg/kg dose of theophylline in a patient who has not
    received theophylline in the previous 24 h will produce an average peak serum

Table 3 *(continued)*
Dosing Titration (as Anhydrous Theophylline)[a,b,c]

theophylline concentration of 10 µg/mL (range 5–15 µg/mL). If dosing with
theophylline is to be continued beyond the loading dose, the above guidelines should
be utilized and serum theophylline concentration monitored at 24-h intervals to
adjust final dosage.

Final dosage adjustment guided by serum theophylline concentration

Peak serum concentration	Dosage adjustment
<9.9 µg/mL	If symptoms are not controlled and current dosage is tolerated, increase dose about 25%. Recheck serum concentration after 3 d for further dosage adjustment
10–14.9 µg/mL	If symptoms are controlled and current dosage is tolerated, maintain dose and recheck serum concentration at 6–12 mo intervals.[d] If symptoms are not controlled and current dosage is tolerated, consider adding additional medication(s) to treatment regimen
15–19.9 µg/mL	Consider 10% decrease in dose to provide greater margin of safety even if current dosage is tolerated.[d]
20–24.9 µg/mL	Decrease dose by 25% even if no adverse effects are present. Recheck serum concentration after 3 d to guide further dosage adjustment
25–30 µg/mL	Skip next dose and decrease subsequent doses at least 25% even if no adverse effects are present. Recheck serum concentration after 3 d to guide further dosage adjustment. If symptomatic, consider whether overdose treatment is indicated (see recommendations for chronic overdosage)
>30 µg/mL	Treat overdose as indicated (see recommendations for chronic overdosage). If theophylline is subsequently resumed, decrease dose by at least 50% and recheck serum concentration after 3 d to guide further dosage adjustment

[a]Patients with more rapid metabolism, clinically identified by higher than average dose requirements, should receive a smaller dose more frequently to prevent breakthrough symptoms resulting from low trough concentrations before the next dose. A reliably absorbed slow-release formulation will decrease fluctuations and permit longer dosing intervals.

[b]For products containing theophylline salts, the appropriate dose of the theophylline salt should be substituted for the anhydrous theophylline dose. To calculate the equivalent dose for theophylline salts, divide the anhydrous theophylline dose by 0.8 for aminophylline, by 0.65 for oxtriphylline, and by 0.5 for the calcium salicylate and sodium glycinate salts.

[c]Dosing recommendation taken from Hendeles L, Weinberger M, Szefler S, et al. Safety and efficacy of theophylline in children with asthma. *J Pediatr* 1992;120:177–183.

[d]Dose reduction and/or serum theophylline concentration measurement is indicated whenever adverse effects are present, physiological abnormalities that can reduce theophylline clearance occur (e.g., sustained fever), or a drug that interacts with theophylline is added or discontinued.

and immunomodulatory effects. Most interesting is the finding that these effects are demonstrable at serum concentrations in the 5–10 µg/mL range, significantly lower that what has been considered necessary for optimal bronchodilator effect (10–20 µg/mL). At the lower serum concentrations, adverse reactions are rare, and routine monitoring of serum theophylline levels is not necessary. Theophylline with both bronchodilator and anti-inflammatory effects is a truly unique drug.

SUGGESTED READING

Barnes, PJ, Pauwels RA. Theophylline in the Management of Asthma: Time For Reappraisal? *Eur Respir J* 1994;7:579–591.

Blake K. Theophylline. In Murphy S, Kelly HW, eds. *Pediatric Asthma, Lung Biology in Health and Disease*. New York, Dekker, 1999, vol 126.

Ellis EF. Theophylline toxicity. *J Allergy Clin Immunol* 1985;76:297–301.

Hendeles L, Weinberger M, Szefler S, et al. Safety and efficacy of theophylline in children with asthma. *J Pediatr* 1992;151:1907–1914.

Kidney J, Dominguez M, Taylor P, et al. Immunomodulation by theophylline in asthma. *Am J Respir Crit Care Med* 1995;151:1907–1914.

May CD. History of the introduction of theophylline into the treatment of asthma. *Clin Allergy* 1974;4:211–217.

Proceedings of the Theophylline Forum, Stockholm. *Clin Exp Allergy* 1996;26(suppl 2):1–59.

Selby C, Engleman H, Fitzpatrick M, et al. Inhaled salmeterol or oral theophylline in nocturnal asthma? *Am J Respir Crit Care Med* 1997;155:104–108.

Vassallo R, Lipsky JJ. Theophylline: Recent advances in the understanding of its mode of action and uses in clinical practice. *Mayo Clin Proc* 1998;73:346–354.

Weinberger M, Hendeles L. Theophylline. In: Middleton E Jr, Reed CE, Ellis EF, et al, eds. *Allergy: Principles and Practice*. St. Louis, Mosby, 1998.

20 Antileukotriene Agents in the Management of Asthma

Sheldon L. Spector, MD

INTRODUCTION

The role of inflammation in asthma has been the main theme of various guidelines on its treatment and the emphasis of the National Asthma Education Program (NAEP). There are several treatment options when selecting anti-inflammatory agents for managing asthma patients. Although inhaled corticosteroids are associated with considerably fewer side effects than oral corticosteroids, and currently are the anti-inflammatory medication of choice, they nevertheless have certain side effects. In the usual doses, they have been shown to be safe and well tolerated. However, with higher doses, they can produce adverse effects such as oral candidiasis, dysphonia, osteoporosis, possible growth retardation and even ocular effects, such as glaucoma and cataract formation.

Cromolyn and nedocromil are other anti-inflammatory agents that have been used in the treatment of asthma, but these medications are less effective than the inhaled corticosteroids. Theophylline also has anti-inflammatory properties. Unfortunately, its potential side effects, its narrow therapeutic range and its requirement for careful monitoring make it second-line therapy, even though previously it was a front-line agent. The antileukotriene agents represent the newest in anti-inflammatory treatment options. They represent the first new class for asthma management that has been introduced in more than 20 yr. The three leukotriene-modifying agents currently available include zafirlukast (Accolate™), montelukast (Singulair™) and zileuton (Zyflo™). There are others in clinical development.

From: *Current Clinical Practice: Allergic Diseases: Diagnosis and Treatment, 2nd Edition*
Edited by: P. Lieberman and J. Anderson © Humana Press Inc., Totowa, NJ

> The National Institutes of Health guidelines for asthma manage-
> ment mention antileukotrienes as alternative agents for treatment
> of mild, persistent asthma.

When the NAEP treatment guidelines came out in 1997, the antileukotrienes were mentioned as an alternative to inhaled corticosteroids, cromolyn, nedocromil or sustained-release theophylline in patients with mild, persistent asthma. More recently, international guidelines suggested their use for moderate asthma. Some investigators have suggested that they be tried in the severe asthmatic patient, since their mode of action is different from that of the inhaled corticosteroids, and it is often difficult to predict responders from nonresponders. This discussion will concern itself primarily with the clinical studies of antileukotrienes and their expanded role in the treatment of asthma.

BIOSYNTHESIS AND POTENCY OF LEUKOTRIENES

Previously identified as slow-reacting substance of anaphylaxis (SRS/A), the leukotrienes are a family of proinflammatory lipid mediators derived from arachidonic acid via the 5-lipoxygenase pathway. Their name is derived from the word *leukocytes* that produced them and the triene-containing chemical structure. The cysteinyl or sulfidopeptide leukotrienes LTC_4, LTD_4 LTE_4 are so named because each contains a thioether-linked cysteine residue.

Another leukotriene, LTB_4, contains a similar lipid lacking the thioether-linked peptide. Many types of inflammatory cells can produce leukotrienes, especially eosinophils, mast cells and macrophages. A number of signals can stimulate the production of leukotrienes, including trauma, infection, allergen and inflammation. These stimuli trigger phospholipase A_2-mediated release of arachidonic acids from nuclear-membrane phospholipids. The nucleus arachidonic acid binds to 5-lipoxygenase-activating protein (FLAP), a membranous protein that presents arachidonic acid to 5-lipoxygenase. The unstable leukotriene LTA_4 is then formed, which, in turn, either is hydrolyzed to LTB_4 or is converted to LTC_4 by LTC_4-synthase, depending on the cell type. After extracellular conversion of LTC_4 to LTD_4, there is subsequent metabolism to LTE_4. The cysteinyl leukotrienes are potent constrictors of airway-smooth muscle, and they also promote mucous secretion and stimulate the infiltration of inflammatory cells into the airway tissue. Although LTB_4 has potent chemotactic effects in certain systems, it does not appear to have as much significance in asthma as do the cysteinyl leukotrienes. Cysteinyl leukotrienes are 1000 times more potent than histamine in eliciting bronchoconstriction following inhalation.

Their relevance in asthma is also suggested by their detection in bronchoalveolar lavage fluid, during both the early- and late-phase allergen challenge. Eosinophils are typically recruited during the early phase and last throughout the late phase. The eosinophils and the later-arriving alveolar macrophage may then contribute to the additional production of leukotrienes.

Leukotriene-modifying agents can be grouped into those that inhibit leukotriene biosynthesis (i.e., 5-lipoxygenase and FLAP inhibitors) and those that block the cysteinyl leukotrienes at the receptor. Pranlukast was the first receptor antagonist to be

> Antileukotrienes have been shown to be effective in exercise-induced asthma, attacks precipitated by allergen challenge, episodes due to the ingestion of nonsteroidal anti-inflammatory agents (NSAIDs) and in chronic asthma.

commercially available in Japan. The only two agents currently available in the United States are zafirlukast and montelukast, which are selective cysteinyl LT_1 antagonists. Zileuton is the only synthesis inhibitor available in the United States, and it blocks the 5-lipoxygenase enzyme.

Various clinical models have been utilized to establish the role of antileukotriene agents in asthma management. These include stimuli that can provoke bronchospasm, such as LTD_4, allergen, exercise, cold air, sulfur dioxide and aspirin. The subject is usually given an antileukotriene agent or placebo before the challenge procedure to mitigate against its bronhoconstrictive effect. One of the first studies employed with any leukotriene modifier at the receptor level was an inhibition of LTD_4-induced bronchoconstriction. A single dose of zafirlukast, for example, can significantly block an LTD_4 challenge immediately and hours after administration; in one study, the dose required to produce bronchoconstriction was more than 100 times greater with zafirlukast than a placebo. Volunteers given pranlukast 400 mg twice a day withstood a 25-fold higher LTD_4 dose, and a 40-mg dose of montelukast shifted the curve 20- to 45-fold in two of six patients with mild asthma. Antileukotriene agents also block both the early- and late-phase response to an allergen challenge. If segmental allergen challenge is utilized, with subsequent bronchoalveolar lavage, zafirlukast can significantly block bronchoalveolar lavage lymphocytes and basophils measured 48 h after antigen challenge.

Montelukast and pranlukast have also inhibited eosinophils using various model systems. A particular challenge of interest is an aspirin challenge in patients who are sensitive to its effect in terms of the production of asthma and rhinitis symptoms. Antileukotrienes prevent an aspirin challenge, which is consistent with the hypothesis that aspirin sensitivity is mediated in some fashion by the cysteinyl leukotrienes. Agents such as zafirlukast have also been given to patients who were undergoing a desensitization procedure with much difficulty, and it allowed for a safe desensitization to occur in such individuals.

ANTILEUKOTRIENES IN CHRONIC ASTHMA STUDIES

Any new agent must undergo the rigors of clinical testing in asthmatic patients to prove effectiveness. Initially, studies are done in mildly ill patients with single doses. In one study of zafirlukast, patients were observed by spirometry for 4 h. By 1 h patients already had significant improvement from baseline, compared to placebo, and it continued for 4 h. Since additional improvement in airway tone was obtained with the subsequent administration of a β_2-adrenergic agonist, such a study emphasizes the different mechanisms of bronchodilation with an antileukotriene versus a β-agonist.

Other studies of acute asthma are under way. Montelukast has been used in the emergency room setting and has been found to provide an acute bronchodilator effect. Until data are published to clarify its role in acute asthma, it is not suggested that these agents be used in this way. There have been many controlled clinical trials confirming the efficacy of antileukotrienes in patients with chronic asthma. Initially there was a 6-wk study using zafirlukast in increasing doses and, subsequently, a 13-wk study with zafirlukast 20 mg twice daily. Although there was somewhat of a dose-response relationship, both studies showed significant improvement in nighttime awakening, morning awakening, daytime symptom score and β-adrenergic agonist usage compared to placebo. There was objective improvement in pulmonary function tests, as measured by peak expiratory flow rate (PEFR) and forced expiratory volume in 1 s (FEV_1). Subgroups of patients with more severe asthma showed somewhat better response, perhaps because they had "more room" to respond. Montelukast has also been shown in a number of studies to improve pulmonary function, daytime and nighttime symptoms and decrease β-agonist usage. There was rapid onset of action, and peripheral blood eosinophil counts were lowered.

Montelukast has also been tried in pediatric studies and, because of favorable results, has an indication in children age 2 yr and above. Zileuton has also undergone successful clinical studies, showing improved pulmonary function and decreased asthma symptoms. It has the ability to reduce the percentage of patients needing supplemental systemic steroids and has been demonstrated to improve quality of life. Unfortunately, its four-times daily administration creates issues of patient adherence.

A number of studies comparing antileukotriene agents with other anti-asthma medications have now been published, either as abstracts or as papers. Antileukotrienes show either equal or greater efficacy than cromolyn and nedocromil. Zileuton had a beneficial effect comparable to theophylline. Both of these agents ideally require blood monitoring—zileuton for its possible liver toxicity and theophylline for its potential dose-related toxicity. Antileukotrienes, as a class, seem to improve quality of life. The safety of these agents has also been studied. Zileuton can produce significantly increased hepatic enzymes, as seen in long-term safety surveillance studies. Since most of these elevations occurred within the first few months of treatment, the package insert suggests liver-function monitoring monthly for the first 3 mo and quarterly thereafter.

By contrast, the incidence of elevated liver-function tests with zafirlukast and with montelukast at clinically effective doses is comparable to that of placebo. Many cases of Churg-Strauss syndrome have been reported in association with zafirlukast and montelukast therapy, especially in patients with severe asthma following reductions in oral steroid usage. The best explanation for the appearance of this unusual syndrome in relationship to administration of these antileukotrienes is the unmasking of a previous condition when oral steroids are tapered because of the introduction of the antileukotriene agent.

To support this assumption, the package insert for fluticasone now contains a warning against the possible appearance of the Churg-Strauss syndrome upon tapering of oral steroids.

ANTILEUKOTRIENES: *Were Do They Fit In Your Practice?*

In the 1997 NAEP guidelines, the two antileukotrienes available at the time, zafirlukast and zileuton, were recommended as first-line anti-inflammatory therapy in patients 12 yr of age or older who have mild, persistent asthma. Since this publication, montelukast became available as an additional agent for use in children ages 2 yr and older, and zafirlukast for children 7 yr and older.

> Antileukotrienes may be steroid sparing, permitting decreased dosing of inhaled corticosteroids.

Recent international guidelines have suggested the use of these agents in moderate asthma as well. This concept expands the suggestion from the 1997 NAEP guidelines.

Although antileukotrienes have a significant bronchodilator effect, they should not be substituted for β_2-adrenergic agonists on either a long-term or short-term basis under definitive studies, confirm their usefulness in this way.

Based on limited data, they are at least as good as and, often better than cromolyn or nedocromil, especially with their ease of use and anticipated improved compliance as oral agents. In one study in which blood monitoring was included, zileuton and theophylline had comparable effectiveness.

There are now studies that have compared the oral antileukotriene agents with inhaled corticosteroid therapy. In one study, montelukast had a quicker onset of action, although a moderate dose of inhaled steroids performed slightly better than montelukast using certain clinical parameters. In other studies, moderate doses of corticosteroid aerosols had an effect comparable to the antileukotrienes. Should a patient be experiencing a side effect from corticosteroid therapy, such as hoarseness or thrush, the antileukotriene may very well be preferred. In fact, patient compliance may be better with an oral agent, especially if "steroid phobia" also exists in the mind of the patient. There are ongoing studies comparing the more potent inhaled corticosteroids or higher doses of inhaled steroids. Such studies will help clarify their use in patients with moderate to severe asthma.

A particularly attractive concept might be to employ inhaled corticosteroids and antileukotrienes together to minimize the dose of inhaled steroids and thereby mitigate possible side effects. Since the mode of action of inhaled steroids and leukotriene modifiers is different, it is not surprising that in one study of patients receiving high-dose inhaled corticosteroids (mean beclomethasone dipropionate dose of 1600 mg/d), the addition of zafirlukast produced significant improvement in pulmonary function and asthma symptoms without affecting the adverse side-effect profile. Other studies have suggested that patients receiving half the dose of inhaled steroid plus an antileukotriene perform as well as those receiving double the dose of the inhaled steroid. In the 9-mo open-label study, either montelukast 10 mg daily or inhaled beclomethasone dipropionate 400 µg daily brought about similar improvement in daytime symptoms, nighttime awakenings, β_2-adrenergic agonist usage and lung function. Over time, once-a-day antileukotrienes may do better than an inhaled steroid taken multiple times throughout the day.

I have used antileukotrienes in patients with chronic cough, with and without underlying asthma, with some success. This may be due to the effect of antileukotrienes on the irritant receptor. Data have also been presented regarding our experience in blocking an allergic reaction to household pets in a controlled study with cat-sensitive individuals. Individuals with exercise-induced asthma placed on a regimen of antileukotrienes can often minimize, or even eliminate, their "p.r.n use" (as needed) of β-adrenergic agonists. All of the available agents have been shown to be effective in exercise-induced bronchospasm.

There also are a few studies that show that the leukotriene blockers improve nasal symptoms, especially stuffiness, and possibly symptoms of sinusitis (according to case reports). Thus, orally administered antileukotrienes have the added advantage of helping associated organ systems. Other studies are under way in conditions in which inflammation is also thought to play a role, including chronic obstructive pulmonary disease, various inflammatory bowel diseases and arthritides and skin disease such as chronic urticaria.

SUMMARY

Although the antileukotrienes cannot be effective in every patient with asthma, they represent an important new class of anti-inflammatory therapy that will help control asthma symptoms in virtually every category of asthma, from the mild to the severe. In a number of studies they decrease daytime and nighttime asthma symptoms, improve pulmonary function and reduce the need for concomitant β-agonists or even inhaled corticosteroids. They also reduce the number of asthma exacerbations and often improve upper airway symptoms, as reflected in improved quality of life. Although every patient with asthma will not respond to the antileukotrienes in view of the heterogeneity of the disease, antileukotrienes represent a welcome addition to our armamentarium, especially in patients with persistent mild to moderate asthma.

SUGGESTED READING

Calhoun WJ, Lavins BJ, Minkwitz MC, Evans R, Gleich GJ, Cohn J. Effect of zafirlukast (Accolate) on cellular mediators of inflammation: Bronchoalveolar lavage fluid findings after segmental antigen challenge. *Am J Respir Crit Care Med* 1998;157:1381–1389.

Grossman J, Smith LJ. Long-term safety and efficacy of zafirlukast in the treatment of asthma: Interim results of an open-label extension trial. *Ann Allergy Asthma Immunol* 1999;82:361–369.

Israel E, Fischer AR, Rosenberg MA, et al. The pivotal role of 5-lipoxygenase products in the reaction of aspirin-sensitive asthmatics to aspirin. *Am Rev Respir Dis* 1993;148:1447–1451.

Liu MC, Dube LM, Lancaster J. Acute and chronic effects of a 5-lipoxygenase inhibitor in asthma: A 6-month randomized multicenter trial. *J Allergy Clin Immunol* 1996;98:859–871.

Nathan RA, Bernstein JA, Bielory L, et al. Zafirlukast improves asthma symptoms and quality of life in patients with moderate reversible airflow obstruction. *J Allergy Clin Immunol* 1998;102:935–942.

National Asthma Education and Prevention Program. Expert Panel Report 2. Guidelines for the Diagnosis and Management of Asthma. Bethesda, MD: National Institutes of Health, National Heart, Lung, and Blood Institute; 1997.

Reiss TF, Hill JB, Harman E, et al. Increased urinary excretion of LTE after exercise and attenuation of exercise-induced bronchospasm by montelukast, a cysteinyl leukotriene receptor antagonist. *Thorax* 1997;52:1030–1035.

Spector SL. Leukotriene activity modulation in asthma. *Drugs* 1997;54:369–384.

Spector SL, Smith LJ, Glass M, "Accolate" Asthma Trialist Group. Effects of 6 weeks of therapy with oral doses of ICI-204,219, a leukotriene D receptor antagonist in subjects with bronchial asthma. *Am J Respir Crit Care Med* 1994;150:618–623.

Suissa S, Dennis R, Ernst P, Sheehy O, Wood-Dauphinee S. Effectiveness of the leukotriene receptor antagonist zafirlukast for mild-to-moderate asthma: A randomized, double-blind, placebo-controlled trial. *Ann Intern Med* 1997;126:177–183.

Virchow J, Hassall SM, Summerton L. Harris A. Improved asthma control over 6 weeks with Accolate (zafirlukast) in patients on high-dose inhaled corticosteroids. *J Investig Med* 1997;45:286A.

21 Cromolyn and Nedocromil
Nonsteroidal Anti-Inflammatory Therapy for Asthma and Other Allergic Diseases

Stephen F. Kemp, MD

CONTENTS

INTRODUCTION
MECHANISMS OF ACTION
CLINICAL EFFICACY
SAFETY, TOXICITY, AND POTENTIAL SIDE EFFECTS
OTHER THERAPEUTIC USES FOR CROMOLYN OR NEDOCROMIL
SUMMARY
SUGGESTED READING

INTRODUCTION

Cromolyn sodium and nedocromil sodium are two nonsteroidal anti-inflammatory medications that are highly effective in the treatment of asthma, allergic rhinitis and allergic eye disease. They are not, however, chemically or mechanistically related to the prostaglandin synthetase inhibitors commonly known as nonsteroidal anti-inflammatory drugs (NSAIDs).

Both cromolyn sodium and nedocromil sodium are water soluble and fat insoluble and are totally ionized at physiological pH. These physical and chemical properties suggest that all biological activities are due to drug interactions with an unidentified surface receptor.

Cromolyn sodium is a derivative of chromone-2-carboxylic acid, whereas nedocromil sodium is a pyranoquinolone (Fig. 1). Despite their chemical and structural differences, they both exert remarkably similar anti-inflammatory actions.

MECHANISMS OF ACTION (TABLE 1)

Both cromolyn and nedocromil apparently exert their effects on the "intermediate conductance" chloride channels of cells. In nonexcitable cells, the rapid release of intracellular calcium opens chloride channels on the cell's surface. This action induces an influx of chloride ions resulting in, for example, degranulation and mediator release

From: *Current Clinical Practice: Allergic Diseases: Diagnosis and Treatment, 2nd Edition*
Edited by: P. Lieberman and J. Anderson © Humana Press Inc., Totowa, NJ

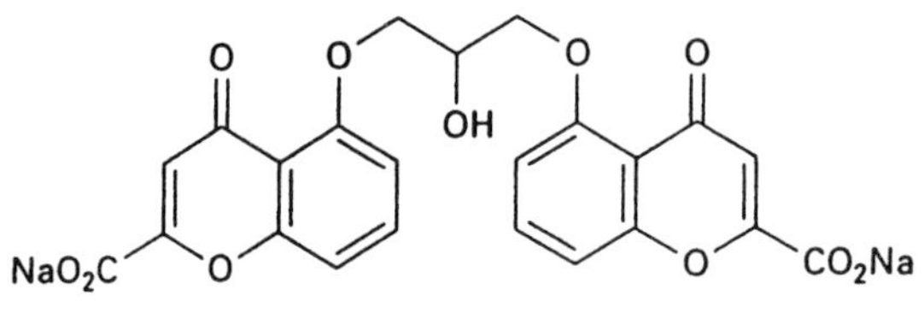

Sodium Cromoglycate

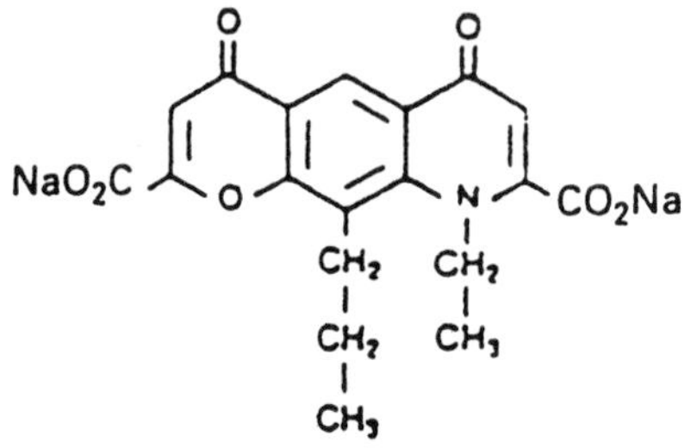

Nedocromil sodium

Fig. 1. Structural formulas of nedocromil sodium and sodium cromoglycate.

from mast cells or depolarization of sensory neurons. Mast cell degranulation depends on the sustained elevation of intracellular calcium following a transient inositol triphosphate–induced increase in calcium caused by the release of calcium from intracellular stores. Cromolyn and nedocromil abolish or inhibit the calcium channel activation that follows the antigen crosslinking of membrane-bound IgE.

By blocking the activity of chloride channel pathways on cells, such as mast cells, eosinophils, epithelial cells, endothelial cells, fibroblasts and sensory neurons, these drugs dampen the inflammatory responses associated with allergic disease. This impairment of chloride channels may be related to drug-induced phosphorylation of a 78-kD protein thought to be associated with the termination of mast cell mediator release. A structurally similar protein interacts with the cellular cytoskeleton, and its phosphorylation by cromolyn may help to explain the inhibitory effects of cromolyn and nedocromil on chloride channels. These drugs may imitate a natural inhibitory process, thus accounting for their lack of toxicity.

In summary, the clinical activity of these drugs apparently derives from their down-regulation of a variety of cells involved in the inflammatory response, both allergic and nonallergic factors. Of particular importance is their ability to down-regulate eosinophil-driven inflammation. Neither cromolyn nor nedocromil has intrinsic bronchodilatory, anticholinergic or antihistaminic activity.

CLINICAL EFFICACY

Asthma

Both cromolyn and nedocromil effectively block the asthmatic response to a variety of stimuli (Table 2). These include not only allergen-induced reactions but also those

Table 1
Mechanisms of Action

1. Block chloride channels, thereby decreasing:
   • Mast cell degranulation
   • Activation of eosinophils
   • Nerve conduction through sensory neurons
2. No intrinsic bronchodilatory, anticholinergic or antihistaminic activity

Table 2
Asthma-Inducing Agents Inhibited by Cromolyn and Nedocromil

Allergens
Chemicals (mediators)
   Adenosine monophosphate
   Hypertonic saline
Neurogenic
   NO_2
   SO_2
   Sodium metabisulfite
   Bradykinin
   Substance P
   Neurokinin A
   Capsaicin
Physical factors
   Fog
   Exercise
   Cold air

related to neurogenic, chemical and physical factors, such as substance P, bradykinin, nitric oxide, sulfur dioxide, sodium metabisulfite, cold air and fog. In addition, they can prevent exercise-induced bronchospasm. The drugs are thus versatile and protect against a wide array of asthma-inducing stimuli.

The key features of cromolyn and nedocromil are outlined in Table 3. Their action is clearly anti-inflammatory. Biopsy and bronchoalveolar lavage studies obtained after provocative challenges or during long-term therapy both demonstrate very significant reductions in inflammatory markers. Both drugs decrease the number of indolent and activated eosinophils found in bronchoalveolar lavage fluid and biopsy specimens of respiratory mucosa. In addition, cromolyn decreases the amount of albumin present in bronchoalveolar lavage fluid.

Numerous in vitro findings complement these in vivo effects. These findings include inhibition of macrophage release of neutrophil chemotactic factor, decreased eosinophil chemotaxis and inhibition of eosinophil and mast cell degranulation, among other activities.

Long-term administration of both drugs produces clear-cut clinical improvement manifested by decreased symptom scores, gradual increases in forced expiratory volume in 1 s (FEV_1), decreased peak flow diurnal variability and decreased bronchial hyperresponsiveness following histamine or methacholine challenge. However, acute

Table 3
Key Features of Use in Asthma

- Anti-inflammatory
- Decreases bronchial hyperresponsiveness
- Blocks early- and late-phase allergic reaction
- Prevents bronchospasm in response to allergic and numerous, non-allergic stimuli
- Maintenance prophylaxis for inhalant allergens
- Major role in mild to moderate persistent asthma
- May potentially be corticosteroid sparing
- Excellent safety profile

administration of cromolyn or nedocromil has no effect on bronchoconstriction induced by directly acting spasmogens such as histamine or methacholine. Both cromolyn and nedocromil decrease bronchodilator use and also reduce the dosage of inhaled corticosteroids necessary to control asthma. These effects are seen in both allergic and nonallergic asthmatics.

Cromolyn and nedocromil are very similar in their clinical effects, and there are no dramatic differences between the two drugs. However, some minor clinical differences are summarized in Table 4.

Both drugs will prevent the early- and late-phase allergic response when they are administered before an allergen challenge. However, nedocromil will prevent the late-phase response when it is administered after an allergen challenge, whereas cromolyn will not. Both drugs exert their effects on nonallergic asthma stimuli. Nedocromil, however, seems to be slightly more effective in blocking asthma caused by nitric oxide, sulfur dioxide, sodium metabisulfite and adenosine monophosphate. In addition, nedocromil may be more effective at inhibiting eosinophil chemotaxis. Specifically, nedocromil, but not cromolyn, inhibits chemotaxis of eosinophils induced by platelet-activating factor and leukotriene B_4.

Whether or not these observations result in clinically detectable differences between the two agents is unclear. However, some evidence suggests subtle clinical differences exist between the two drugs:

1. Nedocromil may have a faster onset of action. It exerted its beneficial effects within a few days in one study, while cromolyn effects may take 2–4 wk.
2. In another study, cromolyn displayed a longer duration of activity in the prevention of exercise-induced asthma.
3. The maintenance dosing frequency required for nedocromil may be less than that required for cromolyn. A twice-daily regimen is effective for some patients taking nedocromil.
4. Nedocromil may be more effective than cromolyn in the treatment of nonallergic asthmatics. The rationale for this statement is its superior effect in blocking nonallergic asthma triggers.
5. Nedocromil may control asthmatic cough more effectively than cromolyn. However, cromolyn may help to reduce the chronic cough associated with angiotensin-converting enzyme (ACE) inhibitors, presumably because of its inhibition of sensory nerve activation.

Table 4
Features Distinguishing Nedocromil from Cromolyn

Nedocromil blocks the late-phase pulmonary response to allergen challenge when administered before or shortly after provocative challenge. Cromolyn is effective only when it is administered before challenge.

Nedocromil inhalation inhibits the release of cytotoxic mediators in aspirin-sensitive asthmatics whose platelets are challenged in vitro with aspirin. Cromolyn inhalation does not.

Nedocromil may be more effective in preventing asthma due to nonallergic triggers, such as NO_2, SO_2, metabisulfite and adenosine monophosphate.

Nedocromil may be more effective in blocking eosinophil chemotaxis.

Nedocromil has a faster onset of action.

Cromolyn may have a longer duration of effect in preventing exercise bronchospasm.

Cromolyn may inhibit angiotensin-converting enzyme (ACE) inhibitor–induced cough because of its inhibition of sensory nerve activation.

Cromolyn may potentially alleviate refractory atopic dermatitis.

Cromolyn may help to alleviate the common cold.

Nedocromil may require less frequent dosing as a maintenance regimen.

Nedocromil is more efficacious than cromolyn in the treatment of vernal keratoconjunctivitis and is effective in patients whose chronic symptoms of allergic conjunctivitis are not controlled fully by cromolyn. Ocular preparations of nedocromil are not commercially available in the United States.

6. A certain percentage of patients will not take nedocromil because of an unpleasant taste. Most patients do not taste nedocromil. No unpleasant taste is associated with inhaled cromolyn.

No consistent difference between cromolyn and nedocromil exists in clinical trials involving subjects with asthma. Some trials report clinical equivalence while others report a relative advantage of one over the other in controlling certain asthma features.

It should be emphasized that neither drug is a bronchodilator. Indeed, both drugs seem to have irritative properties that will cause cough or wheeze in some patients whose asthma has not been adequately controlled. As a practical point, therefore, a brief therapeutic course of corticosteroids may be necessary to control active asthmatic inflammation before initiation of these drugs.

Both drugs are indicated for maintenance control of mild to moderate persistent asthma and may additionally help to reduce the dependency on inhaled corticosteroids in severe, persistent asthma. Nedocromil is available in the United States only as a metered dose inhaler (MDI). Cromolyn is available as both an MDI and a nebulizer solution. Therefore, cromolyn may be used in infants and small children who cannot use an MDI.

The initial dosage frequency for both cromolyn and nedocromil is four times daily once acute asthmatic inflammation is controlled. Dosage reductions are almost always possible for maintenance therapy. Prophylactic administration prior to allergen exposure, such as a visit to a relative who resides with a pet to whom the patient is allergic, is a unique therapeutic use for both drugs. Both should be administered before exposure and every 4 h during exposure. Both drugs effectively prevent exercise-induced bronchospasm when administered immediately prior to strenuous exercise. Better efficacy has been reported for cromolyn when it is inhaled slowly from a large-

> Perhaps the key features of cromolyn and nedocromil are their superb safety profile and the fact that both have anti-inflammatory activity.

volume (700 ml) holding chamber than from more rapid conventional inhalation. These results may be related to more homogeneous pulmonary distribution.

Allergic Rhinitis

Both nedocromil and cromolyn are effective agents in the therapy of both seasonal and perennial forms of allergic rhinitis. However, this discussion will be limited to the use of cromolyn, since nasal preparations of nedocromil are not commercially available in the United States. Cromolyn is available in an aqueous form, both with and without prescription, for the therapy of allergic rhinitis. As with asthma, cromolyn administration prevents both the early and late nasal responses to allergen and decreases both activated and indolent eosinophils found in nasal secretions and biopsies.

As in asthma, nasal cromolyn should be administered once the rhinitis is reasonably controlled, and it should be given prior to exposure. Thus, therapy for seasonal allergic rhinitis should be initiated before the allergy season begins. This drug can be highly effective in blocking symptoms resulting from isolated allergy exposure when it is administered immediately before mowing the lawn or visiting a relative with a pet.

It is important to remember that cromolyn is a preventive agent that needs to be used regularly during allergen exposure. It has no immediate effect. Its initial dose is two sprays four times daily, but this dosage frequency potentially can be reduced after the first 2–3 wk of therapy.

The safety profile of nasal cromolyn is excellent. Therefore, it is an excellent drug for use in children for whom nasal corticosteroids are considered undesirable. Nonetheless, nasal corticosteroids have a superior therapeutic effect compared to nasal cromolyn. Moreover, additional medications are usually necessary to achieve an acceptable clinical response to cromolyn, especially when congestion is a troublesome nasal symptom.

Allergic Eye Disease

Cromolyn may be effective in the management of several allergic eye diseases. All of these disorders appear to involve mast cells and eosinophils. These conditions include seasonal allergic conjunctivitis, vernal keratoconjunctivitis, atopic keratoconjunctivitis and giant papillary conjunctivitis. Nedocromil is more efficacious than cromolyn in the treatment of vernal keratoconjunctivitis and is effective in patients whose chronic symptoms of allergic conjunctivitis are not controlled fully by cromolyn. Ocular preparations of nedocromil, however, are not commercially available in the United States.

Seasonal Allergic Conjunctivitis

Ocular cromolyn therapy is virtually as effective as oral antihistamines for seasonal allergic conjunctivitis. It reduces itching, stinging and photosensitivity. Therapeutic response in seasonal allergic conjunctivitis may be related to allergen–specific IgE antibody levels.

As with other allergic diseases, the drug should be started when the patient is relatively free of symptoms. It is administered at a dose of 1–2 drops four times daily. Ocular cromolyn is not effective acutely. However, it can also be used prophylactically before specific allergen exposure.

VERNAL KERATOCONJUNCTIVITIS

Vernal keratoconjunctivitis is recurrent, bilateral, interstitial inflammation of the conjunctivae that occurs more frequently in warm, dry climates. Most affected patients develop symptoms before puberty, and symptoms usually resolve by 25 yr of age. Symptoms of severe itching, tearing, burning, mucoid discharge and photophobia may occur perennially, but are characteristically worse during spring and summer months. Abnormalities may include giant papillae on upper tarsal conjunctivae, corneal plaques, scarring and decreased visual acuity.

Several studies indicate that ocular cromolyn is effective for vernal keratoconjunctivitis. Beneficial effects seem to occur within 1 wk of initiating therapy and are manifested by decreased pruritus and mucous secretion. The dosage is 1–2 drops four times daily. Lodoxamide is generally more effective, however.

ATOPIC KERATOCONJUNCTIVITIS

Atopic keratoconjunctivitis is the ocular counterpart to atopic dermatitis. However, only a small percentage of patients with atopic dermatitis develop atopic keratoconjunctivitis. Associated symptoms include severe itching, burning, mucoid discharge and photosensitivity. Cataracts and keratoconus may develop. Double-blind placebo-controlled crossover studies have shown beneficial effects of cromolyn on discharge, photophobia, papillary hypertrophy and both limbal and corneal changes. In addition, dosage reductions for topical corticosteroids have been reported.

GIANT PAPILLARY CONJUNCTIVITIS

Evidence suggests that giant papillary conjunctivitis is triggered by an inflammatory response to any foreign substance, such as a contact lens or ocular prosthesis, that irritates the upper tarsal conjunctiva. Because pathological changes are similar to those seen in allergic eye disorders, cromolyn has been employed. A reduction in symptoms and increased tolerance to contact lens wear have been demonstrated in many patients. The dose is the same as for other ocular disorders. Affected patients should discontinue contact lens wear while the condition persists and should consider switching to disposable contact lenses once it resolves.

OTHER THERAPEUTIC USES FOR CROMOLYN OR NEDOCROMIL

Atopic dermatitis is an inflammatory, IgE-mediated skin disease characterized by intense pruritus, xerosis and scaly, licheniform rash with a characteristic anatomical distribution. Therapy is directed at avoidance of inciting stimuli, moisture retention, emollients, antipruritics and topical corticosteroids.

One report of a placebo-controlled, randomized, crossover study suggests that topical cromolyn may potentially benefit patients for whom the above therapeutic methods have failed. Cromolyn prepared in an emollient base was applied to the skin of children and adolescents with moderate to severe atopic dermatitis. All subjects concomitantly applied a midpotency topical steroid. Objective severity decreased significantly in the cromolyn-steroid group compared to the group treated with steroid alone. The study authors posit an additive anti-inflammatory effect based on the different mechanisms of action employed by corticosteroids and cromolyn.

Other reports have proposed that intranasal cromolyn or nedocromil (not commercially available in the United States as an intranasal preparation) may benefit the common cold. The causative viruses or atypical bacteria may produce a variety of inflammatory mediators, including histamine, cytokines, leukotrienes and nitric oxide. Compared to placebo, both cromolyn and nedocromil provide swifter resolution and reduced severity of symptoms in nonallergic subjects. Both drugs also reduce symptoms of virus-induced asthma exacerbations.

Systemic mastocytosis, a disease characterized by mast cell proliferation in multiple organ systems, usually features urticaria pigmentosa (brownish macules that transform into wheals upon stroking) and recurrent episodes of flushing, tachycardia, pruritus, headache, syncope, abdominal pain or diarrhea. Since it inhibits mast cell degranulation, orally administered cromolyn has some efficacy in mastocytosis, particularly for symptoms involving the gastrointestinal tract. However, cromolyn does not reduce plasma or urinary histamine levels in patients with mastocytosis.

SAFETY, TOXICITY, AND POTENTIAL SIDE EFFECTS

Nedocromil and cromolyn are two of the safest drugs available for treatment of allergic diseases. They possess little, if any, toxicity. Local irritation is the most common side effect. Nedocromil is perceived by some patients to have an unpleasant taste, which may limit its use.

SUMMARY

Both nedocromil sodium and cromolyn sodium are useful anti-inflammatory drugs in the therapy of allergic diseases. These diseases include asthma, allergic rhinitis and allergic ocular disorders. Additional therapeutic uses have been proposed. Nedocromil and cromolyn are both available in the United States for asthma therapy, but only cromolyn is available for the treatment of the other conditions.

Both drugs are indicated for use in mild to moderate persistent asthma and may permit dosage reductions in inhaled steroids in more severe asthmatics. They effectively reduce symptoms, improve lung function and decrease bronchial hyperreactivity. In addition, both can be used prophylactically prior to isolated allergen exposures. They are particularly useful in children for whom inhaled corticosteroids are considered undesirable. Both drugs should be administered initially once the underlying illness is relatively well controlled, and both must be used regularly for maintenance therapy. Neither drug has intrinsic bronchodilatory, antihistaminic or anticholinergic activities. Therefore, neither drug is useful for the treatment of acute symptoms. In fact, they may transiently worsen symptoms associated with acute ocular, nasal or pulmonary inflammation. Both drugs have excellent safety profiles, and no consistent, severe adverse reactions occur with either drug.

SUGGESTED READING

Barnes PJ, Holgate ST, Laitinen LA, Pauwels R. Asthma mechanisms, determinants of severity and treatment: The role of nedocromil sodium. *Clin Exp Allergy* 1995;25:771–787.

Edwards AM. Sodium cromoglycate (Intal) as an anti-inflammatory agent for the treatment of chronic asthma. *Clin Exp Allergy* 1994;24:612–623.

Holgate ST. A rationale for the use of nedocromil sodium in the treatment of asthma. *J Allergy Clin Immunol* 1996;98:S157–160.

Johnston SL. Cromolyns: treatment for the common cold? *Clin Exp Allergy* 1996;26:989–994.

Laube BL, Edwards AM, Dalby RN, Creticos PS, Norman PS. The efficacy of slow versus faster inhalation of cromolyn sodium in protecting against allergen challenge in patients with asthma. *J Allergy Clin Immunol* 1998;101:475–483.

MacLeod JDA. The treatment of allergic eye disease: Has sodium cromoglycate had its day? *Clin Exp Allergy* 1999;29:436–438.

Moore C, Ehlayel MS, Junprasert J, Sorensen RU. Topical sodium cromoglycate in the treatment of moderate-to-severe atopic dermatitis. *Ann Allergy Asthma Immunol* 1998;81:452–458.

National Asthma Education and Prevention Program. Expert Panel Report 2: Guidelines for the Diagnosis and Management of Asthma. Bethesda, MD, National Institutes of Health. National Heart, Lung, and Blood Institute. Publication No. 97-4051, 1997.

Norris AA, Alton EWFW. Chloride transport and the action of sodium cromoglycate and nedocromil sodium. *Clin Exp Allergy* 1996;26:250–253.

Spector S. Ideal pharmacology for allergic rhinitis. *J Allergy Clin Immunol* 1999;103:S386–387.

22 Anticholinergic Agents in Respiratory Diseases

Juan L. Rodriguez, MD

CONTENTS

INTRODUCTION

The origin of the anticholinergic agents is found in the belladonna plants from which atropine and scopolamine are derived. In ancient times, extracts of these plants were used as poisonous agents because of their potent physiological effects. The first recorded use of belladonna alkaloids for the treatment of respiratory diseases comes from India where the smoke of burning jimsonweed (Datura stramonium) was used to treat asthma symptoms. British settlers in India introduced the use of belladonna alkaloids into western medicine in the 19th century. Atropine was isolated in its pure form by Mein in 1831. Although found to be useful for the treatment of respiratory conditions such as asthma and disorders of gastrointestinal motility, these substances were limited by their toxicity, including the effects on the heart and the undesirable side effects such as dry mouth, urinary retention and pupillary dilation. Recently there has been an effort to develop anticholinergic substances with little or no undesirable side effects. These efforts have led to the development of quaternary ammonium compounds of atropine such as ipratropium bromide that share with atropine beneficial effects on the respiratory tract with few undesirable effects. The addition of the quaternary ammonium structure makes this medication poorly absorbable through the mucosa of the respiratory and gastrointestinal tract (Fig. 1). This property confers its low potential for side effects.

From: *Current Clinical Practice: Allergic Diseases: Diagnosis and Treatment, 2nd Edition*
Edited by: P. Lieberman and J. Anderson © Humana Press Inc., Totowa, NJ

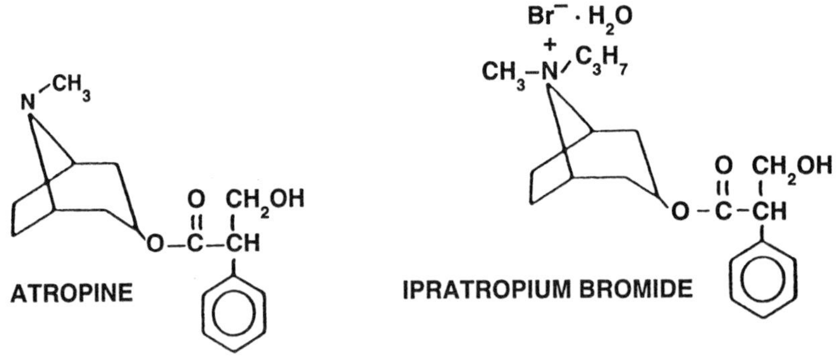

Fig. 1. Structures of atropine and ipratropium bromide.

THE PARASYMPATHETIC NERVOUS SYSTEM AND THE AIRWAYS

The airways are under parasympathetic control via the vagus nerve. Fibers from the vagus nerve synapse with the postganglionic nerves located in the tracheal smooth muscle. Parasympathetic nerves have effects at the level of smooth muscle, airway ciliary epithelia and mucous glands. Fibers from these postganglionic nerves directly innervate bronchial smooth muscle and glands where acetylcholine is released and its activity mediated via muscarinic receptors. There are five types of muscarinic receptors (M1–M5). The lung contains only M1, M2 and M3 receptors, and the nose contains M1 and M3 receptors. The physiological activity mediated by these receptors is shown in Table 1. Bronchial smooth muscle contains M2 and M3 receptors. Bronchial smooth muscle constricts under the influence of acetylcholine binding with the M3 receptor. Acetylcholine also stimulates M2 receptors, located in the postganglionic nerve endings, that decrease further release of acetylcholine via a negative feedback mechanism. This dual effect of acetylcholine explains why nonspecific blockage of muscarinic receptors could promote smooth muscle relaxation (via M3 antagonism), a desirable effect in asthma, and at the same time promote smooth muscle contraction by blocking M2 receptors and allowing for more acetylcholine release. Most of the parasympathetic innervation of the airways occurs in the upper branches of the respiratory tract with little innervation beyond the terminal bronchioles. This suggests that the parasympathetic activity takes place at the level of the trachea and the large- and middle-sized bronchi, with less influence on small airways and alveoli.

Lung mucous glands and the airway ciliated epithelium appear to be under parasympathetic control. When the airway is mechanically stimulated the increase in secretions observed is a reflex response mediated by the parasympathetic innervation. This effect is abrogated by atropine. Increased mucous production is seen in asthma and chronic obstructive pulmonary disease (COPD), and the glandular hypertrophy seen in these conditions may be due in part to chronic cholinergic stimulation. This effect on mucous secretion is mediated by the activity of acetylcholine on M3 receptors. Excessive mucus contributes to the obstruction of the airways seen in these conditions. The clearance of mucus and secretions from the airways depends on the beating of cilia. Atropine appears to decrease ciliary clearance of mucus, but ipratropium does not have this effect, giving this compound an advantage over atropine in the treatment of asthma and COPD.

Table 1
Location and Function of Muscarinic Receptors in the Airways

Receptor	Location	Function
M1	Alveoli, glands, ganglia	Enhances transmission
M2	Postganglionic nerves	Negative feedback
		Reduces transmission
M3	Smooth muscle lung	Contraction smooth muscle
	Glands	Secretion mucous and serous glands

THE ROLE OF THE PARASYMPATHETIC NERVOUS SYSTEM IN ASTHMA

Denervation of the lungs has been utilized in the past in the treatment of asthmatics. Some studies reported impressive results. In asthmatics, the unstimulated airway tone is increased compared to normal controls. This increased tone can be completely blocked by ipratropium, suggesting a vagally mediated mechanism. Nonspecific airway hyperresponsiveness is characteristic of most patients with asthma. It is believed that the response to many nonspecific stimuli such as exercise, cold air and sulfur dioxide is partially vagus nerve–mediated because they can be blocked by the intravenous administration of atropine or with the use of adequate doses of inhaled anticholinergic agents in humans. Intravenous or inhaled atropine blocks antigen-induced increases in airway resistance in allergic asthmatics in a dose-dependant fashion. Some studies, on the other hand, have concluded that cholinergic mechanisms are not important in allergic asthma. However, in these studies, low doses of inhaled anticholinergics were used, suggesting inadequate vagal blockade. In exacerbations of asthma due to viral infections, vagal mechanisms play an important role. Evidence suggests that in humans the hyperresponsiveness seen in naturally occuring viral infections could be blocked by atropine. This implies a role for increased acetylcholine release as a contributor to hyperresponsiveness. This is most likely due to a loss of function of the M2 inhibitory receptors at the parasympathetic nerve endings allowing for increased acetylcholine release. In nocturnal asthma and in stress-associated bronchospasm, vagally mediated bronchoconstriction also plays a role.

ANTICHOLINERGIC DRUGS IN RESPIRATORY DISEASES

Atropine was the first anticholinergic used to treat respiratory diseases such as asthma. Its role in respiratory diseases is limited by its side effects such as urine retention and dry mouth. It remains widely employed, mostly in anesthesia, where it is used to reduce secretions of the upper airways and to reduce laryngospasm. It is still found in some oral preparations used in the treatment of rhinitis. Ipratropium bromide (Atrovent), a quaternary ammonium derivative of atropine, is the anticholinergic currently indicated for use in the treatment of COPD, allergic and nonallergic rhinitis and the rhinorrea of the common cold. It is also utilized in the treatment of asthma because of its bronchodilatory properties. Table 2 compares ipratropium bromide and atropine characteristics. It is available in an aqueous nasal spray for rhinitis, in an aqueous nebulizer solution for use in COPD and in a metered dose inhaler either alone

---

- Anticholinergic (antimuscarinic) drugs exert their effect at the target organ to block secretion and smooth-muscle contraction in the respiratory tract
- Ipratropium bromide is the only anticholinergic agent available in the United States at this time
- Approved indications for ipratropium bromide are:
    Upper respiratory infection
    Perennial rhinitis
    Maintenance therapy of chronic bronchitis and emphysema
- It can also be useful in:
    As a maintenance bronchodilator in select cases of asthma
    In management of exacerbations of asthma and chronic
        obstructive pulmonary disease in combination with a
        β-adrenergic
    Gustatory rhinitis

---

or in combination with albuterol (Combivent). Its inhibition of rhinorrea makes it a useful medication for the symptomatic relief of allergic and nonallergic rhinitis, gustatory rhinitis (onset of rhinorrea induced by eating hot and spicy foods) and the common cold, conditions for which it is also indicated. It is available as a nasal spray in two concentrations. The 0.03% concentration delivers 21 μg of ipratropium per spray, and the dose recommended in chronic rhinitis is two sprays in each nostril two or three times a day. For the treatment of the common cold, it is available in a dose of 0.06%, and the recommended dose is two sprays per nostril three to four times a day. In the treatment of rhinitis, it can be used in conjunction with a topical corticosteroid nasal spray and with an antihistamine (Table 3). It has a rapid onset of action, usually within a few hours. Caution should be taken not to spray it inadvertently in the eyes as it may cause temporary blurred vision.

Other muscarinic receptor antagonists include oxitropium bromide, a derivative of scopolamine, and tiotropium bromide, developed as a long-acting and more bronchoselective anticholinergic agent. None of these agents is currently available for use in the United States.

ANTICHOLINERGIC DRUGS IN ASTHMA AND COPD

When ipratropium is compared to β_2-adrenergics in asthma, the adrenergic agents show superior bronchodilation. The bronchodilatory activity of ipratropium is more gradual, although more sustained, than that of albuterol. Thus, ipratropium should not be used alone as a bronchodilator in asthma. However, ipratropium in combination with a β_2 adrenergic agent such as albuterol produces better bronchodilation than either agent alone when delivered by nebulization in the setting of acute severe asthma, especially in the pediatric population. A recent study suggests that among children with a severe exacerbation of asthma presenting to the emergency department with a peak flow of <50% of predictive value, the addition of ipratropium bromide to albuterol and corticosteroid therapy significantly reduces the hospitalization rate. This effect was not seen in those with a moderate (peak flow rate between 50 and

Table 2
Comparison of Ipratropium Bromide and Atropine

Ipratropium Bromide	Atropine
Synthetic analog of atropine	Botanical origin
Water soluble	Water soluble
No absorption from respiratory tract	Absorbed from respiratory tract
No central nervous system effect	Central nervous system activity
No decrease in mucociliary clearance	Decreased mucociliary clearance

Table 3
Ipratropium Bromide in Chronic Rhinitis

Approved use	Indicated for symptomatic relief of rhinorrhea in allergic and nonallergic perennial rhinitis
Formulations	Available as a 0.03% solution for perennial rhinitis Available as a 0.06% solution for the common cold
Dosing	The recommended dose for rhinitis is two sprays in each nostril of the 0.03% solution two or three times daily For the common cold the recommended dose is two sprays in each nostril of the 0.06% solution three to four times daily
Side effects	Well tolerated by most patients Avoid contact with eyes
Other uses	Useful in gustatory rhinitis

70% predicted) exacerbation. Another study in children with mild and moderate asthmatic exacerbations failed to demonstrate an additive bronchodilatory effect of ipratropium when added to repeated albuterol treatments. Studies of the effectiveness of combination therapy using albuterol and ipratropium bromide in adults with an acute exacerbation of asthma have produced conflicting results. A recent study of adult asthmatics presenting to the emergency department with acute exacerbation of asthma showed that a single dose of ipratropium and albuterol in combination conferred additional bronchodilation as compared to albuterol alone. The patients who exhibited most benefit from the addition of ipratropium were those who had consumed the least inhaled β_2-agonist before presentation and not those with the most severe asthma. Recent guidelines published by the National Asthma Education Program Expert Panel recommend the addition of ipratropium bromide to high-dose β_2-agonist by nebulization in severe exacerbations of asthma with FEV_1 or peak flows below 50%. Since there are asthmatic patients who are going to respond with significant bronchodilation to anticholinergic blockade, a trial with ipratropium should be considered to identify those patients who would benefit from regular treatment in stable asthma. This may be especially true in elderly asthmatic patients with a component of chronic, fixed obstruction or those with long-standing asthma. However, it is important to recognize that most asthmatics do not require or respond to ipratropium in stable

Table 4
Ipratropium Bromide in COPD and Asthma

Approved use	Approved in United States only for treatment of chronic bronchitis and emphysema
Formulations	Metered dose inhaler and solution for nebulization Available in combination with albuterol in metered dose inhaler (Combivent)
Dosing	Starting dose of metered dose inhaler: 2 puffs 4 times/d Solution for nebulization: 2.5 cc 3 to 4 times/d
Use in asthma	In combination with a β-agonist may be beneficial in maintenance treatment of some asthmatics and in acute exacerbations of asthma Solutions of ipratropium bromide and albuterol are compatible and may be mixed for use in nebulizer

asthma. Except in elderly asthmatics, its use is not recommended as routine treatment for stable asthma according to recently published guidelines by the National Asthma Education Program Expert Panel. Another group of asthmatics that may benefit from regular use of ipratropium includes those taking concomitant β-blocking medications for other indications. Patients whose asthma is triggered by emotional distress may also respond well to anticholinergic blockade.

It is quite clear that ipratropium is a superior bronchodilator compared to β-agonist in patients with chronic bronchitis and emphysema, and it is the bronchodilator of choice in these conditions. It offers greater relief of airflow limitation and hyperinflation than albuterol. Its use is indicated for maintenance treatment of bronchospasm associated with COPD. A combination of Atrovent and albuterol (Combivent) in a metered dose inhaler is now available in the United States and is indicated for the treatment of COPD. Each actuation of Combivent delivers 18 μg of ipratropium and 103 μg of albuterol sulfate. As in the case of asthma, the combination of ipratropium and albuterol offers significantly better bronchodilation in COPD patients than either ipratropium or albuterol given separately. Ipratropium is also available as a solution for nebulization, and it can be administered mixed with albuterol in the nebulizer (Table 4).

CONCLUSIONS

New quaternary anticholinergic agents are useful medications to use in the treatment of respiratory conditions of the upper and lower respiratory tract. Their unique mechanism of action and the paucity of side effects give these agents an important role as adjunct therapy in the management of COPD, acute severe asthma and rhinitis.

SUGGESTED READING

Ducharme F, Davis GM. Randomized controlled trial of ipratropium bromide and frequent low doses of salbutamol in the management of mild and moderate acute pediatric asthma. *J Pediatr* 1998;133:479–485.
Garrett JE, Town GI, Rodwell P, Kelly A. Nebulized salbutamol with and without ipratropium bromide in the treatment of acute asthma. *J Allergy Clin Immunol* 1997;100:165–170.

Ikeda A, Nishimura K, Koyama H, Izumi T. Bronchodilating effects of combined therapy with clinical dosages of ipratropium bromide and salbutamol for stable COPD: Comparison with ipratropium bromide alone. *Chest* 1995;107:401–405.

Meltzer EO, Spector SL, eds. Anticholinergic therapy for allergic and nonallergic rhinitis and the common cold. *J Allergy Clin Immunol* 1995;95 (no 5, pt 2):1065–1152.

Qureshi F, Pestian J, Davis P, Zaritsky A. Effect of nebulized ipratropium on the hospitalization rates of children with asthma. *N Engl J Med* 1998;339:1030–1035.

23   Glucocorticoid Therapy in Asthma

Joseph D. Spahn, MD *and Stanley J. Szefler,* MD

CONTENTS

INTRODUCTION

Glucocorticoid (GC) therapy remains one of the most valuable treatment methods in the management of both the acute and chronic manifestations of asthma. GCs have been used in the treatment of asthma for the past 50 yr. Initial studies evaluating the effect of cortisone on asthma revealed significant improvements in asthma symptoms and pulmonary function. Unfortunately, much of the early enthusiasm for oral GC use was dampened with the realization that long-term use of this medication resulted in multiple adverse effects. The subsequent development of highly effective inhaled GC preparations has revolutionized asthma care. By virtue of high topical to systemic potency, inhaled GC therapy has proven to be safe and effective in the treatment of asthma. This chapter will provide a broad overview of the structure, mechanisms of action, pharmacokinetics, efficacy, adverse effects and current issues associated with GC therapy in asthma.

CHEMISTRY

Synthetic GCs are cortisone-based molecules that have undergone structural modifications designed to enhance their potencies and prolong their durations of action. Anti-inflammatory GCs have a 17-hydroxyl group and methyl groups at carbons 18 and 19 (Fig. 1). Further modifications to the basic steroid structure have increased the anti-inflammatory while decreasing mineralocorticoid effects; however, it has not

From: *Current Clinical Practice: Allergic Diseases: Diagnosis and Treatment, 2nd Edition*
Edited by: P. Lieberman and J. Anderson © Humana Press Inc., Totowa, NJ

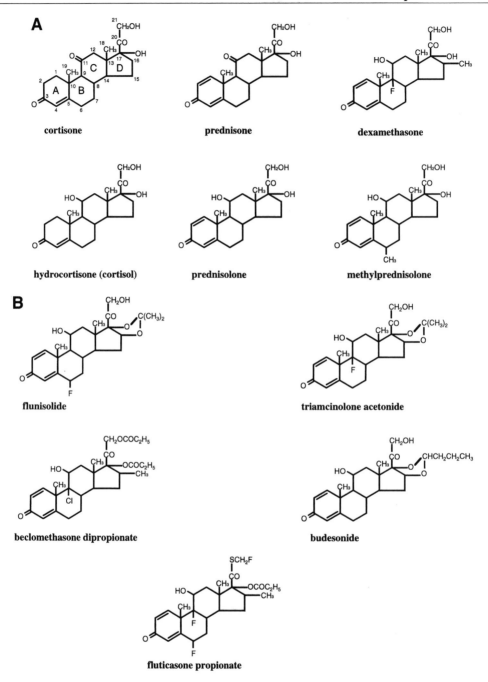

Fig. 1. Molecular structures of commonly administered systemic glucocorticoids (**A**) and available inhaled glucocorticoids (**B**) used in the treatment of asthma. Carbon nomenclature and ring nomenclature are noted for cortisone.

been possible to separate the unwanted metabolic effects while retaining the desired anti-inflammatory properties of the synthetic glucocorticoids that are systemically administered.

Table 1
Mechanisms of Glucocorticoid Action in Asthma

I. Inhibitory Effects
   A. Inhibition of leukocyte adhesion/migration
   B. Inhibition of leukocyte activation, function and survival
      1. T-lymphocytes
      2. Eosinophils
      3. Monocyte/macrophages
   C. Inhibition of the production of cytokines important in the differentiation, proliferation and activation of inflammatory cells
      1. IL-2, IL-3, IL-4, IL-5
   D. Inhibition of the production and/or release of inflammatory mediators
      1. Lipid mediators (platelet activating factor, leukotrienes, prostaglandins)
      2. Cytokines (IL-1, IL-6, TNF_α)
      3. Eosinophil-derived cytotoxic proteins such as eosinophil cationic protein (ECP), major basic protein (MBP)
II. Positive Effects
   A. Stimulation of lipocortin expression
      Inhibition of arachidonic acid metabolite synthesis
   B. Vasoconstrictive properties
      Decreased edema
      Less extravasation of pro-inflammatory mediators
   C. Potentiation of β-adrenergic receptor
      Heightened response to β-agonists

MECHANISMS OF ACTION

Over the past 10 yr, it has become increasingly clear that asthma is an inflammatory airways disease. Given that inflammation plays an important role in the pathogenesis of asthma, drugs that interfere with the inflammatory response should be effective in the treatment of this disease. Thus, it is not surprising that, by virtue of their anti-inflammatory properties, GCs have become the cornerstone of asthma therapy. Recent studies have shown GCs to act at several levels of the inflammatory response (Table 1), with their primary effect coming mainly from their ability to inhibit the expression and/or production of molecules involved in the initiation and maintenance of the inflammatory response. Specifically, they inhibit the up-regulation of adhesion molecules on endothelial cells that are required for the adhesion and subsequent migration of inflammatory cells to sites of inflammation. They also inhibit the production of cytokines involved in inflammatory cell recruitment, activation and proliferation. GCs also display potent vasoconstrictive properties. By decreasing capillary permeability at sites of inflammation, less plasma exudation occurs, resulting in a reduction in the concentration of inflammatory and chemotactic factors and ultimately in a decrease in the inflammatory response. Another salutary effect of GC therapy that is especially relevant to asthma is the up-regulation of β-adrenergic receptors on airway smooth muscle cells.

Table 2
Potential Drug Interactions with Systemic Glucocorticoids

Glucocorticoid	Drugs that Increase Clearance	Drugs that Decrease Clearance
Methylprednisolone	Carbamazepine	Ketoconazole
	Phenobarbital	Troleandomycin
	Phenytoin	Erythromycin
	Rifampin	Oral contraceptives
Prednisolone	Antacids (decrease absorption)	Ketoconazole
	Carbamazepine	Oral contraceptives
	Phenobarbital	
	Phenytoin	
	Rifampin	
Dexamethasone	Carbamazepine	
	Phenobarbital	
	Phenytoin	

ORAL GC THERAPY

Pharmacokinetics

The pharmacokinetics of GCs can influence dosing strategies; however, in general, GC dosing regimens are not dependent upon pharmacokinetic parameters, dosing being empirical or based on the patient's history of prior response. Exceptions to this are when gross abnormalities of absorption or elimination, as with some drug interactions (e.g., anticonvulsants), result in a clinically significant reduction of systemic GC exposure. In this scenario, clinical response to treatment would be expected to be diminished. Prednisone, prednisolone and methylprednisolone are all rapidly and nearly completely absorbed following oral administration, with peak plasma concentrations occurring within 1–2 h. Of interest, prednisone is an inactive pro-drug that requires biotransformation of the 11-ketone group to an 11-hydroxyl group. This conversion to prednisolone (its active form) occurs via first-pass hepatic metabolism.

Once absorbed, GCs bind to serum proteins with prednisolone binding to transcortin, albumin and α_1-acid glycoprotein while methylprednisolone binds primarily to albumin. GCs are metabolized in the liver into inactive compounds. The rate of metabolism or clearance of a GC can be altered by drug interactions and disease states. Hyperthyroid patients require higher GC doses because of enhanced clearance and metabolism. With hypothyroid patients, slowed elimination is a concern; however, this has not been well studied. Cystic fibrosis results in enhanced clearance of prednisolone. GC elimination may also be altered by numerous concomitant medications (Table 2). Drug interactions may result in either reduced or enhanced clearance, and consequently an increased risk for adverse effects or a diminished therapeutic response. The anticonvulsants, phenytoin, phenobarbital and carbamazepine, cause an increased rate of elimination for dexamethasone, prednisolone and methylprednisolone. Of note, methylprednisolone clearance is most significantly affected. Rifampin, like the above anticonvulsants, enhances the clearance of GCs and can result in diminished therapeutic effect and breakthrough asthma symptoms in the steroid-dependent patient.

In contrast to anticonvulsants and rifampin, other medications can reduce GC elimination. Significant reductions of clearance have been noted with concomitant ketoconazole administration. The macrolide antibiotics, erythromycin, troleandomycin, and clarithromycin, can also delay GC clearance; however, this effect is limited to methylprednisolone. Clearance rates can be reduced from 50–70% with the above macrolides. In addition, a 50% reduction of prednisolone elimination can be expected with coadministration of oral contraceptives.

If a drug interaction that increases clearance is identified, one can simply increase the GC dose. Alternatively, a "split" dosing regimen may be considered with two thirds of the total daily GC dose administered in the morning and the remaining one third administered in the afternoon. This strategy may provide for a more normal plasma concentration vs time curve and could result in better responsiveness. If these changes offer no benefit, a change to a GC with a longer half-life, such as dexamethasone, could be another option.

Pharmacodynamics

Pharmacodynamics is the study of drug action and can be measured with regard to onset of action, peak effect, duration of effect and offset of action. GCs are somewhat unique in that a number of steps at the molecular level are required for them to exert their biological effects. These likely contribute to the slow onset and slow dissipation of effects that characterize GC actions. This principle is consistent with observed responses of patients with asthma following systemic administration of GCs. In asthmatics given a single dose of 40 mg of prednisolone, onset of improved pulmonary function was observed 3 h after administration, with maximal effect at 9–12 h post dose followed by gradual return to near baseline values at 36 h post dose. Of interest, studies have demonstrated that larger doses merely extend the duration of effect rather than the maximal intensity of response. Smaller doses of GCs given more frequently appear to provide more effectiveness than single large doses. Thus, the frequency of dosing may be more important than actual dose administered. With systemically administered GCs, comparisons of low and high doses for acute severe obstruction have not always shown a clear benefit with high-dose therapy (as discussed later).

Efficacy of Oral GC Therapy in Asthma

EFFECT ON BRONCHIAL HYPERRESPONSIVENESS (BHR)

BHR or airway "twitchiness" is an important feature of asthma. Although not absolute, BHR has been shown to correlate with disease severity, frequency of symptoms and need for treatment. Although the precise relationship remains elusive, airway inflammation is thought to contribute to BHR. Oral GCs can attenuate BHR with high-dose prednisone therapy shown both to improve pulmonary function and lessen BHR in adults and children with asthma. Reductions in bronchoalveolar lavage (BAL) fluid eosinophil counts and reductions in the number of inflammatory cells expressing pro-inflammatory cytokines have also been associated with diminished BHR following a short course of high-dose prednisone. These observations suggest that GCs, by inhibiting cytokine synthesis, inhibit airway eosinophilia and subsequently lessen BHR.

- Glucocorticoids (GCs) are the most effective therapy for allergic disease.
- In asthma, topical GCs decrease bronchial hyperresponsiveness when given long term.
- In therapy of acute exacerbations of asthma, the early institution of systemic GC therapy can prevent emergency room visits and hospitalization.
- In patients with chronic severe asthma who require regular systemic GC therapy, all other treatments should be maximized and the lowest dose sufficient for control should be established through regular monitoring visits.

EFFECTS OF SYSTEMIC GC THERAPY ON ACUTE EXACERBATIONS OF ASTHMA IN ADULTS

Numerous studies have evaluated the effect of GC therapy in acute asthma. Most have demonstrated efficacy, while a minority have not. The reader is also encouraged to read the review by McFadden (*see* Suggested Reading) that nicely summarizes the studies evaluating the efficacy of GC therapy in acute asthma. Studies in the emergency room have shown that a single dose of iv methylprednisolone can decrease the need for subsequent hospitalization. In studies evaluating the effectiveness of iv GC therapy in hospitalized patients, the majority of studies have shown GC therapy superior to placebo as measured by improvement in pulmonary function. Despite widespread use, the optimal dose of GC in the acute setting has not been firmly established. In one of the few studies that have attempted to determine a dose response, 40 mg of methylprednisolone was equally effective as 125 mg administered every 6 h for 72 h in a group of patients admitted with status asthmaticus (*see* Fanta et al.). A study that evaluated three doses of prednisolone (0.2, 0.4 and 0.6 mg/kg/d) for 2 wk in asthmatics requiring a prednisolone burst as a result of worsening asthma symptoms found the highest dose to be the most effective (*see* Webb). Of note, a plateau in effect by day 8 was observed for all 3 doses of prednisolone. The author concluded that an 8-d course of prednisolone is sufficient for treating acute asthma and that the time course of response to prednisolone therapy is not dose dependent.

There is also no consensus regarding the duration of GC treatment for acute asthma. Since duration of treatment is in part related to the severity of the initial episode, recommendations for the length of treatment must be tailored to the individual case. With that in mind, it has recently been recommended to treat patients admitted in status asthmaticus with at least 36–48 hr of iv therapy with transition to oral GC therapy when tolerated. The duration of the oral GC taper will depend on the individual's response, but should span 4–12 d. Short courses of GC administered in the outpatient department have also been shown to decrease the rate of asthma relapse.

In summary, although most studies have shown systemic GC to be highly effective therapy in acute asthma, a clear consensus on the optimal type, dose, route of administration (oral vs intravenous) and duration of treatment does not exist. A number of protocols outlining systemic GC therapy in acute asthma have been published. Keep in mind that therapy should be tailored to the individual patient's condition. The National Heart, Lung, and Blood Institute (NHLBI) published its revised guidelines established by an expert panel of asthma specialists (*see* Suggested Reading). This document recommends prednisolone, prednisone or methylprednisolone 120–180 mg/d in 3 or 4 doses for 48 h, then 60–80 mg/d until peak expiratory flow rate (PEFR) reaches 70% of predicted or personal best. McFadden, in his analysis of GC therapy in acute asthma, provides a more complete dosing schedule (*see* the review by McFadden). He recommends administering methylprednisolone 40 mg iv every 6 h or prednisone 60 mg orally every 6–8 h for 36–48 h with a taper to 60 mg prednisone/day when the FEV_1 approaches 50% of predicted. This dose is held for the next 4 d prior to instituting a taper in 4-d intervals reaching 0 mg in 12 d.

ACUTE ASTHMA IN CHILDREN

There have been several studies evaluating the efficacy of systemic GC therapy in children. As with the studies in adults, the majority have shown systemic GC therapy to be effective in the treatment of acute asthma in children with improvements in PEFR, FEV_1, and PaO_2, decreased frequency of wheezing, or fewer episodes of relapse. Studies evaluating the effect of a single dose of GC (parenteral or oral) in the emergency department setting have uniformly found this therapy superior to placebo in decreasing the number of children who ultimately require admission. As all clinicians who care for children know, iv administration of GC requires placement of an indwelling venous catheter, often a difficult task to perform in an agitated wheezing toddler. Thus, oral GC therapy is an alternative to iv GC therapy in children. The liquid forms of prednisone (Prelone®, Pediapred®) can be administered to infants and young children who cannot swallow pills. In addition, the liquid form is very quickly absorbed with peak serum levels occurring within 1 h compared to 2 h with tablets.

An important study published in 1987, evaluated whether early intervention with oral steroid therapy during an acute asthma exacerbation would prevent further progression of asthma symptoms (*see* Harris). This study evaluated the effect of a short course of high-dose oral prednisone therapy (30–40 mg twice daily for 7 d) vs placebo in 41 children with an acute asthma exacerbation. All patients randomized to receive prednisone improved during the week of treatment, with only one relapse noted following discontinuation of therapy. In contrast, 42% of those randomized to receive placebo developed worsening asthma symptoms requiring rescue intervention. Somewhat surprisingly, a sizable percentage of patients receiving placebo improved at the same rate as those who received prednisone. Unfortunately, there were no reliable distinguishing characteristics that could have served as predictors of those patients who required GC therapy to prevent worsening of their asthma compared to those who improved spontaneously. Thus, since continued symptoms often lead to emergency care and/or hospitalization, the above study supports the use of oral steroid therapy early for acute exacerbations.

As is the case for adults, issues such as the optimal GC dose, duration of treatment and route of administration in children remain largely empirical and depend largely on the severity of the acute exacerbation. As orally administered GCs are rapidly absorbed and are usually as effective as iv GCs, oral therapy can be used in many cases. Hospitalized children who require high flow rates of oxygen to adequately treat hypoxemia are obvious candidates for iv GC therapy. In this situation, methylprednisolone sodium succinate (Solu-Medrol®) 1–2 mg/kg as a loading dose followed by 0.5–1 mg/kg every 4–6 h can be administered. Once oral medications are tolerated, a switch to oral prednisone can be made at a dose of 2 mg/kg/d in 2 divided doses for an additional

2–4 d followed by a taper to 1 mg/kg/d administered in a single morning dose for an additional 2–4 d prior to stopping. For outpatient management of acute exacerbations, we usually recommend a short course of prednisone 2 mg/kg/d in 2 divided doses for 2–3 days followed by reduction to 1 mg/kg in a single morning dose for an additional 2–3 d. Of note, the revised NHLBI guidelines recommend administering prednisone, prednisolone or methylprednisolone, 1 mg/kg/dose every 6 h for 48 h, then 1–2 mg/kg/d (maximum dose 60 mg/d) in 2 divided doses until PEF is 70% of predicted or personal best.

EFFICACY OF ORAL GC THERAPY IN THE MANAGEMENT OF CHRONIC ASTHMA

Inhaled GC therapy has allowed the majority of patients with asthma to maintain good control of their disease. When used appropriately, inhaled GC therapy has allowed a significant number of patients with severe asthma to reduce or even discontinue their maintenance oral steroid. Unfortunately, a small number of asthma patients continue to require regular use of oral GC despite high-dose inhaled GC therapy and are commonly referred to as steroid-dependent asthmatics. Given that daily administration of oral GC therapy results in multiple adverse effects, investigators began evaluating the effectiveness and adverse-effects profile of intermittently administered oral GC therapy (*see* Harter et al.). Harter and colleagues were the first to make the important and insightful observation that the therapeutic effects of steroids appeared to persist longer than their metabolic effects. Given this observation, they studied several dosage schedules and found that a single morning dose of oral GC administered every other day was the most effective in optimizing asthma control while minimizing adverse effects. This is a hallmark study, since it set the standard for using alternate-day steroids in patients with severe asthma.

There are several management issues to consider when caring for patients with steroid-dependent asthma. First, all other asthma therapy should be optimized, including inhaled GC, long-acting β-agonists and/or theophylline and judicious use of short-acting β-agonists. Second, the diagnosis of asthma should be firmly established. Third, factors such as inappropriate inhalation technique and poor compliance with asthma medications, environmental control (in atopic patients), gastroesophageal reflux and sinusitis, which can contribute to poor asthma control, should be considered and, if present, adequately treated. Lastly, given the inevitable development of potentially severe steroid-associated adverse effects, every attempt should be made to determine the lowest possible oral steroid dose to be administered, and if at all possible, it should be administered on alternate days.

To determine the need for, and lowest possible required oral GC dose (i.e., steroid threshold), a gradual taper of the GC should be attempted with close monitoring of the patient's symptoms (nocturnal episodes of wheezing/shortness of breath, degree of exercise-induced bronchospasm, frequency of inhaled bronchodilator use) and pulmonary function (PEFR monitoring, spirometry). The daily oral GC dose can be tapered by 5 mg/wk until 20 mg on alternate days is reached or until breakthrough asthma symptoms or declining pulmonary function is observed. Since most of these individuals will be adrenally suppressed, the taper is then slowed with weekly reductions in the oral GC dose by 2.5 mg every other week with periodic measurement of morning cortisol levels to assess adrenal recovery. If during the GC taper, the patient develops increasing asthma symptoms and/or diminished pulmonary function, a

Table 3
Adverse Effects Associated with Systemic Glucocorticoid Use

Cardiovascular effects
- Hypertension, atherosclerosis

Dermatolic effects
- Dermal thinning/increased skin fragility
- Acne
- Striae
- Hirsutism

Endocrinological effects
- Adrenal suppression
- Growth suppression and delayed sexual maturation in children
- Weight gain, development of cushingoid habitus
- Diabetes mellitus

Hematological effects
- Lymphopenia, neutrophilia

Immunological effects
- Diminished immunoglobulin G (IgG) levels
- Loss of delayed-type hypersensitivity (DTH)
- Potential for increased risk of opportunistic infection/severe varicella infection

Metabolic effects
- Hypokalemia, hyperglycemia, hyperlipidemia

Musculoskeletal effects
- Osteoporosis/vertebral compression fractures
- Aseptic necrosis of bone (hips, shoulders, knees)
- Myopathy (acute and chronic forms)

Ophthalmaolgical effects
- Cataracts, glaucoma

Psychological/Neurological effects:
- Mood swings, psychosis
- Steroid withdrawal syndrome
- Pseudotumor cerebri

beneficial steroid effect is documented and a threshold dose is defined. If the threshold dose is >20 mg in adults (or >10 mg in children) on alternate days, consideration for alternative asthma medications may be indicated. If a beneficial effect of long-term oral GC therapy is not derived, every attempt should be made to safely taper the patient off oral GC therapy completely. If this can be accomplished, many of the debilitating adverse effects associated with oral GC therapy can be prevented.

Adverse Effects of Systemic GC Therapy

As all nucleated cells in the body have a common GC receptor, all are potentially affected by GC therapy and thus susceptible to the development of untoward effects. These effects can occur immediately (i.e., metabolic effects) or can develop insidiously over several months to years (i.e., osteoporosis and cataracts). In addition, some adverse effects are limited to children (growth suppression), while others appear to require interaction with other drugs (nonsteroidal anti-inflammatory agents and medications for peptic ulcer disease). Most adverse effects appear to depend on dose and duration of treatment, although this has not been uniformly noted. Table 3 lists many of the common adverse effects associated with long-term GC use.

OSTEOPOROSIS

Osteoporosis, a significant and common adverse effect, is often overlooked secondary to its insidious onset and the insensitivity of conventional diagnostic methods. All patients who have been receiving >7.5 mg prednisone (or equivalent) daily for at least 6 mo are at risk for developing osteoporosis. Although the etiology of GC-induced osteoporosis is complex, decreased calcium absorption and decreased renal reabsorption are major factors. In addition, GCs inhibit osteoblast function, resulting in decreased bone growth, while stimulating osteoclast activity resulting in bone resorption. Trabecular bone (ribs, vertebrae) appears to be more affected by GCs than cortical bone. Factors that increase the likelihood of the development of osteoporosis include inactivity, sex hormone deficiency, a diet deficient in calcium and concurrent use of drugs such as furosemide and anticonvulsants, and excessive thyroid hormone replacement.

Because demineralization of bone is not detectable on conventional radiographs until a significant degree of bone mineral density is lost, the diagnosis of osteoporosis is best made by documenting decreased bone mineral density with a bone densitometer. Further assessment of osteoporosis in the steroid-dependent asthmatic includes 24-h urine calcium measurement that provides useful information regarding the extent of GC-induced renal calcium loss. Biochemical markers such as serum osteocalcin (a marker of osteoblast activity) and urinary hydroxyproline (a marker of bone resorption) may eventually become routinely followed, but at present insufficient information is available to apply these markers for general clinical practice.

Treatment of osteoporosis, as is the case for all steroid-induced adverse effects, consists of attempting to decrease the oral GC dose and/or frequency, increasing calcium intake to 1000–1500 mg of elemental calcium per day supplemented with at least 400 IU/d of vitamin D (Table 4), and increasing physical activity (especially gravity-dependent activities such as walking). Avoidance of activities such as heavy lifting, high-impact aerobics and contact sports (football, wrestling) is recommended as these activities can result in compression fractures of the vertebral bodies (bending, lifting, contact sports) in addition to fractures of the long bones (contact sports). If hypercalciuria is present, hydrochlorothiazide can be used alone or in combination with a potassium-sparing diuretic. Patients with severe osteoporosis may require treatment with a remitive medication.

MYOPATHY

Two distinct types of myopathy can occur with systemic GC therapy. An acute, severe myopathy associated with short-term high-dose parenteral GC therapy has been reported in patients hospitalized with severe asthma exacerbations. Fortunately, this presentation is rare with several other conditions contributing, including intubation with mechanical ventilation, concurrent use of muscle relaxant therapy (paralysis) and possible accelerated disuse atrophy. Affected patients often have markedly elevated serum creatine phosphokinase (CPK) levels and diffuse necrosis of skeletal muscle on biopsy. Recovery begins after GC withdrawal, but more than 6 mo may be required for complete recovery.

Table 4
Management of Glucocorticoid-Induced Osteoporosis

Minimize oral glucocorticoid dose to ≤20 mg in adults and ≤10 mg in children (prednisone
  or equivalent) on alternate days
Increase calcium (Ca^{2+}) intake to 1000–1500 mg elemental Ca^{2+}/d
  Increase dietary calcium intake by eating foods high in calcium
  Consider additonal calcium in the form of a calcium supplement[a] such as:
    Calcium carbonate (40% elemental Ca^{2+})
      Oscal® 500 contains 500 mg elemental Ca^{2+}/tablet
      Tums® contain 200 mg elemental Ca^{2+}/chewable tablet
    Calcium citrate (21% elemental Ca^{2+})
      Citracal® 950 contains 200 mg elemental Ca^{2+}
    Calcium gluconate (9% elemental Ca^{2+})
  Vitamin D supplementation—400 IU/d
Increase physical activity
  Gravity-dependent activities, such as walking/low-impact aerobics, are most effective
Avoid heavy lifting, contact sports and high-impact aerobics
Consider diuretic therapy with hydrochlorothiazide if 24-hr urinary Ca^{2+} excretion is high
Other agents used for severe osteoporosis (with consultation from endocrinologist)
  Calcitonin
  Bisphosphonates
  Calcitriol
  Sodium fluoride
  Estrogen (indicated for postmenopausal osteoporosis)

[a]Note that Ca^{2+} is in the form of a salt; thus, the amount of elemental Ca^{2+} will be a percentage of the
total weight of the tablet unless the label specifies the amount of elemental Ca^{2+}/tablet.

More commonly encountered is the insidious development of proximal muscle
atrophy. As with the other previously described adverse effects, those patients receiving
daily steroids or large alternate-day doses for prolonged periods are at greatest risk.
Isokinetic muscle testing of hip flexor strength appears to be the most sensitive and
objective measure of proximal muscle weakness. Enzymes of muscle origin such as
CPK, aldolase and lactate dehydrogenase (LDH) are almost never increased, and biopsy
of affected muscle reveals atrophy rather than necrosis. To correct and/or prevent
GC-induced myopathy, every attempt should be made to taper the GC dose and a
program designed to improve muscle strength initiated.

CATARACTS

  Posterior subcapsular cataracts (PSC) are a well-described complication of long-
term GC use with an incidence of up to 29%. The mechanism(s) involved in the
development PSC is not clear, but may involve disturbances of carbohydrate metabolism
or "dehydration" of the lens. GC-induced cataracts are often small, but can at times
significantly affect visual acuity, requiring surgical intervention. Although the development of cataracts appears to be related to the daily dose, cumulative dose and duration
of treatment, there is a significant degree of variability with respect to individual
susceptibility to cataract formation. It is unknown whether GC dose reduction will
result in regression or disappearance of the cataract, although some studies suggest

that if recognized early, regression can occur. A yearly ophthalmological examination to determine the presence of cataracts is recommended for all patients receiving maintenance oral GC therapy.

GROWTH SUPPRESSION

Growth suppression is the GC-associated adverse effect that causes the most concern for clinicians caring for children. Regular daily therapy, frequent short courses or high-dose alternate-day GC therapy often results in suppression of linear growth. Doses of prednisone as small as 0.1 mg/kg administered daily for as short a period as 3 mo have resulted in significant suppression of linear growth. When GC is administered on alternate days, the degree of suppression may be less, but significant growth suppression can still occur. Complicating the issue of GC-induced growth suppression is the finding that asthma itself can impair growth. This is a significant issue, especially as it pertains to whether long-term inhaled GC therapy is associated with growth suppression (*see* later). As daily or high-dose alternate-day GC therapy for extended periods can result in permanent growth retardation, every effort should be made to decrease the amount of oral GC to less than 20 mg on alternate days. If the child's oral GC dose cannot be tapered to ≤20 mg on alternate days, treatment with recombinant growth hormone can be considered. Growth hormone therapy can increase linear growth in children receiving long-term GC therapy, but the response is dependent on the dose of growth hormone administered: The higher the daily dose of prednisone, the less effective growth hormone therapy is.

ADRENAL INSUFFICIENCY

Patients with adrenal suppression as a consequence of long-term oral GC therapy are at risk of developing acute adrenal insufficiency at times of stress such as surgical procedures, gastroenteritis resulting in dehydration or trauma. Patients who develop acute adrenal insufficiency can have dehydration, shock, electrolyte abnormalities, severe abdominal pain and lethargy out of proportion to the severity of their presenting illness. This is a medical emergency and requires prompt diagnosis and rapid treatment with iv hydrocortisone (2 mg/kg initially followed by 1.5 mg/kg every 6 h until stabilization is achieved and oral therapy is tolerated) and vigorous fluid replacement with normal saline if dehydration and hypotension are present. All patients undergoing long-term high-dose GC therapy should be considered adrenally suppressed and should wear a medical alert bracelet that identifies them as being at risk for acute adrenal insufficiency. All adrenally suppressed individuals should be given hydrocortisone at the time of any surgical procedure (1–2 mg/kg) and every 6 h thereafter for the next 24–48 h, with a switch to their usual oral GC dose when oral medications are tolerated. The same recommendations are to be followed at other times of acute stress. Complete recovery from adrenal suppression can take from 6 mo to 1 yr after cessation of long-term GC use. Thus, all patients with a history of long-term GC use should be considered adrenally suppressed and should be managed as such for up to 1 yr following cessation or significant reduction of oral GC therapy.

OTHER ADVERSE EFFECTS

Other common adverse effects of long-term GC therapy include increased appetite with weight gain and the development of a cushingoid habitus consisting of a moon facies, buffalo hump, central obesity with wasting of the extremities, atrophy of the skin with the development of striae and hirsutism. Psychological disturbances from increased emotional lability to frank psychosis can occur, as well as hypertension, peptic ulcer disease, atherosclerosis, aseptic necrosis of bone and diabetes mellitus. Long-term GC use can also result in immunological attenuation with loss of delayed-type hypersensitivity, diminished IgG levels without change in functional antibody response, potential for reactivation of latent tuberculosis infection and possible increased risk for infection, especially the development of severe varicella.

INHALED GC THERAPY

Effective and safe forms of inhaled GC were first introduced in the early 1970s with the development of drugs and delivery devices that provided optimal topical to systemic potency. By effectively delivering small quantities of a potent GC directly into the airway, inhaled GC therapy maximizes the beneficial effects while minimizing the systemic effects associated with long-term GC use. Although these medications had been available for 25 yr, their use, especially in pediatric patients, had been limited to those patients with severe asthma. As our understanding of asthma has changed, with increasing emphasis on airway inflammation even in mild asthma, inhaled GCs are now considered first-line therapy in all patients with persistent asthma (*see* Revised NHLBI Guidelines).

Efficacy of Inhaled GC Therapy

As mentioned previously, bronchial hyperresponsiveness (BHR) is an important feature of asthma. Studies evaluating the effect of inhaled GC therapy in asthma have consistently demonstrated a favorable effect on BHR in both adults and children. Decreases in BHR from two- to seven-fold have been reported within 6 wk of instituting inhaled GC therapy. Of significance, the decreases in BHR have been associated with fewer asthma symptoms, improved pulmonary function, less need for supplemental β-agonist use and fewer exacerbations requiring oral GC therapy.

Recent studies using bronchoscopy and bronchial biopsy have demonstrated reductions in airway inflammation after institution of inhaled GCs. Specifically, significant reductions in the number of inflammatory cells, the number of cells expressing pro-inflammatory cytokines and the number of activated inflammatory cells have been noted. In addition, inhaled GC therapy has recently been shown to be effective in decreasing the thickness of the basement membrane of asthmatics. Basement membrane thickening is a characteristic finding in chronic asthma, and although its role in the pathophysiology of asthma is unclear, it may contribute to the development of chronic and potentially irreversible airflow obstruction. In summary, long-term administration of inhaled GC therapy results in reductions in BHR, symptoms and need for supplemental β-agonist use. Associated with this is improved pulmonary function and suppression of the inflammatory response characteristic of asthma.

Given the relatively rare occurrence of asthma hospitalizations and life-threatening events, epidemiological studies have been performed to help determine whether inhaled GC therapy is associated with reduced asthma morbidity. In the last year, such studies have demonstrated a protective effect of inhaled GC on hospitalization for acute asthma. Donahue et al. (*see* Suggested Reading), found asthmatics receiving inhaled GC to be 50% less likely to be hospitalized with acute asthma compared to those not

---

Use of GCs in Asthma

- Inhaled GCs are now considered first-line therapy in mild, moderate and severe asthma.
- The exact dose and type of inhaled GC must be tailored to the patient, over time.
- In acute asthma exacerbations systemic GCs (e.g., oral) usually are needed.
- When asthma is not under control, higher does of inhaled GC are needed. Over time, when asthma is under control, lower doses of inhaled GC are usually possible.
- In a few "steroid-dependent" asthmatics, oral and inhaled GCs are needed daily for control.
- The risk of side effects of GC increases with dose.

---

receiving inhaled GC. Using frequency of as-needed β-agonist therapy as a surrogate marker of disease severity, they found GC to confer even greater protective effects in patients requiring more than eight canisters of albuterol/year with a 70% reduction in the rate of hospitalization noted. In one of the few studies that sought to determine whether routine use of inhaled GC was associated with less risk for death due to asthma, Ernst et al. (*see* Suggested Reading), found subjects using ≥1 canister/month of beclomethasone dipropionate (BDP) to be one tenth as likely to die or have a near-fatal asthma exacerbation compared to asthmatics not receiving an inhaled GC.

INHALED GCs AS FIRST-LINE THERAPY

Inhaled GCs were initially reserved for use in patients with moderate to severe asthma, but as our understanding of this disease has advanced, inhaled GCs are now recommended for individuals with mild persistent asthma. Whether inhaled GC therapy should be first-line therapy in children with mild asthma remains a topic of debate. Those who favor the use of inhaled GC therapy in mild asthma argue that since this medication reduces airway inflammation, BHR and need for supplemental β-agonist therapy, it should be used in all patients with mild persistent asthma or asthma of greater severity. Given that inhaled GC therapy is not without the potential for adverse effects, and that adequate long-term studies evaluating bone demineralization and growth delay have yet to be completed, others argue that its use should be reserved for those with more frequent symptoms, i.e., those with moderate to severe persistent asthma.

Two relatively recent studies, one in children and the other in adults, evaluated the efficacy and adverse effects of budesonide in mild asthma. Both studies found budesonide therapy effective in decreasing asthma symptoms and supplemental β-agonist use and improving pulmonary function. In addition, the childhood study found doses of budesonide of ≤400 µg/d not to result in growth suppression over a 3.5-year period (*see* Agertoft and Pedersen), although higher doses did. An intriguing finding from this study was the observation that the longer the child had asthma before institution of budesonide therapy, the less significant the response to budesonide therapy. A similar result was seen in the study of adult asthmatics (*see* Haahtela et al.). In this study, one half of the study population was treated with budesonide for 2 yr, and the other was treated with regularly administered terbutaline. Not surprisingly, the group receiving budesonide had significant improvement in pulmonary function while those receiving terbutaline actually had gradual worsening. The study was then extended for an additional year, at which time those who were taking terbutaline received budesonide while those initially taking budesonide either received a smaller dose (400 μg/d compared to 1200 μg/d) or were administered placebo. The pulmonary function of those asthmatics who were given budesonide therapy after 2 yr of placebo therapy improved, but not to the same extent as in those patients who received budesonide at the time of diagnosis. The results from both studies suggest that the longer the time from the initiation of symptoms and subsequent treatment with inhaled GC the less effective the therapy will be. Although this suggestion is speculative, the loss of response may be due to the development of some degree of irreversible airflow obstruction secondary to airway remodeling.

INHALED GC AND ASTHMA REMISSION

Over the past several years, increased attention has been directed to whether long-term inhaled GC therapy can induce asthma remissions. The recent observation that early institution of inhaled GC results in the greatest potential for restoration of normal lung function further supports the concept that inhaled GC therapy can be a disease-modifying agent. Another intriguing aspect of the Haahtela study discussed previously came from the observations they made when the asthmatics who had received high-dose budesonide therapy for 2 years were rerandomized to receive either placebo or low-dose budesonide for 1 yr. Approximately three fourths of patients randomized to low-dose budesonide maintained good asthma control despite receiving one third of the original dose. In contrast, the majority of the subjects re-randomized to placebo therapy developed worsening asthma symptoms. Of interest is that a sizable minority of patients (approximately one third) treated with long-term budesonide therapy appeared to sustain a prolonged remission. This finding suggests that in a subpopulation of asthmatics, long-term inhaled GC therapy may indeed have a disease-modifying effect. Further research in this area is greatly needed.

TYPES OF INHALED GCs

There are currently five inhaled GC preparations available for use in the United States: beclomethasone dipropionate (BDP) marketed as Vanceril® or Beclovent®, both of which deliver 42 μg per actuation, and Vanceril-DS® (84 mg/actuation); triamcinolone acetonide (TAA) marketed as Azmacort®, which delivers 200 μg from the canister but only 100 μg per inhalation from the built-in spacer device; flunisolide (FLN) marketed as AeroBid®, which delivers 250 μg per actuation; fluticasone propionate (FP) marketed as Flovent, which is available in 3 doses: 44, 110 and 220 μg/actuation; and budesonide (BUD) marketed as Pulmicort® (200 μg/actuation). Recommended dosages for both adults and children for all of the inhaled GCs are listed in Table 5. BUD and FP are thought to be "second"-generation inhaled GCs in that they appear to have greater topical-to-systemic potencies. BUD and FP have recently been shown to have oral GC-sparing effects in adults with steroid-dependent asthma. Few if any studies have attempted to compare the clinical efficacy of the available inhaled GCs. As a result, it is difficult to make judgments regarding which drug is the most potent,

Table 5
Dosage Guidelines Presented in the *National Asthma Education Program Expert Panel Report 2:*
Estimated Comparative Daily Dosages

Glucocorticoid	Low dose	Medium dose	High dose
ADULTS			
Beclomethasone dipropionate	168–504 µg	504–840 µg	>840 µg
42 µg/puff	(4–12 puffs)	(12–20 puffs)	(>20 puffs)
84 µg/puff	(2–6 puffs)	(6–10 puffs)	(>10 puffs)
Budesonide Turbuhaler	200–400 µg	400–600 µg	>600 µg
200 µg/dose	(1–2 inhalations)	(2–3 inhalations)	(>3 inhalations)
Flunisolide	500–1000 µg	1000–2000 µg	>2,000 µg
250 µg/puff	(2–4 puffs)	(4–8 puffs)	(>8 puffs)
Fluticasone propionate	88–264 µg	264–660 µg	>660 µg
MDI: 44, 110, 220 µg/puff	(2–6 puffs–44 µg) or	(2–6 puffs–110 µg)	(>6 puffs–110 µg) or
	(2 puffs–110 µg)		(>3 puffs–220 µg)
Triamcinolone acetonide	400–1,000 µg	1000–2000 µg	>2,000 µg
100 µg/puff	(4–10 puffs)	(10–20 puffs)	(>20 puffs)
CHILDREN			
Beclomethasone dipropionate	84–336 µg	336–672 µg	>672 µg
42 µg/puff	(2–8 puffs)	(8–16 puffs)	(>16 puffs)
84 µg/puff			
Budesonide Turbuhaler	100–200 µg	200–400 µg	>400 µg
200 µg/dose	(1 inhalation)	(1–2 inhalations)	(>2 inhalations)
Flunisolide	500–750 µg	1000–1250 µg	>1250 µg
250 µg/puff	(2–3 puffs)	(4–5 puffs)	(>5 puffs)
Fluticasone propionate	88–176 µg	176–440 µg	>440 µg
MDI: 44, 110, 220 µg/puff	(2–4 puffs–44 µg)	(4–10 puffs–44 µg)	(>4 puffs–110 µg)
	or	or	
		(2–4 puffs–110 µg)	
Triamcinolone acetonide	400–800 µg	800–1200 µg	>1200 µg
100 µg/puff	(4–8 puffs)	(8–12 puffs)	(>12 puffs)

although several studies have found FP to be roughly two times as potent as BDP. In addition, high-dose FP therapy (≥1000 µg/d) has been shown to result in two to four times greater suppression of adrenal function than equivalent doses of budesonide. Thus, it appears as if FP may be more potent than the other inhaled GC products on the market both in terms of efficacy and potential for systemic effects at high doses. With the possible exception of FP, the differences between the products come mainly from the amount of drug delivered per actuation.

Just as there have been few studies comparing the bioequivalence of the various inhaled GC compounds, few studies have compared the bioequivalence of inhaled and oral GCs. In one study, 2000 µg of inhaled BUD was found to be as effective as ~40 mg of daily prednisone in terms of improving asthma control, whereas 1840 µg/d was equivalent to ≥ 15 mg/d of prednisone in terms of its systemic effects (*see* Toogood, 1989). This observation reiterates two important points: (1) inhaled GC have a higher topical to systemic ratio and (2) high-dose inhaled GC therapy can result in significant systemic effects.

Dose/Frequency of Use

The dose of inhaled GC chosen is largely dependent on the clinical situation. The more severe or poorly controlled the asthma, the higher the initial dose. We often begin with high-dose inhaled GC therapy in an attempt to optimize pulmonary function and clinical symptoms. Once the patient's asthma is improved, we then taper the dose, following clinical symptoms and pulmonary function closely. The ideal inhaled steroid dose should be large enough to control asthma symptoms yet small enough to avoid the potential for adverse systemic effects. In the past, inhaled GCs were frequently administered three to four times daily, but the recent trend has been to dose these drugs twice daily. Adherence rates increase significantly when a drug can be delivered twice daily as opposed to four times daily. Studies of patients with moderate to severe asthma that have evaluated the effectiveness of twice-daily compared to four-times daily therapy (same total daily dose administered) have demonstrated enhanced efficacy when the GC is administered four times daily. In contrast, studies in mild asthmatics have failed to show improved efficacy of the more frequently administered drug. Thus, when deciding upon how often to administer an inhaled GC, one must consider the clinical situation, keeping in mind that compliance rates decrease significantly when the drug is administered more than twice daily. If the patient's asthma is poorly controlled, high-dose GC therapy should be administered four times daily with the patient's dose (both frequency of administration and amount administered) decreased as asthma control improves.

Adverse Effects of Inhaled GC Therapy

Adrenal Suppression

Inhaled GC therapy can result in suppression of the hypothalamic-pituitary-adrenal (HPA) axis. The degree of suppression is largely dependent on the dose and frequency of the inhaled GC delivered, the duration of treatment, route of administration and time of day the drug is administered. The preponderance of data would suggest doses of 400 µg/d or less are not associated with changes in the HPA axis, but as the inhaled dose is increased to above 1000 µg/d, HPA axis suppression clearly occurs. Although FP is thought to have systemic effects comparable to the other inhaled GCs at doses recommended for the treatment of mild and moderate asthma (176–440 µg/d), the same cannot be said regarding high-dose FP therapy (≥1000 µg/d). A number of studies have demonstrated significantly greater HPA axis suppression with FP compared to equivalent doses of budesonide. This is an important and possibly unique observation for FP. Thus, high-dose FP should be used only in patients with severe, poorly controlled asthma or in patients with steroid-dependent asthma. Whether or not modest reductions in HPA axis are of clinical relevance remains to be determined.

Growth Suppression

Growth suppression is the steroid-associated adverse effect that causes the most concern for clinicians caring for children. Whether clinically significant growth suppression can occur with long-term inhaled GC therapy remains controversial, with some studies suggesting that doses of as little as 400 µg/d of BDP can result in suppression of linear growth. Unfortunately, almost all of the studies that have attempted to determine the effect of inhaled GC on growth have been limited, making definitive conclusions regarding growth suppression difficult. Many studies have been criticized as growth was not the primary outcome variable. Most also have methodological flaws in that they

---

Effect of Inhaled GC Therapy Upon Growth

- Recently the FDA has required warning labels about possible effects on growth in children on all prescriptions of inhaled GC.
- While it is debatable that long-term growth suppression will occur with use of inhaled GCs, some studies have shown that short-term suppression can occur in some children.
- It is well to remember that asthma causes significant morbidity and is a life-threatening condition. For overall control, inhaled GCs are usually a safe and most effective anti-inflammatory asthma prevention treatment.
- As with any therapy, before prescribing it physicians must weigh any potential risk with the known benefit.

---

fail to adequately assess pubertal status, lack baseline growth velocity data, display significant differences in baseline height or age between the different treatment groups or lack appropriate untreated control groups. Complicating this issue further is the long-known but often overlooked observation that asthma, especially poorly controlled asthma, can adversely affect growth.

There have now been several controlled studies demonstrating short-term growth suppression using moderate doses of BDP. In all of the studies, 7 mo to 1 yr of BDP therapy (336–400 µg/d) resulted in a loss of 1–1.5 cm of growth compared to the control group. Of potential significance, one of the studies suggested that the growth-suppressive effect of BDP appeared to be greatest during the first 3 mo of therapy (*see* Simons et al.). The growth curve for BDP appeared to parallel that of the other treatment groups from 3 mo on. In addition, not all studies have demonstrated growth suppression with inhaled GC therapy. Long-term (22 mo) budesonide (600 µg/d) therapy was not shown to display any suppressive effect on growth in a Swedish study published several years ago. In this study, growth rates among the male asthmatics were found to be significantly decreased compared to age-matched nonasthmatic controls, but when the growth rates between the asthmatics treated with placebo vs budesonide were compared, those treated with budesonide displayed better growth (–0.44 cm/yr for budesonide vs –0.70 cm/yr for placebo).

A large, 5-yr randomized, multicenter study sponsored by the National Institutes of Health, the Childhood Asthma Management Program (CAMP), is an ongoing study that is designed to answer many of the questions regarding inhaled GC use in childhood asthma. This study, in which over 1000 children have been randomized to receive placebo, nedocromil, or budesonide, is designed to measure the natural history of childhood asthma. In addition, it will significantly enhance the field of our current knowledge in terms of both the efficacy and adverse effects of the two study medications.

OSTEOPOROSIS

Despite the fact that osteoporosis can be a debilitating complication of oral GC therapy, there have been a paucity of studies evaluating the effect of inhaled GC on bone metabolism, and more importantly, bone mineral density (BMD). Some studies have found significant reductions in BMD of the femoral neck of asthmatics treated with inhaled GC compared to age-matched controls, with significant inverse correlations found between BMD and the dose duration (product of the average daily dose of inhaled GC in grams and the duration of therapy in months) of inhaled GC therapy. Of note, other studies have failed to demonstrate any deleterious effect on BMD.

Given the discrepancy in results among the above studies, Toogood et al. sought to differentiate between the effect of inhaled GC compared to the potential effect of other variables such as past or current oral GC use, age, physical activity level and postmenopausal state on bone density. They found inhaled GC therapy to result in a dose-dependent reduction of BMD with a decrease of approximately 0.5 standard deviation for each increment of inhaled GC dose of 1 mg/day. Of surprise, a larger lifetime exposure to inhaled GC was associated with a more normal BMD. The authors speculated that this "protective effect" was due to reconstitution of BMD following conversion from oral to inhaled GC therapy. Lastly, postmenopausal women receiving estrogen-replacement therapy were likely to have normal bone density. They concluded that the daily dose, but not the duration of therapy, adversely affects bone density, and that estrogen therapy may offset inhaled GC effects on bone demineralization in postmenopausal women. In summary, many factors appear to contribute to the development of osteoporosis, including dose, frequency of administration and duration of use in addition to time of use above a "threshold" dose. Information is needed on how to manage steroid-induced osteoporosis, especially in cases in which long-term use of high-dose inhaled GCs is indicated to manage severe persistent asthma.

CATARACTS/GLAUCOMA

Recent reports have suggested that long-term inhaled GC therapy can be associated with the development of cataracts and/or glaucoma. These large epidemiological studies found weak, but statistically significant, associations between inhaled GC therapy and either cataracts or glaucoma. Of note, these studies evaluated elderly individuals with mean ages of 65. In addition, the studies failed to provide any indication of clinical significance or visual impairment. In 1998, Agertoft and Pedersen reported on slit-lamp evaluations in 157 asthmatic children receiving budesonide for an average of 4.5 yr and in 111 age-matched, asthmatic controls. Only one posterior subcapsular cataract was identified; this was in a child receiving budesonide, but the cataract had been diagnosed 2 yr before the child underwent budesonide therapy. The authors concluded that long-term treatment with budesonide in children is unlikely to cause cataracts and that ophthalmological surveillance is probably not warranted.

OTHER ADVERSE EFFECTS

A number of other adverse effects have been associated with inhaled GC therapy, including hypoglycemia, development of cushingoid features, opportunistic infections, dermal thinning and psychosis. Most adverse effects are from case reports; few controlled studies have evaluated their potential significance.

SUMMARY

GC therapy has become an important pharmacological method in asthma therapy. While potent and generally effective, systemic GCs are not without risks for development of serious adverse effects, especially when used in high doses for prolonged periods. Fortunately, inhaled GC products have been developed that greatly minimize the adverse systemic effects while retaining beneficial airway effects. Many previously steroid-dependent asthmatics have been tapered off oral GC therapy following institution of inhaled GC therapy. As with oral GC therapy, high-dose inhaled GC therapy has been associated with adverse systemic effects, and it is still unclear whether long-term administration of inhaled GC will result in growth suppression and osteoporosis. Thus, the clinician must balance the therapeutic effects of both inhaled and oral GC with the risks for adverse effects. Obviously, using the lowest possible effective GC doses as well as maximizing other therapeutic methods are means by which this goal can be achieved. Early recognition and appropriate management are other methods to minimize GC-induced adverse effects. With the principles set forth, specifically maximization of therapy, early recognition and appropriate management of adverse effects, the potential severe complications of GC therapy can be minimized.

ACKNOWLEDGMENT

We would like to acknowledge the valuable contribution to the first edition of this chapter by Alan Kamada, PHARMD. Supported in part by the National Institutes of Health, Heart, Lung, and Blood Institute, Grant HL-36577. Dr. Szefler is the Helen Wohlberg and Herman Lambert Chair in Pharmacokinetics.

SUGGESTED READING

Agertoft L, Pedersen S. Bone mineral density in children with asthma receiving long-term treatment with budesonide. *Am J Respir Crit Care Med* 1998;157:178–183.

Agertoft L, Pedersen S. Effects of long-term treatment with an inhaled corticosteroid on growth and pulmonary function in asthmatic children. *Respir Med* 1994;88:373–381.

Donahue JG, Weiss ST, Livingston JM, et al. Inhaled steroids and the risk of hospitalization for asthma. *JAMA* 1997;277:887–891.

Ernst P, Spitzer WO, Suissa S, et al. Risk of fatal and near fatal asthma in relation to inhaled corticosteroid use. *JAMA* 1992;268:3462–3464.

Expert Panel Report 2: Guidelines for the Diagnosis and Management of Asthma. National Institutes of Health, National Heart, Lung, and Blood Institute. *NIH* publication No. 97-4051, 1997.

Fanta CH, Rossing TH, McFadden ER. Glucocorticoids in acute asthma: A critical controlled study. *Am J Med* 1983;74:845–851.

Haahtela T, Jarvinen M, Kava T, Kiviranta K, et. al. Effects of reducing or discontinuing inhaled budesonide in patients with mild asthma. *N Engl J Med* 1994;331:700–705.

Harris JB, Weinberger MM, Nassif E, Smith G, Milavetz G, Stillerman A. Early intervention with short courses of prednisone to prevent progression of asthma in ambulatory patients incompletely responsive to bronchodilators. *J Pediatr* 1987;110:627–633.

Harter JG, Reddy WJ, Thorn GW. Studies on an intermittent corticosteroid dosage regimen. *N Engl J Med* 1963;269:591–596.

McFadden ER Jr. Dosages of corticosteroids in asthma. *Am Rev Respir Dis* 1993;147:1306–1310.

Robinson D, Hamid Q, Ying S, Bentley A, Assoufi B, Durham, Kay AB. Prednisolone treatment in asthma is associated with modulation of bronchoalveolar lavage cell interleukin-4, interleukin-5, and interferon-γ cytokine gene expression. *Am Rev Respir Dis* 1993;148:401–406.

Simons FER, and the Canadian Beclomethasone Dipropionate-Salmeterol Xinafoate Study Group. A comparison of beclomethasone dipropionate, salmeterol, and placebo in children with asthma. *N Engl J Med* 1997;337:1659–1665.

Toogood JH, Baskerville JC, Markov AE, et al. Bone mineral density and the risk of fracture in patients receiving long-term inhaled steroid therapy for asthma. *J Allergy Clin Immunol* 1995;96:157–166.

Toogood JH, Baskerville J, Jennings B, Lefcoe NM, Johansson S-A. Bioequivalent doses of budesonide and prednisone in moderate and severe asthma. *J Allergy Clin Immunol* 1989;84:688–700.

Webb JR. Dose response of patients to oral corticosteroid treatment during exacerbations of asthma. *Br J Med* 1986;292:1045–1047.

24 Environmental Control of Respiratory Irritants and Allergens

Edward M. Zoratti, MD

INTRODUCTION

We are continuously exposed to a broad spectrum of airborne allergens and irritants that are present in the air we breathe. Contact with these airborne substances frequently triggers respiratory tract symptoms in patients with underlying asthma, bronchitis and rhinoconjunctivitis. Although outdoor-air quality receives a great deal of attention, average Americans spend more than 90% of their time indoors. Therefore, the indoor environment is likely to have the most significant impact on susceptible patients when respiratory irritants and allergens are present.

Even patients who do not have allergic disease may develop bothersome respiratory tract and ocular irritation when exposed to sufficiently high concentrations of airborne particulate matter or volatile substances that are capable of producing an inflammatory response when contacting the mucosal surfaces of the eyes, nose, pharynx, trachea and lungs. However, the respiratory and conjunctival surfaces of allergic and asthmatic patients are often chronically iirritated because of their underlying inflammatory disease. These inflamed tissues respond to very low concentrations of airborne irritants with excessive mucous production, nasal congestion, sneezing attacks, nasal and ocular itching or bronchoconstriction.

Compared to respiratory irritants, the airborne concentration of an allergen that is required to trigger symptoms in sensitized individuals may be miniscule. For example, exposure to an environment containing as little as 10 µg of dust mite allergen per gram

From: *Current Clinical Practice: Allergic Diseases: Diagnosis and Treatment, 2nd Edition*
Edited by: P. Lieberman and J. Anderson © Humana Press Inc., Totowa, NJ

of settled housedust can result in an asthma attack in an already allergic patient. Even lower concentrations of allergen (2 µg/g) may lead to developing dust-mite sensitivity in susceptible infants.

Therefore, it is important that measures be taken to control the environment of allergic patients and nonallergic patients with recurrent rhinitis, conjunctivitis or bronchitis. The potential benefits of minimizing irritant and allergen exposure include lower symptom frequency and severity, lower medication requirements and decreased risk of allergic sensitization. The rationale for employing a variety of low-cost, safe and simple methods to reduce exposure to common indoor irritants and allergens will be the focus of this chapter.

ENVIRONMENTAL CONTROL OF IRRITANTS

The air inside a patient's home or workplace often contains a variety of substances that can be classified as irritants based on their noxious effects on mucous membranes such as those of the conjunctiva and respiratory tract. Sufficient exposure to these irritants results in ocular burning, itching and redness, as well as symptoms of rhinitis, bronchitis and, in susceptible asthmatic patients, bronchoconstriction.

Irritant exposure will cause symptoms in all patients if the exposure is intense. However, in a subset of individuals, including most patients with allergies and asthma, the threshold of tolerance to these substances is very low because of chronic inflammation in the target organs.

In this section, we will focus on the common irritants that are present in the home or workplace, including environmental tobacco smoke, vapors from household products and nitrogen dioxide (NO_2).

Environmental Tobacco Smoke (ETS)

Nearly everyone in the United States has some degree of exposure to "secondhand" or "environmental" tobacco smoke (ETS). The Environmental Protection Agency estimates that exposure to ETS is associated with approximately 3000 lung cancer deaths annually and up to 60,000 deaths due to ischemic heart disease. However, the adverse effects of ETS on respiratory health are much more common. Although rarely fatal, these adverse effects significantly impact the quality of life in patients with recurrent bronchitis, asthma, rhinitis, conjunctivitis and middle ear disease.

Tobacco smoke is a mixture of a large number of pollutants contained in both airborne particles and vapors that are capable of irritating the conjunctiva and respiratory tract. This ultimately leads to swelling, excessive mucous production and impaired airway ciliary function. These effects of ETS on the respiratory tract are related to both the concentration and duration of exposure to ETS. The only effective method to control ETS is by minimizing cigaret, cigar or pipe smoking in the home and other locations, such as the school or workplace, that the allergic patient frequently visits. Helpful "partial" controls include limiting smoking to outdoors or only in well-ventilated areas or areas of the home that are equipped with an efficient exhaust fan. Many times, improving ventilation by enhancing fresh air exchange into the home or workplace will result in readily apparent improvement. However, in subjects with underlying severe asthma, rhinitis and conjunctivitis, even minimal smoke exposure can result in exacerbation of their symptoms, and strict smoke avoidance is necessary.

Efforts to control ETS exposure typically involve difficult behavior changes for the patients, their families, friends and coworkers. The primary care provider can play a role in supporting environmental control for tobacco smoke by helping to facilitate this sometimes-painful process in several ways. First, the provider can supply information to the patient and others to underscore the dangers of secondhand smoke, making it clear that environmental change is necessary. Next, advice regarding environmental manipulation or a list of local resources that can aid with the procurement and installation of devices to improve ventilation or minimize ETS in the home or workplace can be provided. In addition, physicians and other health care professionals should provide appropriate materials and medications that support smoking cessation efforts by patients, family members or coworkers who have an earnest desire to do so. Finally, all health care providers should be active advocates for legislation that limits cigaret consumption in public areas.

Recent reports (*see* Suggested Reading) should provide confidence to both health care providers and patients that the considerable effort required to minimize ETS exposure will be met with clinical improvement. One such report investigated the effect of minimizing ETS exposure in a patient population that typically has intensive exposure to cigaret smoke and a high incidence of respiratory tract symptoms. The first report involves the recent California law prohibiting smoking in bars and taverns that has resulted in rapid improvement in reported respiratory tract symptoms among bar and tavern workers in that state. Another longitudinal study has documented clear benefit of reduced ETS exposure specifically among subjects with asthma. Although ETS exposure is often difficult to measure, these and other studies point to the important role that minimizing exposure can play in improving respiratory health.

Environmental Control of Household Irritants Other Than Tobacco Smoke

A diverse group of airborne pollutants has detrimental effects on respiratory health primarily by inducing irritation of the mucous membranes. Because of the enormous number of substances that can potentially act as respiratory irritants, we will limit this section to typically encountered household products.

Some of the most commonly encountered irritants within a home include cosmetics, perfumes, household cleaning agents and a variety of adhesives, paints, and sealants typically used for hobbies and do-it-yourself projects. Some of these products give off a noticeable odor and are easily recognized as "triggers" for respiratory and ocular symptoms because of the short time-frame between exposure and symptom onset. Other items such as air fresheners, potpourri and incense, are utilized in a fashion leading to long-term low-level exposure, and a high index of suspicion is required to identify these as significant triggers. Fortunately, once these items are identified, most can be easily avoided, replaced with less noxious alternatives or used only in well-ventilated areas.

Formaldehyde and small amounts of other volatile organic compounds (VOCs) that may be released from building materials may also trigger respiratory symptoms. Other VOCs may be found in household solvents and personal hygiene products such as perfumes, hair sprays, nail polish and nail polish remover that may evoke sudden respiratory difficulty in susceptible patients. Although these compounds are often continuously detectable in the home, their effects on respiratory health are debatable at the low concentrations that are typically present. However, in high concentrations

Table 1
Common Household Irritants and Environmental Control Recommendations

Common Irritants and Their Sources	Control Recommendations
Environmental tobacco smoke: Some Harmful Components of Smoke 　Carbon Dioxide 　Nicotine 　Benzene 　Formaldehyde 　Acrolein 　Particulate matter	Aid patient and family members in efforts 　to cease smoking "Necessary" smoking should be confined to 　outdoors (preferably) or in well-ventilated 　areas Susceptible patients should avoid cigaret- 　smoke–laden areas of the home or workplace Air cleaners equipped with a HEPA filter may 　be helpful for small areas like bedrooms Ensure adequate ventilation and add exhaust 　devices or modify air exchange if required.
Volatile organic compounds (VOCs): Examples and Sources 　Formaldehyde (building materials) 　Carbon tetrachloride (solvents) 　Toluene (paints, sealants) 　Aldehydes (perfuming agents)	Identification of source and adequate sealing 　of VOC containers or removal from home Increase ventilation in confined areas or 　throughout home when nonremovable 　source materials are suspected. Vapor-proof door seals between living areas 　and garage or work areas that contain irritant 　substances Activated charcoal filter masks for unavoidable 　exposure as occurs in the workplace.
Nitrogen dioxide: Sources 　Natural gas ranges or artificial 　　fireplaces 　Wood-burning stoves or fireplaces 　Tobacco smoke 　Kerosene or propane space heaters	Identification of the source and removal 　if possible Improve exhaust system for appliance Improve ventilation where appliance is located Substitute electrical devices if possible

these compounds have known significant respiratory irritant properties. Interestingly, the trend in homebuilding over the last several decades has been a progressive march toward airtight and energy-efficient housing. This trend has led to a situation in which the air in some homes and commercial buildings may contain extremely high concentrations of indoor pollutants, including VOCs. This poor air exchange has been potentially linked to a variety of building-related illness, including the "sick-building syndrome."

Nitrogen dioxide is another indoor pollutant that has been linked to poor asthma control as well as to irritant effects on the eyes, nose, throat and lungs. The primary source of this compound is inadequately vented gas cooking ranges, artificial fireplaces or space heaters that burn kerosene or natural gas. Nitrogen dioxide is also a product of wood burning or cigaret smoking within the home.

The recommended environmental control measures for these common household air pollutants, including VOCs and nitrogen dioxide, are similar to those discussed for environmental tobacco smoke (Table 1). Successful environmental control can be

Table 2
Commonly Encountered Indoor Allergens

Potential Sources of Allergens	Specific Examples
Insects/arachnids	Cockroaches and dust mites
Household pets	Cats, dogs, rodents, rabbits
Indoor molds	*Penicillium, Aspergillus* and *Cladosporium*
Pollens/molds transferred indoors	Grass, weed and tree pollen
Wild rodents	Rats, mice
Furniture components	Horse hair- or Kapok-stuffed furniture
Foods and drugs	Steam from seafood, penicillin "powder," psyllium,
Latex-containing articles	Rubber gloves, rubber balloons

accomplished only with a high index of suspicion and knowledge of common sources for these irritants. Removal of sources of VOCs such as solvents, building materials and some personal care products should be most effective. Likewise, adequate venting of wood burning stoves and gas ranges can control levels of nitrogen dioxide. Finally, increasing fresh air exchange can be an effective method of decreasing any indoor irritant, since the source of most of these compounds is inside the home, and the concentration gradient favors improvement of the indoor environment with ventilation.

ENVIRONMENTAL CONTROL OF INDOOR ALLERGENS

A variety of biological sources are capable of generating airborne proteins in the home that can lead to allergic sensitization (Table 2). The situation with indoor allergens is different in several ways from the previously discussed "irritants." First, since extremely small levels of these proteins (microgram amounts) can trigger symptoms in sensitized subjects, even more intensive environmental control measures are appropriate for allergic patients. Second, even intermittent exposure to an allergen has a "priming" effect leading to a "twitchiness" of the airways, resulting in recurrent bronchospasm and nasal congestion in response to subsequent encounters with allergens and irritants at levels that previously were too low to act as symptom triggers. Finally, a single, short-lived exposure to an allergen not only can lead to immediate bronchospasm, rhinitis or conjunctivitis but it also has been associated with a sustained "late-phase" response with symptom-onset beginning 6–8 h after allergen encounter.

Physicians addressing patients with a chief complaint consistent with the typical symptoms of seasonal allergic rhinoconjunctivitis frequently appreciate the effects of environmental allergens. However, a body of evidence has accumulated that implies that indoor allergens have an important role in chronic asthma. First, it is estimated that 60–80% of patients with asthma have evidence of allergic sensitization to inhaled allergens. Likewise, IgE-mediated sensitization to common allergens is a strong risk factor for asthma, with the severity of allergic sensitization correlating with the severity of asthma and bronchial hyperresponsiveness. In addition, inhalation of allergen results in immediate bronchoconstriction followed by subsequent airway inflammation leading to chronic, recurrent asthma. Finally, asthma symptoms, peak flow measurements and bronchial responsiveness to methacholine all improve when patients are able to avoid inhaled allergens.

The expected benefits of allergen avoidance include improved symptom control, lowered medication requirements and lowering of the symptom threshold to subsequent allergen exposure. This section will focus on the clinically important indoor allergens and the environmental control measures that can limit exposure to these proteins.

Environmental Control for Dust Mite Allergy

House dust is a mixture of soil particles, small fibers, skin scales and products derived from household animals, insects, bacteria and fungi. Within this mixture live tiny eight-legged acarids (related to the spider) named dust mites.

Dust mites are considered among the most clinically important indoor allergens throughout the world. The body of the dust mite as well as its fecal particles contains large amounts of the primary allergenic proteins named Der p 1 and Der f 1. It is the inhalation of these particles that can lead to initial immune recognition leading to allergic sensitization and subsequently to the recognizable symptoms of allergic rhinoconjunctivitis and asthma. In fact, it has been shown that as little as 2 µg of these allergenic proteins per gram of house dust can result in sensitization, and 10 µg of protein per gram of dust is sufficient to trigger acute bronchospasm in previously sensitized individuals.

The importance of environmental control in the management of dust mite allergy is underscored by the fact that a high level of dust mite exposure has been identified as a risk factor for the development of asthma. Furthermore, several studies among dust-mite–sensitive asthmatics have shown that moving them to dust-mite-free–living conditions results in dramatic improvement of their asthma.

Our knowledge of the biology and life cycle of dust mites can be exploited to design rational environmental control measures (Table 3) that can be recommended to dust mite allergic patients or those at high risk for sensitization.

The first factor to consider, is that an individual's greatest exposure to dust mite typically occurs while sleeping in bed. In fact, house dust obtained from bedding contains a higher concentration of dust mite allergen than dust collected from other areas of the home. Furthermore, an average of 8 h each day is spent breathing air that is in proximity to bedding surfaces. This close physical contact with a surface that is the source of allergen exposure is particularly important for dust mite allergy because the particles that contain the relevant allergenic proteins are "heavy" and remain airborne for only a few minutes after they are propelled into the air by mechanical disruption of their reservoir (the bed). Therefore, the area of the home that should be the focus of dust mite environmental control recommendations should be the bedroom and specifically, the bed itself.

Other factors to consider are the conditions that promote dust mite growth and reproduction. Dust mites thrive when provided with an adequate food source. It appears that pillows and bedding provide an excellent living environment with a "built-in" food source for the dust mite. In fact, human skin scales are among the mite's preferred diet, leading to their scientific name dermatophagoides (skin eater). Frequent bedding changes and laundering are important to clear the bedding of accumulated allergen and human skin. In addition, washing objects in hot water can also kill dust mites.

The mattress and pillows serve as large reservoirs of dust mite. Multiple studies have shown that encasing the mattress, box springs and pillows in impermeable covers

Table 3
Dust Mite Environmental Control Recommendations

Factor Influencing Dust Mite Exposure	Environmental Control Response
Most dust mite exposure occurs in the bedroom	First-line avoidance measures should focus on modifying the bed and the bedroom environment
Limiting "food sources" can minimize dust mite growth	Removal of nonwashable dust collectors in the bed such as stuffed toys and feather-fill pillows, along with frequent laundering of the bedding is recommended
The mattress, box springs and pillows are frequently large reservoirs of dust mite allergen	Encasement of these items in allergen-impermeable covers will immediately lower allergen exposure
Humid environments favor mite growth	Lower indoor humidity to ≤50% and consider removing damp carpets, upholstered furniture
Dust mites are temperature sensitive	Launder in hot water (130° F) weekly. Freezing small items may be effective
Respirable mite allergen particles remain airborne for 10 min after disturbing an environment	Avoid vacuuming or wear dust mask for housecleaning. Air cleaner is unlikely to be helpful.
Some patients may exhibit refractory symptoms that persist in spite of medications and other environmental control attempts	Carpet and upholstered furniture removal or use of acaricides may be suggested with understanding that efficacy is questionable

results in an immediate and dramatic fall in dust mite exposure. This effect can be sustained by weekly washing of the remaining bedding in hot water.

The use of feather-containing pillows and comforters should also be discouraged since these items usually cannot tolerate frequent laundering and tend to harbor large amounts of mite allergen. However, recent studies have shown that when laundering is avoided for extended periods, dust mite accumulation may be higher in polyester-filled than in feather-filled pillows. Regardless of the type of pillow used, the clinician's recommendations should include either using allergen-impermeable pillow covers or frequent washing in hot water.

The requirement for the use of hot water during laundering is due to the fact that dust mites do not tolerate temperature extremes and thrive at ambient temperatures of 65–80°F. To be completely lethal to dust mites, laundering would need to involve somewhat higher temperatures than those considered safe or practical. However, a recommendation to employ water temperatures of approximately 130°F will achieve a several-log decrease in viable mites. The fact that dust mites do not survive cold temperatures can also be exploited. Although I am not aware of any specific studies, many pediatric allergists suggest a weekly trip to the freezer for stuffed toys or other mite-laden objects that are "critical" for a child to sleep with.

Common Indoor Allergens in Different Situations in United States	
Situation	*Allergen*
Most homes	House dust, mites
Home in mountain	Animal (e.g., cat)
Eastern inner city	Cockroach
Summer cottage	Mold and mites
School	Animals (from home)
Damp basement	Mold
Basement bedroom	Mites

One other factor that is important for dust mite survival is humidity. An ideal environment for mite growth can be found in upholstered furniture, carpeting, beds and other objects where the ambient humidity is 60%, along with moderate temperatures and an ample source of fibers and human skin for food. The use of air conditioning and dehumidifiers to keep the indoor humidity 50 % has been promoted as a method to decrease mite growth. Unfortunately, successful mite control with dehumidification has been shown only in studies performed in areas of very high humidity such as in tropical areas. Nonetheless, in highly mite-sensitive individuals, dehumidification in addition to removal of carpets, stuffed animals, upholstered furniture and other "dust collectors" in the bedroom may be a reasonable recommendation while one is awaiting the results of studies that should clarify the utility of such a combined environmental control approach.

Finally, dust mite allergen is present on relatively large (10–25 μ) particles that remain airborne for a period of only 10 min after mechanical disturbance has propelled them into the air. Dust mite allergic patients can minimize their exposure to these airborne particles by avoiding recently vacuumed areas of the home or areas where a "cloud " of dust has been raised by disruption of dust reservoirs. Practical advice should include having a nonallergic person perform these tasks if possible. When this is not practical, the use of a dust mask can minimize exposure. In addition, the use of microporous filters or "double bag"-equipped vacuum cleaners is advisable. The large reservoirs of dust mite combined with the short time that mite allergen particles are airborne make the use of air filtration devices of little value.

My routine approach to the mite-sensitive patient is to advise the use of impermeable covers for mattresses, box springs and pillows in all cases. In addition, I suggest weekly laundering with hot water for all bedding (including the pillow if the patient chooses not to encase it), the removal of stuffed or feather-containing items as universal recommendations. In the case of severe or refractory symptoms in highly sensitive subjects I will also discuss dehumidification and the removal of upholstered furniture and carpeting in the bedroom.

A number of agents that can be sprinkled onto carpeting and other dust mite reservoirs in an attempt to kill dust mites (acaricides), or agents designed to denature mite proteins (such as tannic acid) have been developed and are commercially available. Unfortunately, I believe that their cost, limited efficacy and inconvenience outweigh the anticipated benefits for most patients. However, this is an area that holds great potential for future success when dealing with environmental control for dust mite allergy.

Finally, a carefully obtained clinical history may point to the presence of significant allergen exposure via other dust-laden articles or in certain areas of the home. Patients often provide a convincing scenario of rapid-onset sneezing episodes or asthma symptom onset within minutes of exposure in these environments. If these factors can be identified, simple avoidance of these exposures can be applied.

Environmental Control for Cockroach Allergy

Cockroach infestation is most common in the inner city and impoverished areas of America as well as the Southeast United States. However, these insects are ubiquitous, and infestation may not be visibly apparent in up to 30% of infested buildings. The allergenic protein from cockroaches can be found in gastrointestinal secretions (saliva and feces), as well as in their outer chitin shell. Therefore, it should be appreciated that eradication of the living cockroaches only partially depletes the reservoir of allergen.

Recent reports have confirmed an association of cockroach allergen exposure and asthma. The National Cooperative Inner City Asthma Study (NCICAS) studied nearly 500 urban children and found that compared to nonallergic subjects, children who were allergic to cockroach and exposed to high levels of allergen in their homes had a threefold higher asthma hospitalization rate. Cockroach allergen has also been long recognized as a trigger for allergic rhinoconjunctivitis.

Total, sustained eradication of cockroaches appears to be a particularly difficult task, and even when accomplished, elevated allergen levels persist for months. Some studies of single-family dwellings report successful cockroach control by extermination followed by rigorous, repeated cleaning that can deny the cockroach its source of food and water. However, success rates in studies performed in inner city apartments and multifamily dwellings have been low. The fact that cockroaches tend to live behind walls and are able to penetrate through narrow cracks in walls and furniture makes them difficult to directly target with insecticides and cleaning solutions.

Fortunately, the recognition of cockroach as an important factor in inner city asthma has spurred a flurry of research and interest in developing successful eradication processes. For the time being, some potentially beneficial methods to keep cockroach allergen at low levels should be advised. These methods include the use of impermeable mattress and pillow covers, since, as with the dust mite, these objects represent a reservoir of allergen that can produce transiently high concentrations of allergen-laden respirable particles in proximity to the patient. In addition, the use of organophosphate or pyrethrin containing insecticides can be an effective approach in single-family housing, especially when applied by a professional exterminator and when careful attention is paid to maintaining a continuous clean, food-free, dry environment. In most studies, the kitchen has been identified as the area most highly contaminated with cockroach allergen and should be the focus of eradication of living insects. However, human exposure is most likely to occur in the bedroom, and this area must also be kept free of food and water that can attract cockroaches. Finally, "bait stations" that attract and trap cockroaches can be used for surveillance to monitor when reapplication of insecticide may be necessary.

Environmental Control for Pet Allergy

Another group of clinically important environmental allergens are airborne proteins derived from household pets. Nearly half of the households in the United States have a pet cat or dog. Astonishingly, one third of all pet-allergic individuals have the offending animal in their home. Although dramatic improvement in allergic symptoms can be achieved by removing pets from the home, many patients do not accept this treatment strategy. A variety of other household pets, including mice, guinea pigs, hamsters, chinchillas, rabbits and other fur-bearing animals, are potentially allergenic. Less commonly, problems have been reported with birds and non-fur-bearing pets. Recently a convincing case of iguana allergy has been reported, although reptiles have generally been considered "allergy safe." Recommended environmental control measures are similar for all fur-bearing animals; however, the focus of the following discussion will be on the most common household pets in the United States—cats and dogs.

CAT ALLERGY

Cats secrete a protein antigen (Fel d 1) derived from their skin and saliva. This protein is responsible for inducing the majority of symptoms in cat-allergic patients. Fel d 1 is released after the secretions dry on the cat's fur and a fraction of this antigen becomes airborne on small particles that may remain buoyant for several hours. The physical characteristics of these small particles allow them to distribute to areas of the home that are distant to where the cat is "kept" and allow the antigen to "stick" to household surfaces and clothing. Several studies have shown that amounts of Fel d 1, which are sufficient to produce symptoms, can be present in homes and other buildings (such as airports, schools and hospitals) where cats have rarely been present. Presumably, this occurs from transfer of antigen that adheres to the clothing of cat owners and subsequently to surfaces outside the home.

Clearly, the most effective method to lower cat-allergen levels within a home is to remove the cat. However, since a significant proportion of cat owners find this unacceptable, alternative methods that focus on "treating the cat" or "removing" accumulated antigen while the cat is still in the home have been proposed.

It is important to note that even when a cat is removed from the home it may take many months for clinical improvement to occur. Studies show that there is a gradual decline in Fel d I after the cat is removed and that even 6 mo later some homes have high concentrations of the protein recovered from household dust samples. It is felt that this is due to allergen that is adherent to surfaces and present in reservoirs such as carpeting, mattresses and furniture. Therefore, it may be important for patients who have removed the cat to institute aggressive cleaning measures such as washing walls, steam cleaning carpeting, removing likely reservoirs and increasing fresh air exchange in the home. One study suggests that these cleaning methods result in more rapid decline of cat allergen levels, and therefore more rapid clinical improvement in patients can be expected.

Several studies have suggested that washing cats with tap water weekly may diminish the amount of allergen that becomes airborne and eventually distributes throughout the home. A recent study concluded that immersing and cleaning the cat with tap water may have a transient effect on lowering the amount of allergen released from the cat, but this beneficial effect had a duration of less than 24 h. It may be that more frequent washing or the use of detergents or allergen-denaturing shampoos may improve this

Sources of Pet Allergens	
Animal	*Source*
Cat	Excretion from body and saliva
Dog	Pelt, especially with shedding
Mouse, rat,	Urine
Gerbil, guinea pig, hamster	Urine
Bird	Feather, egg, feces

seemingly "logical" approach to cat allergy. However, further studies are required before a practical and effective method of cat washing can be promoted. On the other hand, investigators at our institution report that many cats quickly acclimate to being washed, and some even seem to enjoy the experience!

A number of commercial products are available that are designed to spray onto and rub into the cat's fur. Some of these sprays reportedly contain substances capable of denaturing proteins, making them incapable of eliciting an allergic response, and are also intended to be used on carpeting in the homes of cats. No convincing studies have been published that prove that these products are effective.

A practice that has been recommended by some veterinarians has been to medicate the cat with subtherapeutic doses of an animal tranquilizer called acepromazine. The rationale for this approach is that it may diminish the amount of Fel d I the animal produces. Such an effect was not apparent in a placebo-controlled study, and this approach to cat allergy cannot be recommended.

Restricting the cat to certain areas of the home may be helpful. Certainly, designating the bedroom a "cat-free" environment at all times is a logical recommendation. However, the presence of the allergen on small particles makes significant exposure likely to occur even in areas of the home that are most remote from the living quarters of the cat. Based on this, the use of room air cleaners with HEPA filters may provide a mechanism to clear airborne allergen in a relatively small area such as a bedroom. One study confirmed a decrease in the amount of airborne cat allergen using such a "safe-room" approach, but clinical symptoms in the test subjects were unchanged.

All cat-allergic subjects should be told to avoid direct contact with the animal and also to avoid furniture and other surfaces that the cat frequently visits. A somewhat curious clinical phenomenon is that patients often state that certain cats seem to be well tolerated and others bring on severe allergic symptoms. There is no evidence to suggest that certain breeds of cats or the length of the cat's hair is correlated with the degree of allergen shedding from the animals. However, it has been shown that the degree of variability in the amount of Fel d 1 that is shed between cats may be greater than 100-fold. Another finding is that male cats appear to produce more Fel d 1 than female cats. However, male castration results in a lowering of Fel d 1 production approximating that of female cats. This information may prove useful when allergic subjects insist on bringing a cat into the home.

DOG ALLERGY

Humans appear to have allergic responses to a variety of proteins that are present in the dander, saliva, urine, and serum derived from dogs. The main identified allergens are dog serum albumin and a protein named *Can f 1*, but more than 20 possible allergens have been identified. There is some dog-breed-specific variability in the production of these allergens, but all dogs have been shown to produce the main allergens. The large number of proteins that are potential allergens and the lack of well-standardized materials for diagnostic and research purposes have impaired adequate investigation of the effectiveness of environmental control for dogs.

However, many of the environmental control methods that were discussed for cat allergy can be recommended to dog-allergic patients and can be modified as more elaborate investigations become available in this area.

OTHER HOUSEHOLD PETS

The popularity of pets such as mice, rats, guinea pigs, hamsters, gerbils and rabbits has made allergy to rodents an increasingly important clinical problem. Most studies of rodent allergy have been done in laboratory workers, but the findings in these studies can be adapted to reduce household allergen exposure as well. One important fact is that the urine of rats, guinea pigs, mice and rabbits contains substantial amounts of allergenic proteins, and these proteins can become readily aerosolized and airborne. Therefore, allergic patients may develop severe symptoms upon contact with urine-contaminated bedding when the cages are cleaned, and this activity should be avoided. Likewise, the pelt of gerbils and hamsters appears to be the primary source of allergen. Routine environmental control measures for all household pets should include increased outside air exchange in the room where the pet is kept, confinement of the pet to a limited area of the home and minimal direct or indirect contact with materials that are likely to be reservoirs of the allergen. Ultimately, removal of the pet from the home may be the only successful solution for highly sensitive patients.

A recent popular choice of household pet is the ferret (*Mustela furo*). This furred animal, related to the weasel, is often identified as the allergic trigger by patients.

Little is known about the source or properties of the allergenic ferret proteins.

Although a decidedly uncommon indoor exposure, allergy to horse and cow can cause severe allergic symptoms in sensitive patients, and allergens can be brought into the home on clothing and other items. Commonsense avoidance procedures are recommended.

Indoor Mold Allergy

Fungi are organisms that are ubiquitous in our environment and may flourish in an indoor environment under the appropriate conditions. Several genera seem to be predominant indoors, including Aspergillus, Penicillium and Cladosporium. In general, fungi grow in damp environments such as basements (particularly in damp carpeting), windowsills, crawl spaces, shower stalls, household dust and in air humidification systems. Household plants can also be a common substrate for mold growth.

These organisms can release a variety of potentially allergenic proteins and glyco-protiens in the form of airborne spores as well as secreted substances that may be aerosolized. Most fungal allergens are not well characterized, but crude extracts of the organisms are potent allergens and can elicit vigorous immediate hypersensitivity responses during skin testing.

Value of an Air Cleaner

Important effect only on small particles that remain airborne for extended periods such as:

- Tobacco particles/smoke
- Mold spores
- Cat allergens
- Other particulate matter ("dust")
- Odors

Little effect on house dust mite or pollen "allergens," which are relatively large and heavy particles that remain airborne for only short periods after disturbance

---

Environmental control measures for mold focus on elimination of obvious mold-contaminated areas and adjusting the climate to minimize mold growth. The most potentially beneficial measure is to have mold-sensitive patients spend as little time as possible in areas that are likely to result in exposure (damp basements, crawl spaces, heavy house dust, bathtubs and shower stalls).

Mold growth may be visible on carpet backing, in bathrooms, on concrete or cement block walls or on damp wood surfaces. In these situations the carpeting should be replaced, and the other areas can be cleaned with bleach-based agents. However, a more appropriate long-term measure would be to decrease the indoor humidity by adjusting the home humidification system or repairing the home's foundation to minimize indoor leaks and seepage.

Mold will frequently contaminate both central humidification and freestanding humidification units that are present in many homes. These systems should be adjusted to avoid excess humidity in the home to minimize mold growth. In some areas the use of a dehumidifier is necessary to avoid high relative humidity within the home. The need for indoor humidification will change with climate, and many homes will not require a humidifier. Finally, areas such as bathrooms and kitchens should be equipped with appropriate exhaust mechanisms to evacuate steam that may be episodically generated by cooking or by running hot water.

USE OF AIR-CLEANING DEVICES AND DUCT-CLEANING SERVICES

Patients with allergies to indoor allergens typically ask whether it would be beneficial to purchase an air-cleaning device. In addition, many patients are approached by a variety of companies that offer to perform procedures to clear the heating-duct system of their homes, claiming that this service will improve their allergy symptoms and respiratory health. Unfortunately, a clear answer to their inquiries pertaining to the true benefit of these interventions cannot be provided. A complex interaction of several factors plays a role in determining the effectiveness of air cleaners on the levels of indoor allergens and irritants. Many of these factors will also impact the likelihood of duct cleaning as an adjunctive intervention for patients with recurrent respiratory symptoms. These factors are discussed below.

Particle Size

Allergens such as pollens and dust mite are present on relatively large particles. These large particles become airborne with considerable disturbance, but rapidly settle back to the surface. Therefore, there is only a short time that the particles are subject to air cleaners (when they are airborne). This leads to a situation in which large amounts of settled antigen cannot be filtered, and the small amount that is filtered will be replaced by newly produced antigen.

Mold allergens, the particulate components of environmental tobacco smoke and a sizable fraction of the cat allergen Fel d *1* are present on small particles. Since these particles remain airborne for extended periods, they would be susceptible to air-cleaning devices capable of filtering small particles. However, at any given time only a minute percentage of the total particles are airborne with an overwhelming amount remaining in large reservoirs that serve to act as a "continuous source" of the airborne allergen.

Type of Air Cleaner

There are three basic classifications of air cleaners:

1. *Mechanical filters* are devices that clean the air by having air pass through porous material where particles are trapped based on their size.
2. *Electrostatic precipitators* impart an electrical charge on particles that subsequently adhere to surfaces of opposite electrical charge.
3. *Chemical filters* are those air cleaners that rely on activated charcoal or other substances to absorb gases and odors.

The most beneficial mechanical filters include those that use a high-efficiency particulate air (HEPA) filter. These are capable of removing the vast majority of particles in the size range of the relevant allergens discussed previously. The main problem, as discussed, is that only airborne allergens will be filtered, and only air from a limited area of the home will be drawn to the filter.

Electrostatic precipitators have been shown to also efficiently filter dust mite feces and pollen-size particles (10–20 μ) and will remove a majority of the particulates generated from cigaret smoke. However, they require frequent cleaning and have the same limitations discussed for the HEPA filters.

The activated charcoal and chemical filters do not appear to be efficient in limited studies testing the capability to absorb formaldehyde or nitrous oxide.

Several studies, which were performed to investigate the effects of air cleaners on clinical symptoms, have been inconclusive. Therefore, I do not believe that air cleaners should be a universal recommendation to all patients for environmental control for indoor allergens or irritants. However, the use of air cleaners in conjunction with other environmental control measures has not been adequately studied. If patients insist on purchasing an air-cleaning device, HEPA filter units appear to be most capable of filtering the relevant particle sizes and can be recommended for small area use.

Ventilation-Duct Cleaning

In recent years, ventilation–duct-cleaning services have been advertised to the public. Although allergens can accumulate in the ventilation ducts in settled dust, the degree to which this dust is responsible for worsening allergic symptoms is unknown, and no controlled studies have been published on the effects of duct cleaning on airborne allergen levels or symptom improvement. A consensus of experts in this area is lacking, and the efficacy of this commonly offered service needs to be studied.

APPROACH TO ADVISING THE PATIENT ABOUT ENVIRONMENTAL CONTROL

Patients with allergic rhinitis and asthma can benefit from sound advice pertaining to environmental control. However, advice needs to be tailored to each patient based on the severity of symptoms, the allergens involved and the patient's motivation and personal circumstances.

History

As with any patient encounter, a careful history is important in developing a sufficient index of suspicion for environmental allergen or irritant exposure. Although this chapter's focus has been on the home environment, careful questioning in regard to the workplace can yield information leading to a diagnosis of exposure to an occupational allergen or irritant. Questioning in regard to hobbies and outdoor activities may also provide clues to symptom-triggering exposures that may not be apparent to the patient. In some cases the presence of environmental allergy is obvious, such as a patient's recognition that "I sneeze, my eyes itch and I wheeze whenever I hold my cat." However, long-time exposure to allergens or irritants more commonly results in the development of subacute or chronic symptoms, and the temporal relationship to environmental exposure can often be missed.

Diagnosis

If the history is obvious and the symptoms are of mild or moderate severity, an empiric trial of appropriate environmental measures, with or without pharmacological treatment, may be indicated. When the history is unclear, or when symptoms are severe, prompt evaluation by an allergist and relevant skin testing should be carried out. Definitive recommendations for environmental control can then be made with confidence.

Where there is a suggestive history, asthma should be confirmed by reversible airway obstruction documented by spirometry; airflow will often show improvement upon repeated testing after bronchodilator administration. Alternatively, longitudinal monitoring of properly performed peak flow measurements may document a temporal relationship between allergen exposure and worsening airway obstruction. In addition, a finding of large daily fluctuations in peak flow measurements are characteristic of asthma.

Recommendations

Recommendations for environmental control need to be tailored so that the patient is not overwhelmed or offended. For instance, most parents of children with mild rhinitis will not find it acceptable to remove all carpeting, use acaricides and take away their child's favorite stuffed toy for control of dust mite exposure. In fact, such extensive recommendations may lead to noncompliance with even the simpler measures of encasing the mattress, removal by feather-filled items and washing bedding in hot water, which may provide significant relief of symptoms.

However, when symptoms are severe or progressing, as in a patient with worsening asthma, prompt confirmation of allergy and more aggressive recommendations for environmental control may be warranted. In many instances, it may be difficult to convince a patient that dust or animal contact is a problem. Many times, a positive skin test will provide a visible message that may be helpful in persuading the patient that exposure to the allergen needs to be minimized.

In most instances, environmental control measures and pharmacotherapy will lead to a good clinical outcome for patients with rhinoconjunctivitis and asthma. . It should be noted that many patients are sensitive to more than one allergen. Multiple allergies often result in symptoms that may not be clearly related to a single, obvious allergen exposure, and the effects of simultaneous exposure to multiple allergens may have additive effects on symptom severity. However, even in patients with multiple allergies, studies have shown beneficial effects when exposure to only one allergen is minimized. These subjects often need objective evaluation of allergic sensitization with skin testing or RAST testing (a method to detect specific IgE in the blood). Finally, in patients with refractory symptoms or extensive pharmacological requirements and known allergy, allergen desensitization therapy should be considered.

SUGGESTED READING

Custovic A, Simpson A, Chapman MD, et al. Allergen avoidance in the treatment of asthma and atopic disorders. *Thorax* 1998;53:63.

Eisner MD, Yelin EH, Henke J, et al. Environmental Tobacco Smoke and Adult Asthma. The Impact of Changing Exposure Status on Health Outcomes. *Am J Respir Crit Care Med* 1998;158:170.

Eisner MD, Smith AK, Blanc PD. Bartenders' Respiratory Health After Establishment of Smoke-Free Bars and Taverns. *JAMA* 1998;280:1909.

Fox RW. Air cleaners. A review. *J Allergy Clin Immunol* 1994:94:413.

Nelson HS, Hirsch R, Ohman JL, et al. Recommendations for the use of residential air-cleaning devices in the treatment of allergic respiratory diseases. *J Allergy Clin Immunol* 1988;82:661.

Platts-Mills TAE, Vervloet D, Thomas WR, et al. Indoor allergens and asthma: Report of a third international workshop. *J Allergy Clin Immunol* 1997;100:S1.

Rosentreich DL, Eggleston, PA, Kattan M, et al. The role of cockroach allergy and exposure to cockroach allergen in causing morbidity among inner-city children with asthma. *N Engl J Med* 1997;336:1356.

Sarpong SB, Wood RA, Eggleston PA. Short-term extermination and cleaning on cockroach allergens Bla g 2 in settled dust. *Ann All Asthma Immunol* 1996;76:257.

Sporik R, Holgate ST, Platts-Mills TA, et al. Exposure to house dust mite allergens (Der p 1) and the development of asthma in childhood. *N Engl J Med* 1990;323:502.

Wood RA, Johnson EF, VanNatta ML, et al. A placebo controlled trial of a HEPA air cleaner in the treatment of cat allergy. *Am J Respir Crit Care Med* 1998;158:115.

25 Allergen Immunotherapy

Roger W. Fox, MD and Richard F. Lockey, MD

CONTENTS

INTRODUCTION

Allergen immunotherapy, a series of allergen vaccine injections over a defined period, results in decreased sensitivity or tolerance to inhaled or injected allergens, which can be measured both clinically and immunologically. Vaccine is used to describe the immune-modifying properties of allergen immunotherapy. Such therapy is used to treat allergic rhinitis (hay fever), allergic asthma and stinging-insect hypersensitivity. During the first half of the 20th century, efficacy of allergen immunotherapy was based primarily on clinical observations. However, over the past 40 yr, scientific investigations of numerous allergens and of the complexities of the allergic reaction have revealed the immunological changes required for successful immunotherapy. This chapter reviews inhalant allergen immunotherapy utilized to treat allergic rhinitis and/or allergic asthma. Immunotherapy for stinging-insect hypersensitivity is covered in Chapter 6.

From: *Current Clinical Practice: Allergic Diseases: Diagnosis and Treatment, 2nd Edition*
Edited by: P. Lieberman and J. Anderson © Humana Press Inc., Totowa, NJ

> **When to Consider Allergen Immunotherapy**
>
> - Individuals with documented appropriate clinical symptoms, and either skin test or in vitro evidence of IgE-allergen-specific antibody.
> - Allergic manifestations of rhinitis, bronchial asthma or stinging insect venom sensitivity.
> - Failure to respond to elimination or control of environmental allergic factors.
> - Failure to respond to symptomatic medication or difficulty/inconvenience of using these medications regularly.

ALLERGENS

Sources of aeroallergens include, but are not limited to, pollen, molds and animal emanations, such as dander, saliva, urine, feces and other animal parts derived from mammals, birds, insects and house dust mites. Aeroallergens are able to induce a specific IgE antibody response. This requires that the aeroallergen is sufficiently abundant in the ambient air to both sensitize and provoke allergic symptoms in an atopic individual.

Ragweed pollen–induced allergic rhinitis is an excellent model for the study of aeroallergen–induced allergic diseases: (1) The pollen is found in the air in sufficient quantities during the predictable fall pollinating season, and ragweed pollen proteins are potent sensitizers; (2) ragweed pollen induces symptoms in the sensitized patient during and immediately following the ragweed pollinating season; and (3) ragweed–induced allergic rhinitis can be diagnosed easily historically and by appropriate in vivo or in vitro testing for specific IgE to ragweed allergens and by provocative challenges.

The immediate effects of allergen exposure are readily observed in the ragweed-allergic patient during the ragweed pollinating season. So too are symptoms in the sensitized patient caused by indoor exposure to allergens such as those derived from dust mites, cat and dog, although patients may suffer with perennial allergic symptoms from such environmental exposures. Such a temporal relationship is evidence for specific allergen sensitivity; however, allergic symptoms also are caused by various overlapping pollen and mold seasons. Therefore, it is sometimes difficult to ascertain which particular allergens are the most important as a cause of allergic disease. The physician must know which pollen, molds and other aeroallergens are most important in a given geographical area in which the patient lives. The American Academy of Allergy Asthma and Immunology has established a North American Pollen Network. Pollen and mold reports in various geographical areas are available by calling the National Allergy Bureau at 1-800-9-POLLEN or 1-877-9-ACHOOO, or by writing to the American Academy of Allergy Asthma and Immunology, 611 East Wells Street, Milwaukee, Wisconsin 53202-3889 (www.AAAAI.org).

ALLERGEN VACCINES

Licensing of allergen vaccines for clinical use in the United States is regulated by the Food and Drug Administration, Center for Biologics Evaluation and Research, Division

Table 1
Summary of Controlled Trials of Immunotherapy

	Grass	Weed	Tree	Molds	Mites	Danders Cat Dog	
Allergic Rhinitis	+ +	+ +	+ +	+	+ +	+ +	+
Asthma	+	+ +	+	+/–	+	+ +	+

– No effect
+ Positive effect
+ + Strong positive effect

of Allergenic Products and Parasitology. Many of the common vaccines used in clinical allergy practice are available as standardized products or are pending standardization. This means that allergen vaccines, as provided by commercial manufacturers, meet standards that assure that the appropriate allergens are included in a given vaccine. However, many allergen vaccines derived from natural sources are not yet standardized, and it is probably not economically feasible or practical to standardize all of them currently available for diagnosis and treatment. Currently, unstandardized allergenic vaccines are labeled on the basis of relative concentration (weight by volume or protein nitrogen units per milliliter) of the respective allergen source.

INDICATIONS FOR ALLERGEN IMMUNOTHERAPY

Allergen avoidance, pharmacotherapy and patient education form the basis for treating allergic rhinitis, conjunctivitis and asthma. Allergen immunotherapy is indicated for patients with these diseases who have demonstrated evidence of specific IgE antibodies to clinically relevant allergens and in whom environmental control and pharmacotherapy have failed. The absolute indication for prescribing allergen immunotherapy depends on the degree to which symptoms can be reduced by allergen avoidance, by medication and the amount, type and length of time medications are required to control symptoms. Immunotherapy, when appropriate, should be used adjunctively with continued environmental control measures and appropriate pharmacotherapy. For stinging-insect–induced anaphylaxis, specific Hymenoptera venom immunotherapy is the treatment of choice.

Controlled clinical studies demonstrate that allergen immunotherapy is effective for patients with respiratory allergies (Table 1). Immunotherapy is specific for the allergen administered, and the content of the treatment vaccine is based on the patient's history and allergy test results. In general, the very young (<5 yr old) and elderly patients (>65 yr old) are not candidates for immunotherapy. The very young patient with respiratory allergic diseases usually responds favorably to environmental control and pharmacotherapy, and an uncooperative child is not the ideal candidate for allergen injections. Theoretically, the young patient may benefit the most by immunotherapy by altering the natural course of a chronic disease. The elderly patient rarely requires immunotherapy for the management of rhinitis and/or asthma, because inhalant allergens usually are not contributing to the respiratory symptoms in this age group. The optimal duration of immunotherapy to achieve the best therapeutic response remains unknown; however, studies indicate that 3–5 yr of immunotherapy is adequate for patients who have had a good therapeutic response.

Table 2
Proposed Sequence of Events for Successful Immunotherapy

Step 1. Suppression of the inflammatory cells' response to allergen prior to measurable immunological changes
    Reduced cellular activation and mediator release
    Rapid changes in target organ mast cells, basophils and eosinophils

Step 2. Production of IgG blocking antibodies
    IgG1 subclass antibodies early in the course
    IgG4 subclass antibodies predominate later in the course

Step 3. Suppression of IgE response to seasonal and other allergens
    Blunting of seasonal rise of IgE
    Gradual decline of specific allergen IgE

Step 4. Alteration of the controlling T-cell lymphocytes
    Down-regulation of TH_2 lymphocyte cytokine profile
    Down-regulation of IgE antibody production and eosinophil activation

Step 5. Reduction of target organ hypersensitivity and mast cell and basophil cellular sensitivity
    Reduced cellular hypersensitivity
    Reduced biological responses

IMMUNOLOGICAL CHANGES INDUCED BY ALLERGEN IMMUNOTHERAPY

The commonly recognized immunological changes that occur secondary to successful allergen immunotherapy (Table 2) include: (1) a rise in serum IgG-"blocking" antibody; (2) blunting of the usual seasonal rise of IgE followed by a slow decline of IgE over the course of immunotherapy; (3) increase in IgG- and IgA-blocking antibodies in the respiratory secretions; (4) reduction in basophil reactivity and sensitivity to specific allergens; (5) reduced production of inflammatory mediators during both early- and late-phase responses to allergen exposure; (6) decreased mast cell numbers and eosinophil recruitment and (7) reduced lymphocyte responsiveness (proliferation and cytokine production) to specific allergens and a shift of T-cell subsets away from a TH_2 type (producing IL-4 and IL-5) in favor of a TH_1-type T-lymphocyte response (interferon-gamma [IFN-γ]).

The hallmark of asthma and allergic rhinitis is allergic inflammation of the mucosa and submucosa, predominantly caused by eosinophils. TH_2 lymphocytes amplify and prolong allergic inflammation and late-phase reactions. TH_1 cytokines, i.e., IFN-γ and IL-2, inhibit production of TH_2 cytokines. Successful immunotherapy is associated with a shift in IL-4/IFN-γ production (from IL-4 to IFN-γ) either as a consequence of down-regulation of the TH_2 response or increase in the TH_1 response.

Not all immunological changes associated with effective immunotherapy occur in all subjects, although there is general correlation between clinical improvement and favorable alterations from baseline immunological parameters. Reduction in biological sensitivity to specific allergens has been demonstrated in allergen immunotherapy trials to such allergens as ragweed, mixed grasses, birch and mountain cedar pollen vaccines; the molds, *Alternaria* spp and *Cladosporium* spp; cat dander and house dust mites. Successful allergen immunotherapy ameliorates, but usually does not completely eliminate, the respiratory symptoms of allergic rhinitis and allergic asthma.

CLINICAL TRIALS AND SCIENTIFIC STUDIES

Allergic Rhinitis: Overview

Many randomized, double-blinded controlled trials for allergic rhinitis due to airborne pollens, animal allergens and house dust mite aeroallergens demonstrate efficacy of allergen immunotherapy based on subjective symptoms scores and medication diaries. Favorable immunological changes include decreased basophil histamine release, reduced skin test allergen reactivity and increased allergen-specific IgG blocking antibody.

POLLEN

Nasal challenge studies enable investigators to measure the allergic response in the upper airway following allergen immunotherapy. Such research demonstrates that there is a dose response to ragweed allergen immunotherapy, i.e., an optimal dose above which little or no additional improvement occurs. The first of these studies involved 12 ragweed-sensitive subjects who received immunotherapy, Antigen E (AgE, now known as Amb a 1, the principal ragweed pollen allergen) injections for 3–5 yr and results were compared to those in 27 untreated control subjects. Nasal provocation studies of treated subjects revealed that AgE immunotherapy decreased the clinical response to ragweed and decreased the allergic inflammatory mediator responses (histamine, prostaglandin D_2 [PGD_2], TAME-esterase and kinins) to an intranasal ragweed challenge. In a later study, 26 previously nonimmunized, ragweed-sensitive subjects were randomized to three different dosage regimens (low to high doses; 0.6–25 (μg AgE/ injection) and their responses to ragweed nasal challenges compared. The low-dose immunotherapy regimen provided no protective effect, whereas the moderate dose and high dose caused significantly reduced mediator release from the nasal mucosa following ragweed nasal challenge. Symptom scores, recorded by the moderate- and high-dose–treated subjects over three ragweed seasons, also improved significantly and correlated with the decreased release of inflammatory mediators. There was no significant difference in the degree of clinical improvement between the moderate- and high-dose groups. An example of a typical immunotherapy schedule needed to achieve an optimal immunotherapy dose is found in Table 3.

Nasal challenges also confirm that such therapy attenuates both the immediate and late-phase allergic responses by decreasing mucosal membrane cellular influx and mediator production. Ragweed immunotherapy for 3–5 yr is required to achieve clinical remission. Both mixed- and single-grass pollen immunotherapy studies for hay fever result in significantly decreased symptom-medication scores during the grass pollen season and responses to grass skin testing and nasal challenge testing. Increases in grass-specific IgG-blocking antibody occurs in subjects successfully treated with mixed-grass immunotherapy. The size of both the immediate- and late-phase skin tests to timothy grass vaccine were diminished in a timothy allergen immunotherapy study.

Mountain cedar tree pollen immunotherapy decreases symptom-medication scores during the cedar tree pollen season, reduces the late-phase skin test reaction to mountain cedar pollen diagnostic vaccine and increases the specific IgG and decreases the seasonal rise in specific IgE during the mountain cedar pollination season. Similar clinical and immunological results were obtained in birch pollen allergen immunotherapy

Table 3
Illustrative Dose Schedule for Short Ragweed Allergen Immunotherapy

Dose	Vial	Dilution of 1:10 w/v concentration	Dose	
			mL	Ragweed Amb a 1 (AgE) (μg)
1			0.05	
2			0.1	
3	D	1:100,000	0.2	
4			0.3	
5			0.4	
6			0.05	
7			0.1	
8	C	1:10,000	0.2	
9			0.3	
10			0.4	
11			0.05	
12			0.1	
13	B	1:1000	0.2	
14			0.3	
15			0.4	
16			0.05	
17			0.1	Desirable Dose
18	A	1:100	0.2	Range of 3–12 μg
19			0.3	
20			0.4	

1:10 Weight by volume (w/v) means that 1 g of pure pollen is diluted in 10 mL of diluent. 1:10 w/v of standardized ragweed vaccine contains 400 μg *Amb a 1* (Antigen E)/mL. Maintenance dose of immunotherapy is administered on a weekly to monthly schedule and can be altered on an individual basis. The above schedule represents a weekly injection schedule (week 1–20). More rapid build-up can be accomplished by giving the injections twice weekly or by utilizing a "rush" immunotherapy protocol that achieves maintenance doses in days rather than weeks.

trials. In addition, birch pollen nasal provocation studies show inhibition of allergic symptoms and reduced chemotactic activities for eosinophils and neutrophils in nasal secretions after allergen immunotherapy.

MITES, MOLDS AND ANIMAL DANDERS

House dust mite allergen immunotherapy results in significantly decreased nasal symptom scores, responses to nasal allergen challenge and the size of the skin test reaction. The same changes in specific IgG and IgE as observed with pollen studies were found. *Alternaria* spp mold immunotherapy produced similar decreases in nasal symptom-medication scores, allergen provocative challenges in the skin and nose, and increased serum IgG. Cat allergen immunotherapy results in reduced nasal symptom scores of subjects exposed to a cat in a study room.

Allergic Asthma: Overview

More than 50 controlled immunotherapy trials have been performed with a variety of allergens for seasonal, perennial and animal-induced asthma. Vaccines of rye grass, mixed grasses, ragweed, birch, mountain cedar, *Alternaria* spp, *Cladosporium* spp, house dust mites, cat, dog and cockroach have been used in these trials. Collective analysis of these studies provides important insight, but comparisons among studies are difficult because of varied study designs. Of these studies, 42 demonstrated significant clinical improvement in treated subjects; 23 of these showed a significant increase in the bronchoprovocation threshold to the allergen used for immunotherapy. Of the trials in which immunological parameters were monitored, 16 demonstrated an increase in allergen-specific IgG-blocking antibody, and one showed a decline in specific IgE. Nine reported decreased skin test reactivity to the allergen used for immunotherapy, and two demonstrated reduced in vitro basophil histamine release following allergen challenge. An overall analysis of controlled studies in the treatment of asthma with allergen immunotherapy indicates clinical efficacy in allergic asthmatics.

A meta-analysis of most published, controlled trials of allergen immunotherapy in asthma reviewed in the *American Journal of Respiratory and Critical Care* in 1995 indicates that allergen immunotherapy is effective in the treatment of allergic asthma, provided that the clinically relevant and unavoidable allergen can be identified. Between 1954 and 1997, 54 published randomized controlled trials satisfied the strict inclusion criteria of the Cochrane Database of Systematic Reviews. There were 25 studies reporting immunotherapy for dust mite allergy, 13 studies of pollen allergy, 8 studies of animal dander allergy, 2 studies of allergy to the mold *Cladosporium* spp and 6 studies that attempted simultaneous immunotherapy for multiple aeroallergens. It was found that allergen-specific immunotherapy significantly reduced asthma symptoms and medication requirements, but there was no consistent effect upon lung function. Allergen immunotherapy reduced allergen-specific bronchial hyperreactivity to a greater extent than nonspecific bronchial hyperreactivity. It is not possible to compare the size of improvement with immunotherapy to that obtained with other therapy for asthma. Immunotherapy must be considered for use when asthma is extrinsic or allergic, and unavoidable clinically relevant allergens are identifiable. The arguments favoring immunotherapy are especially strong in the case of younger patients requiring year-round medical management. If allergen immunotherapy is utilized, it should be administered in sufficiently high doses of vaccine to maximize the benefits. With these optimal doses, there is the expectation of a reduction in medication requirements and symptom scores in the majority of treated patients.

The National Heart, Lung, and Blood Institute (NHLBI) in 1997 sponsored an expert panel to establish guidelines for the diagnosis and management of asthma. This national asthma education and prevention program states that 75–85% of asthmatic patients are allergic, and immunotherapy should be considered in such patients when avoidance of allergens and treatment with appropriate medications does not control the disease.

POLLEN

Allergic asthmatic subjects often experience increased bronchial hyperactivity during a specific pollen season. The effect of birch pollen allergen immunotherapy on bronchial reactivity, as measured by methacholine provocation, was investigated in subjects with birch pollen asthma induced during the birch pollen season. Untreated subjects had increased bronchial hyperreactivity to methacholine, whereas those receiving birch pollen immunotherapy did not. In addition, eosinophil cationic protein, an inflammatory mediator derived from eosinophils in the bronchoalveolar lavage fluid, was decreased in subjects receiving birch pollen immunotherapy. Other studies using mixed grasses, cedar, birch, mugwort and ragweed pollen vaccine immunotherapy demonstrate reduced bronchial responses to methacholine or histamine.

The benefits of immunotherapy are specific for the allergen(s) used in treatment. Some studies have shown that single-pollen allergen immunotherapy, such as derived from one grass species, may provide incomplete relief of asthmatic symptoms because of multiple grass sensitivity or because other sensitivities exist, for example, to molds. Similarly, a highly purified standardized ragweed allergen vaccine containing only a single protein allergen, such as ragweed AgE or Amb a 1, may provide incomplete relief of symptoms in ragweed-sensitive asthmatic subjects because they are sensitized to several ragweed proteins and not just AgE.

The IgE immune response of asthmatic subjects is different in the polysensitized vs the monosensitized subject. Patients sensitized to a single allergen have significantly lower total serum IgE levels than those allergic to multiple allergens. The lymphocytes from the polysensitized subject, when challenged with allergen, release significantly more IL-4 (favors IgE production) and CD23 (low-affinity IgE receptor) in vitro than those from the monosensitized subject, although the lymphocyte IFN-γ in vitro production is the same in both groups.

A double-blind placebo–controlled study during the pollen season compared the efficacy of immunotherapy in monosensitized (orchard grass pollen) and polysensitized (multiple pollen, including orchard grass) asthmatic subjects. Subjects allergic to grass pollen were treated with an optimal maintenance dose of a standardized orchard grass pollen vaccine, whereas those allergic to multiple pollen species, including grass, received the same biologically equivalent dose of all standardized allergens to which they were sensitized. The results indicated that monosensitized subjects with orchard grass pollen allergy, but not polysensitized subjects, were significantly protected during the respective pollen season during this study. Higher doses of standardized vaccines over a prolonged treatment schedule are probably required to demonstrate efficacy in polysensitized allergic patients.

A 5-yr study of the role of immunotherapy in ragweed-induced asthma was published in 1993. Clinical parameters (symptom diary scores, medication usage, peak expiratory flow rate (PEFR) measurements and physician evaluations) and other end points (skin test sensitivity, serological parameters and bronchial sensitivity to ragweed and methacholine) were monitored. A standardized, maintenance dose of ragweed vaccine containing Amb a 1, 10 μg/injection, was used to immunize ragweed-sensitive subjects. Both clinical and objective parameters improved, again demonstrating that the use of an appropriate therapeutic dose is necessary to achieve a good clinical response.

Creticos et al. in 1996 examined the efficacy of allergen immunotherapy for asthma exacerbated by seasonal ragweed exposure; 64 patients completed 1 yr of the study treatment, and 53 completed 2 yr. These patients were not exclusively ragweed sensitive. The immunotherapy group had reduced hay fever symptoms, skin test sensitivity to ragweed, sensitivity to bronchial challenges and increased IgG antibodies to ragweed

---

Role of Allergen Immunotherapy in Asthma Management

- A consideration in asthmatics who are allergic: 80% of children over age 2 yr; 50% of adults.
- A possible therapy in asthmatic, with concomitant significant allergic rhinitis—uncontrolled with environmental allergen elimination, plus rhinitis medication.
- An adjuvant therapy in moderate–severe asthmatics who are not well managed with environmental allergen elimination plus asthma medication.

---

as compared with the placebo group. The seasonal increase in IgE antibody to ragweed allergen was abolished in the immunotherapy group after 2 yr. Patients received doses of 4 µg/injection of Amb a 1 the first year and 10 µg/injection the second year. Although positive effects were observed in the immunotherapy asthma group, the clinical effects were limited. Both groups (immunotherapy and placebo) had some improvement in asthma symptoms during the study.

Adkinson et al. in 1997 performed a controlled trial of immunotherapy for asthma in allergic children. A placebo-controlled trial of multiple-allergen immunotherapy in 121 allergic children with moderate to severe perennial asthma was conducted over 2 yr. The median medication score decline was not significantly different between the immunotherapy group and the placebo group. The number of days patients received oral corticosteroids were similar in the two groups. There was no difference between the groups in the use of medical care, symptoms or peak flow rates. Partial or complete remission of asthma occurred in 31% of the immunotherapy group and 28% of the placebo group. The median PC20 for methacholine increased significantly in both groups, but there was no difference between the two study groups. Optimal doses of immunotherapy, ranging from 4.3–26 µg/injection, resulted in a mean 8.8-fold increase in the levels of allergen-specific IgG to *Dermatophagoides pteronyssinus* and *D. farinae* mites, short ragweed, oak and grass. A 61% mean reduction in wheal diameters by prick skin testing to each respective allergen was observed. The group that benefited from immunotherapy was made up of children with milder disease (no inhaled corticosteroids) and younger children (<8.5 years) with a shorter duration of disease. The data indicate that there is no discernible benefit from immunotherapy in allergic children with perennial asthma who already are receiving appropriate and optimal medical treatment from asthma experts.

MITES

Several studies of immunotherapy with vaccines of standardized aqueous *D. pteronyssinus* and/or *D. farinae* house dust mites demonstrate significant benefit. A study by Bousquet et al. (15) revealed that among subjects allergic only to *D. farinae*, children show significantly greater improvement than do adults. As expected, patients with severe, chronic asthma (FEV$_1$ ≤ 70% of predicted), other perennial allergen sensitivities, aspirin intolerance or chronic sinusitis achieve the least benefit from immunotherapy.

A later study by Bousquet et al. (16) analyzed immunotherapy to *D. pteronyssinus* in 74 mite-allergic asthmatics. It demonstrated a significant dose-dependent increased tolerance to the standardized *D. pteronyssinus* allergen, Der p 1, on bronchial allergen challenge in each of the immunized groups vs no change in the control group. A significant reduction in histamine bronchoprovocation hyperresponsiveness also was observed, with the greatest reduction in the highest-dose group. The rate of systemic reactions was lowest in the low-dose and highest in the high-dose group, and since the 7 μg and 21 μg/injection schedules were equally effective, the 7 μg/injection dose was recommended as the appropriate target dose.

DANDERS

Several controlled studies found that cat and dog immunotherapy effectively increases the threshold dose of cat or dog dander vaccine, respectively, needed to induce a positive bronchial challenge in subjects with cat- or dog-specific allergic asthma. Such therapy also results in a reduction of symptoms after dander exposure in a challenge room. Many subjects are given cat or dog immunotherapy, at their own request, in an effort to better tolerate the presence of a pet in their home. However, confirmation of clinical efficacy, under such circumstances, is needed, and elimination of the animal from the environment in which the subject lives is the preferable mode of therapy. There is increasing evidence that the allergens of fur-bearing pets are ubiquitous in many homes and other indoor locations, even where no animals reside. It is being passively introduced into these locations because of the prevalence of such animals in US homes. Including cat and/or dog allergens in the vaccine of a patient with positive skin tests to cat and/or dog may become more commonplace.

MOLDS

Molds that trigger asthma are numerous, diverse and contain multiple allergens, and mold vaccines available for use in the US are not standardized. Controlled immunotherapy trials with standardized vaccines of *Alternaria* spp and *Cladosporium* spp demonstrate efficacy in the treatment of asthma. One such trial of 1 yr of treatment with *Alternaria* spp resulted in ablation or a reduced late-phase response upon *Alternaria* spp allergen challenge in 8 of 10 subjects. Increased concentrations of allergen and methacholine also were required to induce bronchial constriction. *Cladosporium herbarium* vaccine immunotherapy produced significant decreases in symptom-medication scores and response to bronchial challenge tests.

REASONS FOR LACK OF BENEFIT FROM IMMUNOTHERAPY

The reasons for lack of benefit from allergen immunotherapy include: (1) inappropriate treatment with such therapy of non-IgE-mediated disease, such as chronic nonallergic rhinitis or vasomotor rhinitis; (2) utilization of low-potency allergen vaccines; (3) administration of inadequate doses of allergen; (4) ineffective environmental control resulting in continued excessive exposure, for example, to cat or dog dander; (5) a coexistent medical problem, such as sinusitis and nasal polyps, which accounts for most of the symptoms; (6) the allergen vaccine lacks important allergens because of undiagnosed or unrecognized sensitivities.

OVERVIEW OF PRACTICAL ASPECTS

Specific allergen immunotherapy is effective treatment for specific patients with allergic rhinitis and allergic asthma. Careful selection of the patient and the relevant

---

Local Reactions to Allergen Immunotherapy

- Redness and swelling (usually dime–quarter sized) are not uncommon and easily managed with an ice pack, with or without an antihistamine.
- Larger reactions may require an antihistamine as well as short-term oral corticosteroids.
- Significant local reactions may require adjustment of subsequent allergen immunotherapy doses.

---

allergen(s) for immunotherapy requires expertise and knowledge about the pathophysiology of allergic diseases and regional outdoor and indoor allergen sources. Allergen immunotherapy is indicated for symptomatic patients in whom an adequate trial of environmental control and avoidance and appropriate pharmacotherapy has failed. Reduction of symptoms and the amount of medications required occurs in patients who received optimal maintenance doses of specific immunotherapy for a 3- to 5-yr period.

DURATION OF IMMUNOTHERAPY

Clinical trials and observations indicate that immunotherapy can be stopped after 3–5 yr of successful therapy. The results of grass, tree and ragweed immunotherapy trials demonstrate efficacy for several years after cessation of such therapy. In one ragweed study, the immunological parameters and nasal lavage mediators remained unchanged 1 yr after the treatment vaccine was stopped. House dust mite immunotherapy administered for 1–6 yr and then discontinued was found to be most effective after discontinuation if it had been administered for at least 3 yr. The effect of immunotherapy on the reduction of the skin test end points at the conclusion of the treatment was correlated with the duration of efficacy after immunotherapy cessation. Efficacy of a 3-yr course of animal dander immunotherapy was assessed 5 yr after its discontinuation, and one-third of these subjects continued to demonstrate tolerance to cat exposure. When relapses occur after the immunotherapy is discontinued, a good response to restarting such therapy occurs more rapidly than occurs during the initial course of immunotherapy.

ADVERSE REACTIONS

Local Reactions

Patients receiving allergen immunotherapy often experience reactions at the site of the injection (erythema and edema) that cause some local discomfort. No adjustment in vaccine dose is necessary for reactions less than 4 mm in size. Large local reactions, 4 cm or greater in diameter, occur less frequently and may cause more discomfort and persist for 24 h or longer. There is a concern that subsequent increases in the dose of the vaccine following a large local reaction may result in a systemic reaction; however, there is little evidence that such local reactions, whatever their size, place the subject at increased risk for a systemic reaction. This local discomfort can be controlled with cold compresses and oral antihistamines. When such reactions occur, the subsequent allergen immunotherapy dose usually is reduced to the previously tolerated dose and

---

Risk of Systemic Reactions to Allergen Immunotherapy

- Risk rate: 1–2000 injections.
- Most reactions begin within 30 min of injection—thus, a minimum of 20–30 min waiting time is advised.
- More systemic reactions occur:
  - In highly allergic patients.
  - With use of pollen-allergen vaccine, especially during the pollen seasons.
  - During initial dose "buildup" phase, especially with accelerated programs.
- The risk of more serious reactions is increased:
  - In allergic asthmatics.
  - With patients taking concomitant β-blocking drugs

---

subsequently increased. If large local reactions persist, the dose either has to be divided into two doses given at separate sites or maintained at the same dose, if tolerated, or decreased. Large local reactions do not predict the onset of a subsequent systemic reaction, and most systemic reactions occur in the absence of previous large local reactions.

Systemic Reactions

Systemic reactions occur rarely; they may range from mild, manifested as generalized pruritus, urticaria or symptoms of allergic rhinitis and conjunctivitis, to life threatening, with upper and lower airway obstruction and/or anaphylactic shock. Fatalities are rare but do occur. A retrospective survey by questionnaire of allergy specialists in the United States for the period 1945–1983 reported 46 fatalities either from skin testing or immunotherapy. The data from 30 questionnaires allowed further evaluation of the fatalities; 6 were caused by skin testing and 24 by immunotherapy. A later extension of this study included reports of an additional 17 deaths between 1985 and 1989. Further reporting has disclosed another 27 fatalities related to immunotherapy through 1995.

The incidence of systemic reactions from immunotherapy over a 10-yr period at the Mayo Clinic was 0.137%; most were mild and responded to immediate medical intervention. There were no fatalities. The estimated fatality rate from allergen immunotherapy in the United States was approximately one per two million injections for the period of 1985–1989. Some factors cited that increased the likelihood of a systemic reaction are an incorrect injection technique or erroneous dose. This type of mishap was not the cause in all systemic reactions. Other observations were (1) mite-sensitive individuals had more immunotherapy-related asthma reactions than those who were pollen sensitive; (2) fewer reactions occurred with maintenance doses than during the build-up phase; (3) excluding the severe or unstable asthmatic from receiving the immunotherapy injections significantly reduced the rate of systemic reactions.

PRECAUTIONS

No allergen vaccine should be considered completely safe for an allergic subject, and immunotherapy should be carried out only by trained personnel who know how to administer immunotherapy injections, to adjust doses and to manage adverse reactions in a setting where appropriate equipment for such management is immediately available. A detailed protocol to adjust for missed injections and for reactions to immunotherapy is necessary. A protocol for the management of anaphylaxis is indicated, and personnel who administer injections should be trained in the appropriate treatment of anaphylaxis. Prompt recognition and immediate administration of epinephrine in systemic reactions are the mainstays of therapy.

Patients at higher risk for severe life-threatening systemic reaction include those with:

1. Unstable or symptomatic asthma
2. Significant seasonal exacerbation of their allergic symptoms, particularly asthma
3. A high degree of hypersensitivity (by skin testing or specific IgE measurements)
4. Accelerated schedules of immunotherapy, particularly during the initial build-up period
5. High dose maintenance regimens in highly sensitive allergic patients
6. Concomitant use of β-blockers (which makes treatment of anaphylaxis more difficult with epinephrine). β-blockers should be discontinued, when possible, prior to initiation of immunotherapy.
7. Injections from new vials

Patients who become pregnant who are already receiving immunotherapy may be maintained at their current or a reduced dose during pregnancy. Immunotherapy should not be started during pregnancy unless a life-threatening situation exists, e.g., Hymenoptera hypersensitivity. Relative contraindications for immunotherapy include: (1) serious immunopathological and immunodeficiency diseases; (2) malignant disease; (3) severe psychological disorders; (4) poor compliance; (5) patients who are noncompliant; (6) severe uncontrolled asthma or irreversible airway obstruction, <70% predicted FEV_1; (7) significant cardiovascular diseases, which increase the potential side effects from epinephrine; (8) children under 5 yr of age; and (9) systemic mastocytosis.

The risk of systemic allergic reactions and fatal reactions should be reduced and, it is hoped, eliminated by (1) avoiding errors in dosing; (2) utilizing preventive protocols to minimize risk, such as measuring peak flow rates in patients with unstable asthma; (3) reducing doses when injections are given from new vials; (4) reducing doses when injections are given during a particularly high pollen or mold-induced seasonal exacerbation; (5) by using standardized allergen vaccines.

Any physician who administers immunotherapy, regardless of specialty, should be present when the injections are given. The patient should be required to wait 20 min following the injection. A longer wait is indicated for high-risk patients. In the event of any adverse reactions or uncertainity about the dose, the allergist should be consulted prior to administration of another dose of allergen vaccine.

TREATMENT OF ALLERGIC REACTIONS: MEDICATIONS AND EQUIPMENT

Physicians prescribing and/or administering such therapy must be aware of the potential risks and institute appropriate clinic procedures to minimize them. Prompt recognition of signs and symptoms of a systemic reaction and immediate use of epi-

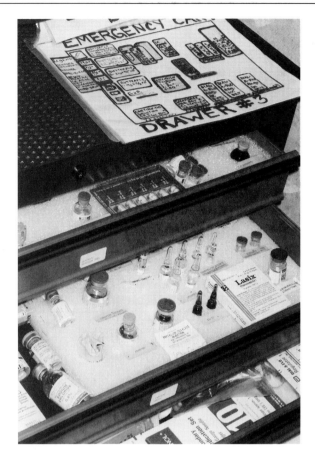

Fig. 1. Emergency medications and supplies as included in a code cart. Office or clinic physicians and staff personnel should be familiar with its contents.

nephrine to treat such a reaction are the mainstays of therapy. The following equipment, medications and reagents should be available: (1) stethoscope and sphygmomanometer, (2) tourniquets, syringes, hypodermic needles and large-bore (14-gage) needles, (3) aqueous epinephrine HCl, 1 : 1000 w/v, (4) equipment to administer oxygen, (5) equipment to administer intravenous fluids, (6) oral airway, (7) antihistamine, (8) corticosteroids and (9) injectable vasopressor. The rare situation in which invasive procedures (electrical cardioversion, tracheotomy, intracardiac injection of drugs) might be essential does not justify the risk of their being available for use under less than ideal circumstances. It is impractical to insist that these procedures be available in every clinic situation.

FUTURE TRENDS IN IMMUNOTHERAPY

New technology and advancement of knowledge in the basic mechanisms and pathophysiology of allergic diseases will completely change allergen immunotherapy in the future. These advances should result in new, safer and substantially more effective methods of manipulating the human immune response. Several approaches may be used: (1) novel delivery systems; (2) allergen fragments or peptides (devoid of

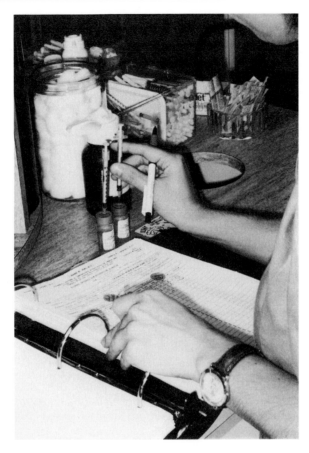

Fig. 2. Careful inspection of the patient's injection dosage sheet and vials of allergen vaccines. Draw up exact amount of the vaccine into a syringe. Document the injection site (right or left arm) and if a local or systemic reaction occurs.

anaphylactic potential) for active immunotherapy; (3) IgE-binding haptens of major allergens for passive saturation of effector cells and induction of blocking antibodies; (4) plasmid DNA immunization; (5) allergen-specific antibodies and antibody fragments for passive therapy, i.e., to be used by inhalation into the nose or lungs and (6) immunotherapy with humanized anti-IgE monoclonal antibody.

SUGGESTED READING

Abramson MJ, Puy RM, Weiner JM. Is allergen immunotherapy effective in asthma? A meta-analysis of randomized controlled trials. *Am J Respir Crit Care Med* 1995;151:969–974.

Adkinson NK, Eggleston PA, Eney D, et al. A controlled trial of immunotherapy for asthma in allergic children. *N Engl J Med* 1997;336:324–331.

Lockey RF, Bukantz SC, eds. *Allergens and Allergen Immunotherapy*, ed. 2, revised and expanded. New York, Marcel Dekker, 1999.

Bousquet J, Michel FB. Specific immunotherapy in asthma: Is it effective? *J Allergy Clin Immunol* 1994;94:1–11.

Bousquet J, Michel FB. Specific immunotherapy in allergic rhinitis and asthma. In: Busse WW, Holgate ST, eds. *Rhinitis and Asthma*. Boston, Blackwell Scientific, 1994, 1309–1324.

Bousquet J, Hejjaoui A, Dhivert H, Clauzel AM, Michel FB. Immunotherapy with the standardized *Dermatophagoideds pteronyssinus* extract. III. Systemic reactions during the rush protocol in patients suffering from asthma. *J Allergy Clin Immunol* 1989;83:797–802.

Bousquet J, Lockey RR, Malling HJ, eds. Allergen immunotherapy: therapeutic vaccines for allergic diseases. Geneva: January 27-29 1997. *Allergy* 1997;53(44 Suppl):1-42.

Bosquet J, Lockey RR, Malling HJ. Allergy immunotherpy: Therapeutic vaccines for allergic diseases. WHO position paper. *J Allergy Clin Immunol* 1998;102:558-562.

Bush RK, Ritter MW. Allergen immunotherapy for the allergic patient. *Immunol Allergy Clin North Am* 1992;12:107–124.

Creticos PS, Reed CE, Norman PS and subcenter investigators of the NIAID study. The NIAID cooperative study of the role of immunotherapy in seasonal ragweed-induced adult asthma. *J Allergy Clin Immunol* 1993;91:226.

Creticos PS, Reed CE, Norman PS, Khoury J, Adkinson NF Jr, Buncher CR, Busse WW, Bush RK, Gadde J, Li JT, et al. Ragweed immunotherapy in adult asthma. *N Engl J Med* 1996;334:501–506.

Durham SR, Till SJ. Immunologic changes associated with allergen immunotherapy. *J Allergy Clin Immunol* 1998;102:157–164.

Fox RW, Lockey RF. Role of immunotherapy in asthma. In: Gershwin ME, Halpern GM, eds. *Bronchial Asthma: Principles of Diagnosis and Treatment*. ed. 3. Totowa, NJ, Humana Press, 1994, pp 365–398.

Joint Task Force on Practice Parameters. Practice parameters for allergen immunotherapy. *J Allergy Clin Immunol* 1996;98:1001–1011.

Lockey RF, Benedict LM, Turkeltaub PC, Bukantz SC. Fatalities from immunotherapy (IT) and skin testing (ST) [see comments]. *J Allergy Clin Immunol* 1987;79:660-667.

Naclerio RM, Proud D, Moylan B, Balcer S, Friedhoff L, Kagey-Sobotka A, Lichtenstein LM, Creticos PS, Hamilton RG, Norman PS, et al. Clinical aspects of allergic disease. A double-blind study of the discontinuation of ragweed immunotherapy. *J Allergy Clin Immunol* 1997;100:293–300.

Norman PS. Immunotherapy: Past and present. *J Allergy Clin Immunol* 1998;102:1–10.

Platts-Mills TAE, Chapman MD. Allergen standardization. *J Allergy Clin Immunol* 1991;621–624.

Platts-Mills TAE, Mueller GA, Wheatley LM. Future directions for allergen immunotherapy. *J Allergy Clin Immunol* 1998;102:335–343.

Stewart GE, Lockey RF. Systemic reactions from immunotherapy. *J Allergy Clin Immunol* 1992;90:567–578.

Van Metre TE, Adkinson NF. Immunotherapy for aeroallergen disease. In: Middleton E, Reed CE, Ellis EF, et al., eds. *Allergy Principles and Practices*, ed. 4. Baltimore, Mosby, 1997, 1489–1506.

26 Controversies in Allergy and Allergy-Like Diseases

Abba I. Terr, MD

CONTENTS

INTRODUCTION
UNCONVENTIONAL THEORIES OF ALLERGY
CONTROVERSIAL METHODS OF ALLERGY DIAGNOSIS
CONTROVERSIAL TREATMENTS FOR ALLERGY
DISCUSSION
SUGGESTED READING

INTRODUCTION

The management of allergic diseases is accomplished most successfully and cost-effectively by the patient's primary care physician in collaboration with a specialist in allergy/immunology. It is critically important to use methods of diagnosis and treatment that are based on sound scientific principles and that have been validated by proper clinical trials. Physicians who treat allergic patients therefore must be aware of the plethora of unproven and controversial methods that are currently promoted by a small group of practitioners, and they should understand the faulty rationale on which they are based. These unproven techniques and their unscientific, or even antiscientific, theories are sometimes deceptively labeled as alternative or complementary forms of medical practice. This implies some measure of efficacy that in fact does not exist.

In contrast to the scientifically rigorous immunopathological foundation underlying our present knowledge of human allergy, the theories advanced by the proponents of the controversial methods described in this chapter lack experimental proof. These theories frequently arise from misinterpretations of chance empirical observations.

UNCONVENTIONAL THEORIES OF ALLERGY

The principal theories on which most of the unproven allergy practices are based are listed in Table 1. So-called *allergic toxemia* is the basis for a number of these practices. It is comprised of two mistaken components. It postulates that allergens are inherently

From: *Current Clinical Practice: Allergic Diseases: Diagnosis and Treatment, 2nd Edition*
Edited by: P. Lieberman and J. Anderson © Humana Press Inc., Totowa, NJ

Table 1
Unproven Allergy Theories

Allergic toxemia
Environmental illness
Food-additive sensitivity
Multiple food allergies
Multiple chemical sensitivities
Candida hypersensitivity

toxic and that virtually any subjective symptom in the absence of objective evidence of pathology can be attributed to allergy. In fact, most allergens are nontoxic in the usual dosage and manner of exposure necessary to either induce or elicit an allergic reaction. The presence or absence of potential toxic properties of an allergen is irrelevant to its ability to evoke an allergic immune response. Furthermore, the manifestations of allergic illness result from inflammation and not toxicity. In contrast, proponents of allergic toxemia in its various forms diagnose this condition not in patients with allergic symptomatology, but rather in patients with multiple vague complaints that usually include fatigue, anxiety, cognitive difficulties with memory and concentration and a variety of physically unexplained pains and other bodily discomforts.

The allergic toxemia concept originated with patients who attributed their multiple medically unexplained symptoms to their diet. This led (i.e., misled) to the idea that multiple food allergies in a single individual can produce an unlimited number of symptoms and that the specific symptoms and implicated foods are variable and changeable. Other ingested substances such as food additives and prescribed medications, particularly antibiotics, are often included as causes of allergic toxemia. To explain unpredictable symptom responses, the concepts of *masking* and *overload* were devised to rationalize the absence or presence, respectively, of unexpected symptoms. The current terminology for unexplained absence/presence of symptoms is *adaptation/deadaptation*. It is clear that these terms are merely descriptive and have yet to be explained by their advocates in a physiologically meaningful way.

Environmental illness and *multiple chemical sensitivities* are names applied to a condition described above as allergic toxemia, but in this case the cause is attributed to numerous common everday environmental chemicals. In most cases these chemicals include pesticides, solvents, perfumes, new carpets, plastic materials, new clothing and virtually any synthetic chemical or commercial product with an odor. Occasionally, electromagnetic fields generated by nearby electric power lines or even household appliances are included as causes of symptoms. Some patients believe that their multisystemic polysymptomatic illness represents hypersensitivity to numerous chemicals, foods and drugs. The term given to this condition is *universal allergy*. Because symptoms in these patients have never been shown to be in fact related to chemicals, the term *idiopathic environmental intolerances* is more accurate. The clinical presentation of this condition is often indistinguishable from that of chronic fatigue syndrome and other controversial subjective conditions.

Periodically over the past century this clinical condition has also been ascribed to the effects of a specific microorganism, usually one that enjoys a normal symbiotic or commensal relationship with the human organism. Formerly called autointoxication

> Perhaps more than any other field of medicine, the practice of allergy has been troubled by proponents of controversial techniques of therapy (many of which have little or nothing to do with allergic disease) that are employed without the support of scientific validation.

> **Unconventional Theories**
>
> The concept of allergic toxemia, environmentally derived illnesses, or sensitivities owing to long-term (low-dose), multiple chemical exposure, which can result in immune "dysfunction," was first proposed 40–50 yr ago. These theories remain unproved today and are unacceptable to the majority of the medical community in the United States.

presumably from normal gastrointestinal microbial flora, this concept has reappeared as a presumptive chronic viral disease. In this case, according to one unproved theory, the persistence of a virus such as the Epstein-Barr virus or human herpesvirus 6 (HHV-6) was postulated to cause chronic "activation" of the immune system. There is no substantiated evidence or even a clear definition of what activation means in this context, and there is no proof currently that persistence of any virus can explain the pattern of symptomatology experienced by such patients. A variant of this theory is the so-called *Candida hypersensitivity syndrome*, attributed to the existence of *Candida albicans* on certain mucous membranes of many healthy individuals. Recently, toxins from indoor molds have been implicated.

CONTROVERSIAL METHODS OF ALLERGY DIAGNOSIS

To select the most appropriate methods for diagnosis and treatment, the clinician should be familiar with the underlying principles of both legitimate and unproved methods. Controversial diagnostic and treatment procedures will be discussed separately (Tables 2 and 3). Some of these procedures are of no proved worth under any circumstance, while others may have a legitimate place in some conditions although not in allergic disease.

The *provocation-neutralization* procedure consists of "testing" the patient with a small amount of a substance in liquid form administered by either intradermal injection or by sublingual drop. The patient records any symptoms or sensations for a period of 10 min thereafter, and any symptom, regardless of its nature or intensity, is taken as indication that the test is "positive." If the patient reports no symptom, the test is repeated using the same test substance at a different concentration until there is a "positive" result. Next, the same substance is tested at lower concentrations until the patient again reports no symptom, at which point the allergy (i.e., the symptom) is said to be "neutralized". The neutralizing dose of the substance is then prescribed as treatment.

Numerous substances are tested, including the common atopic allergens, food extracts, chemicals, drugs and hormones. Because each test substance must be administered separately to elicit symptoms, testing to multiple substances is extremely

Table 2
Unconventional Diagnostic Methods

Provocation–neutralization
Cytotoxic test
Pulse test
Applied kinesiology
Electrodermal testing

Table 3
Unconventional Treatment Methods

Neutralization
Food avoidance
Chemical avoidance
Vitamins and other supplements
Enzyme-potentiated desensitization
Acupuncture
Homeopathy

time consuming. It has been shown, however, that patients cannot distinguish test extracts from placebo controls by this procedure, so the basis of a positive test is merely the power of suggestion. It is therefore worthless for diagnosis, and there is the potential danger that delivery by the sublingual route of an allergen to a patient with a true IgE-mediated allergy might cause life-threatening angioedema of the buccal mucosa or even systemic anaphylaxis.

The *cytotoxic test* consists of applying a drop of the patient's blood onto a microscope slide containing a minute quantity of a food or drug. The unstained blood sample is then inspected microscopically for alterations in the morphology of the leukocytes, which is claimed to indicate allergy to the food or drug. There is no standardization for criteria indicating a positive result, time of incubation, pH, temperature or any other variable that might affect leukocyte viability. There is no reasonable theory linking changes in blood leukocyte appearance and allergic disease. There have been no studies to correlate the result of this test with a rigorous independent proof of allergy, such as the double-blind, placebo-controlled oral food challenge.

The *pulse test* for food allergy is performed by measuring the pulse rate of the patient before and after food ingestion. Remarkably, advocates of this "test" have claimed at various times that an increase, a decrease, or either, is diagnostic of food allergy. There is no independent verification that a pulse change correlates with allergy, nor is there a cogent theory to explain such a phenomenon. The pulse test is an example of a valid medical diagnostic procedure—quantitation of the pulse rate—being misused as an allergy test.

Applied kinesiology is a purported system of health practice that is based on the bizarre concept that a variety of diseases, especially allergy, cause a reduction in the strength of skeletal muscle. The diagnosis of food allergy consists of subjectively testing the ability to resist the forced movement of the patient's outstretched arm during exposure of the patient to a food. Incredibly, the exposure to the presumed food allergen is usually carried out by placing the food in a container that the patient simply holds

> • Allergens are not toxic: The allergic disease is the patient's
> immune/inflammatory response to the allergen.

during the muscle-strength testing. Not surprisingly, there is no experimental proof of either the diagnostic efficacy of the procedure or validation of its theory.

The suggestive power of a mechanical or electrical apparatus in medical diagnosis is illustrated by *electrodermal diagnosis*. In this case a device to measure the electrical resistance of the skin is inserted into a circuit that includes a metal container of a food item and a probe applied to the patient's skin. The probe presumably explores various points on the body surface, and a change in the galvanic resistance of the skin is believed to indicate allergy to that food. The use of a computer-generated printout gives the "results" an aura of high-technology precision.

CONTROVERSIAL TREATMENTS FOR ALLERGY

Treatment regimens that are based on unsubstantiated theories of allergy or unreliable diagnostic tests are clearly not in the patient's best interest. Those discussed here are listed in Table 3. The fact that a patient might seemingly benefit from a particular form of treatment, especially if the illness is largely or completely subjective, does not validate the treatment. Clinical efficacy and safety can be evaluated only by a properly designed and executed controlled trial with appropriate measurements and analysis.

The controversial forms of allergy "treatment" described here have either failed critical tests of efficacy and safety or they have not been evaluated, because of the lack of any compelling reason to do so.

Neutralization therapy is an extension of the provocation-neutralization testing procedure described earlier in this chapter. The so-called neutralizing dose of the test substance is prescribed for self-administration by the patient either to relieve current symptoms or to prevent symptoms when they are believed to be imminent because of an anticipated environmental exposure. The treatment is also recommended on a regular schedule as an ongoing maintenance program. The neutralizing solution is taken by either sublingual drops or subcutaneous injections. There is no evidence of any therapeutic result other than a placebo response.

Avoidance therapy is frequently recommended as a feature of most controversial forms of allergy practice, as it is in conventional practice. The differences, however, are profound with respect to the underlying rationale and the extent and consequences of the recommended program The unreliable diagnostic tests that have been described here invariably "uncover" an extensive list of nonexistent allergies, leading to the unnecessary elimination of numerous foods and the avoidance of environmental items that are ubiquitous in today's world. Extreme elimination diets are obviously dangerous, so proponents of the concept of multiple food allergies usually advise their patients to eat (or to avoid eating) specific foods on a prescribed schedule, usually as a four-day or five-day rotational diet. Proponents of the rotational diet also claim—without substantiation—that such a diet actually prevents the development of food sensitivities. *Chemical avoidance* for patients with so-called multiple chemical sensitivities may be so extreme that major lifestyle changes are necessary to avoid any possible exposure

> • Provocation-neutralization of subjective symptoms should not be confused with the well-established method of objective bronchial provocation challenge.

to all synthetic products and all items that can be detected by odor. Fortunately, most of those individuals in whom multiple food and chemical sensitivities have been diagnosed eventually compromise on these extreme recommendations.

Dietary supplements are frequently a component of these irrational approaches to allergy management. Although there is neither theoretical nor experimental evidence that allergy pathogenesis involves a deficiency of any nutrient, clinicians and others who promote any of these "alternative" programs usually advise their patients to take supplemental vitamins, minerals, amino acids, chemical antioxidants or some combination of these.

A number of unmedical, unscientific and unproven systems of practice offer to help persons with a variety of illnesses, including allergy. The most prevalent today are *acupuncture, chiropractic, homeopathy* and *naturopathy*, but there is also a long list of boutique "therapies" such as *crystal therapy* and *herbalism*. In general, each of these treatment-based systems employs a similar if not identical treatment procedure, regardless of the nature of the disease. Needless to say, needling of the skin, spinal manipulation, ingestion of herbs or any of the other maneuvers embraced by these entities are inconsistent with the known mechanisms of allergy, and proponents of them cannot cite any evidence of effectiveness.

Many of the unconventional treatments discussed above are recommended for patients with presumed allergy in whom the existence of a true hypersensitivity disease is questionable. Recently, an unproved "modification" of allergen immunotherapy for patients with atopic allergy has surfaced. It is called *enzyme-potentiated desensitization*, and it consists of a single preseasonal subcutaneous injection of a conventional pollen extract mixed with a minute quantity of the enzyme β-glucuronidase. It is claimed to be superior to the usual extended course of immunotherapy that requires graduated increasing doses of allergen leading to a successful long-term maintenance program. Although a single low-dose injection of an allergen is certainly less likely than conventional immunotherapy to cause a systemic reaction, there is no evidence that enzyme-potentiated desensitization favorably affects atopic disease, whereas there are now dozens of well-controlled clinical trials confirming efficacy of the conventional high-dose form of treatment.

DISCUSSION

The superficial similarity of many of these unproven methods to scientifically based procedures of diagnosis and treatment of allergic diseases is an opportunity for exploitation by their proponents and a trap for the unwary clinician. The allergic population is very large, and the primary care physician is the first medical contact for most of them. Practitioners of these unconventional procedures are readily available both within and outside the medical profession. They often advertise their services with promises that most physicians cannot and do not make. Only by knowing the specifics of these methods and their claimed theoretical basis can the clinician make

> • Diagnosis of allergic disease is based on history and physical
> examination; identification of the relevant allergens requires a
> valid test for the immune response.

an informed decision and give proper advice to the patient about their use. Some of the more common ones are described here.

With the exception of sublingual allergen administration, the methods reviewed in this chapter are not likely to pose an immediate hazard to health. Rather, their danger is more subtle, pervasive and profound. An incorrect diagnosis made by an unreliable test creates the risk that another disease—physical or psychiatric—remains undiagnosed and untreated. Diagnosing allergy in a person who truly has none may create a lifelong disability characterized by unnecessary avoidance behavior. An extreme form of this unfortunate iatrogenic phenomenon is seen in patients who accept the idea that they have multiple sensitivities to foods and/or chemicals. Some of these individuals live a life of social and material isolation from which they may never recover.

Most allergists would agree that it is far easier to treat an allergy than it is to disabuse a patient of his or her fear of an allergy that does not exist.

The problem of unconventional methods in allergy is of concern to a number of professional societies. In particular, the American Academy of Allergy Asthma and Immunology has published position statements about many of these procedures. These publications also provide literature citations to appropriate studies and evaluations that document their lack of effectiveness.

SUGGESTED READING

American Academy of Allergy and Clinical Immunology Executive Committee. Position Statement: Idiopathic environmental intolerances. *J Allergy Clin Immunol* 1999;103:36.

David TJ. Unorthodox allergy procedures. *Arch Dis Child* 1987;62:1060.

Ferguson A. Food sensitivity or self-deception? *N Engl J Med* 1990;323:476–478.

Golbert TM. A review of controversial diagnostic and therapeutic techniques employed in allergy. *J Allergy Clin Immunol* 1975;56:170.

Grieco MH. Controversial practices in allergy. *JAMA* 1985;253:842.

Kay AB. Alternative allergy and the General Medical Council. *Br Med J* 1993;306:122–124.

McKenna PJ. Disorders with overvalued ideas. *Br J Psychol* 1984;145:579–585.

Selner JC, Staudenmayer H. The relationship of the environment and food to allergic and psychiatric illness. In: Young S, Rubin J, eds. *Psychobiology of Allergic Disorders*. New York, Praeger, 1985.

Terr AI. Unconventional theories and unproved methods in allergy. In: Middleton E, Jr, Reed CE, Ellis EF, eds. *Allergy; Principles and Practice*, ed. 5. St Louis, Mosby, 1998.

27 The Patient with 'Too Many Infections'

Diagnostic Approach

Mary E. Paul, MD
and William T. Shearer, MD, PHD

CONTENTS

INTRODUCTION

The cornerstone of the practice of primary care medicine is the ability to recognize unusual or distinct manifestations of disease and to separate these from those that are routine or expected. Immunodeficiency should be suspected immediately when a patient has an opportunistic infection or the features of one of the immunodeficiency syndromes. However, the primary care provider must more commonly grapple with the question, How many routine infections are too many? Answering this question involves the consideration of factors that influence immune function such as environment and age. This chapter provides an overview of the immune deficiency disorders, the differential diagnosis to be considered for the patient with recurrent infection and a diagnostic approach for the patient suspected of having immunodeficiency.

PRESENTATION

Age influences immune function. The immune system of a newborn is functionally inferior to that of an older child. For example, infants and toddlers < 2 yr old routinely mount a poor antibody response to the polysaccharide antigens found on encapsulated organisms like pneumococcus and Haemophilus influenzae. Serum immunoglobulin concentrations as a whole are lower in the infant than in the older child and adult. Also,

From: *Current Clinical Practice: Allergic Diseases: Diagnosis and Treatment, 2nd Edition*
Edited by: P. Lieberman and J. Anderson © Humana Press Inc., Totowa, NJ

Subjects to Consider with Parents of Child with 'Too Many Infections'

- Age of child and onset of infections
- Type/location of infections
- Number of infections
- Failure to thrive
- Family history of serious infections or early death
- Exposure of child to other children
- Atopic disease symptoms that may mimic infections
- Signs of cystic fibrosis, AIDS, GE reflux

---

the infant and young child have not yet developed the memory immune responses that occur as a result of exposure and infection. For the premature infant, the immaturity of the immune system is magnified. Neutrophil function is depressed. Serum concentrations of immunoglobulin G (IgG) antibody are often further reduced for the preterm infant because two thirds of transplacental transmission of IgG antibody occurs in the third trimester.

While the infant gains in immune function with age, the elderly lose immune function with further aging. The primary immune response weakens. Naive T-cells are replaced by memory cells. Further T-cell changes include the accumulation of cells with signal transduction defects and changes in the predominant cytokine profile produced by T-cells. Regulation of monocyte-macrocyte function changes. The end result is a dysregulation of immune function and an increased risk for infection and malignancy.

Environment dramatically impacts the incidence of infection. Infants frequently exposed to infection as in a day-care setting will have more infections than infants who are not exposed. Passive cigaret smoke inhalation also predisposes to illness, including otitis media, pneumonia and bronchitis. Hygiene of the patients and of caretakers and family members impacts the frequency of such infections as impetigo and furunculosis. For the allergic patient, exposure to indoor allergens such as dust mites and molds often worsens congestion and predisposes to sinusitis and otitis.

The expected frequency of infection varies with the type of infectious organism. No one with normal immunity should have even a single infection with an opportunistic organism. However, we are all subject to viral upper respiratory tract infections (URI). The question of expected frequency of recurrent upper respiratory tract infections is not easily answered. Many individuals experience six to eight respiratory infections per year. This number is increased in children who are exposed to an older sibling or to other children in school. Normally, respiratory infections are mild and last only a few days, and recovery is complete between infections.

In contrast, chronic or severe infection, including chronic bronchitis, otitis, mastoiditis and sinusitis, is often found in individuals with immunodeficiency. Infections may be difficult to clear with oral antibiotics, resulting in prolonged duration of infection and dependency on antibiotics. Unexpected complications may result from infections in the immunodeficient host.

FAMILY HISTORY

The family history is helpful to explore for an individual with recurrent infections. Primary immunodeficiency disorders often run in families. Many are inherited as a result of mutations in genes on the X chromosome, and others are autosomal recessive in inheritance. Autoimmune processes, history of early infant deaths and recurrent infections in other family members are red flags in the family history for a primary immunodeficiency disorder.

THE IMMUNODEFICIENCY DISORDERS

For the sake of ease of discussion, dividing the immunodeficiency disorders into categories of primary and secondary disorders is helpful. The genetic abnormalities that result in the disorder have been described for many of the primary immunodeficiency disorders, and examples of these disorders, the genetic lesion and typical presentation are listed in Table 1. In general, the primary immunodeficiency disorders result from inherent defects in immunity. The secondary immunodeficiency disorders occur when normal immunity is disrupted.

Secondary causes of disruption in immune function must be considered when one is evaluating for immunodeficiency; secondary disorders occur much more commonly than the primary disorders (Table 2). For the individual with recurrent sinusitis and pnuemonia, disorders resulting in impairment of mucous clearance from the respiratory tract such as cystic fibrosis and ciliary dysfunction should be considered. Similarly, the chronic congestion associated with perennial allergic rhinitis can predispose to upper respiratory tract infection. Opportunistic infection and wasting are hallmark findings of the acquired immunodeficiency syndrome (AIDS); however, recurrent bacterial infection is not uncommon in human immunodeficiency virus (HIV) infection, especially in children. Disorders that result in the loss of protein in the stool or urine should be considered in evaluation of hypogammaglobulinemia. Recurrent infection of a single site should trigger an evaluation for a structural or anatomical problem that may have occurred during development, may be due to surgery or may be secondary to trauma. Also, foreign bodies, for example nasogastric tubes and intravenous catheters, predispose to infection. Specific systemic diseases that result in immunodeficiency are listed in Table 2.

Antibody Disorders

The immunodeficiency disorders primarily affecting antibody production usually do not result in recurrent infection until after maternal antibody wanes at 6–12 mo of age. Bruton or X-linked agammaglobulinemia typically occurs at this time in infancy with recurrent infection with encapsulated bacterial infections. Infections may include pneumonia, otitis, sinusitis, septic arthritis, or gastrointestinal tract infections, or they may be systemic, such as septicemia or meningitis. Cases of vaccine-derived polio from the live polio vaccine have been described. Boys with this disorder do not produce antibody because of the absence of mature B-cells. The defect resides in a gene, labeled the *btk* gene for Bruton tyrosine kinase, that is located on the X chromosome. Bruton tyrosine kinase is necessary for B-cell differentiation. Antibody levels are very low to absent, and the markers on peripheral blood lymphocytes indicating mature

Table 1
Examples of Genetic Defects Known to Cause Primary Immunodeficiencies

Disorder	Chromosomal Location	Known Affect on Immune Responses	Typical Clinical Findings
X-Linked agammaglobulinemia	Xq22	Absence of Bruton's tyrosine kinase results in arrest of B-cell development	Recurrent, serious pyogenic infections
X-linked hyper-IgM syndrome	Xq26	CD40 ligand (CD154) is not expressed on T cells	Recurrent, serious pyogenic infections. Also opportunistic infections
DiGeorge anomaly	22q11.2, 10p13	Absence of thymus	Hypocalcemic seizures due to hypopara-thyroidism, cardiac disease, abnormal facies, opportunistic infection
X-linked SCID	Xq13	Absence of the common γ chain of the receptor for cytokines 2, 4, 7, 9, 15	Failure to thrive, opportunistic infection, rash
SCID–CD8 lymphocytopenia (*Zap*-70 Deficiency)	2q12	Deficiency of T-cell kinase involved in thymic T-cell maturation and in intracellular signal transduction	Failure to thrive, opportunistic infections, rash
SCID- T-B+NK+	5p13	Defective IL-7 receptor expression	Failure to thrive, opportunistic infection, rash
*Jak*3 deficiency	19p13.1	Disruption of T-cell intracellular signal transduction	Failure to thrive, opportunistic infection, rash
Adenosine deaminase deficiency	20q13.11	Lymphopenia and poor T-cell function due to toxic effect of adenosine metabolites	Opportunistic infection, poor growth, skin rash
Purine nucleoside phosphorylase deficiency	14q13.1	Abnormal purine metabolism	Opportunistic infection, poor growth, skin rash
X-linked lymphoproliferative syndrome	Xq25	Unregulated stimulation of B-cells by EBV leading to malignant transformation	Lymphadenopathy, hepatosplenomegaly, recurrent opportunistic infections
Wiskott-Aldrich syndrome	Xp11.22–p11.23	WASP is abnormal; abnormalities are seen in the cytoskeleton structure of T-cells and platelets	Thrombocytopenia with bleeding and bruising, eczema, recurrent infection with encapsulated organisms
Ataxia-telangiectasia	11q22–23	Defective DNA-dependent kinase involved in cell cycle control and DNA recombination. Specific etiology of immune system defects still under study	Chronic sinopulmonary disease, cerebellar ataxia, malignancy oculocutaneous telangiectasia
Chronic granulomatous disease	Xq21.1 (gp91^{phox}), 16q24 gp22^{phox}), 7q11.23 (gp47^{phox}), 1q25 (gp67^{phox})	Phagocytes cannot generate respiratory burst because of lack of a component needed for oxidative metabolism	Deep-seated infection, abscess especially with catalase-positive organisms
Leukocyte adhesion deficiency 1	21q22.3 (CD18)	Absence or poor up-regulation of adhesion molecules	Recurrent serious bacterial infections, especially on mucosal surfaces or wound sites; poor wound healing, lack of pus
Hyper IgE syndrome	Proximal 4g	Lymphocytes have poor response to IL-12 resulting in decreased IFN-γ production	Eczema, mucocutaneous conditions, and pulmonary and skin abscesses

Table 2
Secondary Immunodeficiency

Category	Examples
Malnutrition	Developing country, associated with chronic disease
Organ system dysfunction	Nephrotic syndrome, protein-losing enteropathy, diabetes mellitus, uremia
Immunosuppressive agents	Corticosteroids, cytotoxic drugs, cyclosporine, radiation
Infectious diseases	HIV infection, mycobacterial infection, EBV infection, cytomegalovirus infection
Infiltrative disease	Malignant disease, histiocytosis, lymphoproliferative disease, sarcoidosis, multiple myeloma
Surgery and trauma	Burns, splenectomy, head injury
Hereditary diseases	Down syndrome, chromosomal instability syndromes, congenital asplenia, hemoglobinopathies, storage diseases, galactosemia

B-cells, namely, CD19 and CD20, are absent. Antibody is important in protection from infection, especially from encapsulated bacteria. However, these patients also are susceptible to central nervous system infection with viruses, especially enteroviruses, that may prove fatal. Chronic viral infection notwithstanding, the prognosis is good for individuals receiving routine antibody replacement therapy.

A more common form of antibody deficiency is due to very low levels of or absence of IgA with normal IgG and IgM, called selective IgA deficiency. The incidence is 1:400–700 individuals. Affected individuals may have recurrent sinopulmonary tract or ear infections that are intractable to usual therapies. Histories that include pressure-equalizing tubes, chronic tympanic membrane perforation, mastoiditis and previous sinus surgery are not uncommon, although some healthy individuals have very low IgA values. Autoimmune diseases and IgG2 subclass deficiency also are associated with selective IgA deficiency.

Hyperimmunoglobulin M syndrome is classically thought of as an antibody production disorder, although the disorder manifests with opportunistic infection with Pneumocystis carinii pneumonia (PCP) and neutropenia as well as with recurrent bacterial infection. For the X-linked form, the problem resides with the T-cell instead of the B-cell and occurs because of failure to up-regulate the CD40 ligand on the activated T-cell. The CD40 ligand, also labeled CD154, is necessary to provide a second signal in T-cell B-cell communication for the B-cell to switch from IgM production to the production of another class of antibody. IgM levels are very high, and IgG and IgA levels are low in this disorder. Inheritance is classically X linked; however, males without the mutation in the CD40 ligand gene and females have been described with

Type of Infections Common in Selected Immunodeficiency Diseases (ID)	
ID	*Infections*
T-cell	Viral/fungal/opportunistic
B-cell	Bacterial
Bruton's	Bacterial after age 1–2 yr
Severe combined immunodeficiency disease (SCID)	Opportunistic
Chronic granulomatous disease (CGD)	*Staphylococcus, Serratia, Aspergillus*
Complement	*Neisseria*
AIDS	Opportunistic
Common variable immunodeficiency (CVID)	Late-onset bacterial, *Giardia lambia*

the disorder. Therefore, another genetic lesion must exist for this disorder. Prognosis is good for individuals given monthly intravenous immunoglobulin (IVIG) infusions, although the incidence of autoimmune disorders and malignant disease are increased.

An antibody deficiency disorder that typically occurs in older children and in adults, called common variable immunodeficiency (CVID), results from waning ability to produce antibody. Typically, encapsulated bacteria cause chronic or recurrent infection of the middle ear or sinopulmonary tract. Bronchiectasis is not infrequent in this disorder. Patients commonly have gastrointestinal complaints, including malabsorption and diarrhea that result from infection or autoimmune disease. Infection with *Giardia lamblia* is common. Other autoimmune problems and lymphoreticular malignant disease are more common than in the general population. Hypertrophy of lymphoid tissues can occur and may be manifest as lymphadenopathy, splenomegaly or occasionally hepatomegaly. Antibody levels, especially IgG and IgA levels, are typically low. This disorder is linked to selective IgA deficiency in that both can be found in the same family. Treatment is with replacement antibody contained in IVIG.

Transient hypogammaglobulinemia of infancy represents a delay in the attainment of normal antibody levels for age. When the immune system is evaluated these infants typically are found to have low antibody levels. Production of antibody to diphtheria and tetanus toxoids and to A and/or B blood group antigens is normal. IVIG is not indicated for this condition, and antibody levels normalize with time.

Four subclasses of IgG exist, namely IgG1–4, and many patients have been reported who have recurrent sinopulmonary infections and a low level of one or more of the IgG subclasses. However, asymptomatic individuals have also been described who have low subclass levels. Most antibodies against polysaccharide antigens are of the IgG2 subclass, and IgG2 subclass deficiency has been found in association with selective IgA deficiency. Antibody synthesis following a challenge of both protein and polysaccharide antigens must be tested to know the clinical relevancy of a low IgG subclass level.

Children have been described with normal IgG and IgG subclass levels who have a specific inability to respond with antibody production following challenge with polysaccharide antigens such as pneumococcal polysaccharide antigens; they are labeled as having antigen-specific antibody deficiency. These children, typically between 3 and 10 yr of age, have recurrent sinopulmonary infections.

T-cell and Combined Disorders

Primary disorders of T-cell function and combined T-cell B-cell defects come in many forms. The Wiskott-Aldrich syndrome is associated with eczema, recurrent infections and bleeding or bruising as a result of thrombocytopenia and poorly functioning small platelets. Antibody production to polysaccharide antigens can be greatly impaired in this disorder, resulting in bacterial infection such as pneumonia, otitis media, sepsis or meningitis. Opportunistic infections, autoimmune cytopenias and vasculitis are also seen. Patients have low levels of IgM and elevated levels of IgE and IgA. The genetic defect is on the X chromosome, and the gene, the Wiskott-Aldrich syndrome protein (WASP) gene, has been identified. The WASP is necessary for the formation of a normal cytoskeletal structure for T-cells and platelets. Also, CD43 is reduced on T-cells and platelets in this disorder. These patients are at high risk for bleeding complications, fatal infections and malignant disease. Transplantion with HLA-matched sibling or matched unrelated bone marrow has been curative.

Individuals with progressive cerebellar ataxia, ocular and skin telangiectasia and immunodeficiency may have ataxia-telangiectasia (AT). AT is autosomal recessive in inheritance, and the genetic defect is located on chromosome 11; the abnormal gene product is thought to be a signal transduction protein. The disorder involves both cellular and humoral immunodeficiency. Antibody production is often poor, and many of the patients benefit from antibody replacement therapy. Autoimmune problems and malignant disease frequently accompany this disorder. Cells from patients have increased sensitivity to ionizing radiation. Defective DNA repair is found, and chromosomal abnormalities are frequent. Long-term prognosis is poor, and most individuals die because of neurological deterioration or malignant disease by the second decade, although some have reached adulthood.

Severe combined immunodeficiency (SCID) usually occurs in the first 6 mo of life with failure to thrive, diarrhea, skin rash and severe infection, sometimes with opportunistic organisms. Thrush is severe and recalcitrant to the usual therapy. Multiple defects have been described resulting in the SCID phenotype. X-linked SCID occurs as the result of abnormal structure or production of a protein, the γ chain of the IL-2 receptor. This protein, called the common γ chain (gammac), is also necessary in the structure of other cytokine receptors, namely IL-4, IL-7, IL-9 and IL-15. The total lymphocyte count is markedly decreased. T-cell development is abnormal in these individuals, and T-cell numbers are very low, as are natural killer-(NK) cell numbers. The thymus is small and rudimentary. B-cell numbers are usually increased. Bone marrow transplantation is necessary for survival. Human leukocyte antigen (HLA)–matched and HLA haploidentical T-cell–depleted bone marrow transplantation have been corrective for the T-cell defect; however, patients still may not make antibody appropriately and require antibody replacement therapy.

In fact, recent studies have shown that X-linked SCID is likely the consequence of absence of signaling from the IL-7 receptor, in particular, due to the absence of gammac. Also, the Janus kinase, *Jak3*, functions in intracellular transduction of signal initiated by the binding of certain cytokines to their receptor containing the common γ chain. *Jak3* deficiency results in autosomal recessive SCID with low T- and NK-cells and the presence of B-cells. Another form of SCID, in which T-cells are absent but both B- and NK-cells are present, has been shown to be due to defective expression of the IL-7 receptor.

Adenosine deaminase (ADA) deficiency is an autosomal recessive disorder in which this enzyme is not produced, and metabolites of adenosine that are toxic to T-cells and T-cell development cause immunodeficiency. Lymphocyte numbers are very low. The diagnosis is made by demonstrating absence of or low levels of ADA, typically in erythrocytes, or in granulocytes if the patient has received red blood cell (RBC) transfusion. In addition to the recurrent and severe bacterial, viral, fungal or parasitic infections, affected individuals have skeletal and rib-cage abnormalities. HLA-identical and HLA-haploidentical T-cell–depleted bone marrow transplantation has been curative for the T-cell defect. Replacement enzyme, namely, injections with polyethylene glycol conjugated, bovine adenosine deaminase, can improve lymphocyte function. Gene therapy has been tried, and research is under way to improve the efficacy of this therapy.

Multiple other T-cell defects have been described that result in SCID. Another enzyme defect, purine nucleoside phosphorylase deficiency (PNP), results in the clinical picture of SCID; however, the attrition of lymphocyte function is slower than in ADA deficiency, and these patients may be several years of age before the disease is noted. PNP levels are low, and lymphocyte numbers are low. Bone marrow transplantation is the current treatment of choice.

Other defects include T-cell antigen receptor defects, the bare lymphocyte syndrome in which major histocompatibility antigens are not expressed on peripheral blood lymphocytes, and cytokine deficiencies. Another type of autosomal recessive SCID is due to mutations in the recombinase activating genes, RAG-1 or RAG-2, needed for antigen receptor formation. *Zap-70* deficiency is a type of severe immunodeficiency characterized by the absence of CD8+ T cells in the peripheral blood. Zap-70 is a T-cell kinase used in intracellular signal transduction and in thymic T-cell maturation.

The X-linked lymphoproliferative syndrome (Duncan disease), which results in unregulated B-cell proliferation to Epstein-Barr virus (EBV), is now known to be due to an X-chromosome defect in the gene that codes for signaling lymphocytic activation molecule (SLAM)-associated protein (SAP) found on T-cells. SAP is an inhibitor of T-/B-cell interactions induced by SLAM.

Phagocytic Defects

Disorders involving phagocytic cells most commonly have recurrent cutaneous abscesses, periodontitis, pneumonia, osteomyelitis or sepsis. The most common problem in this category of immunodeficiency is neutropenia. Neutropenia is often the result of decreased production of neutrophils due to medication use, such as antibiotic use, or to infection, such as viral infection. Other acquired causes of neutropenia include autoimmune diseases, aplastic anemia, toxins, antineutrophil antibodies, glycogen storage disease type IB and infiltrative disorders such as neoplasia or myelofibrosis. Notable viral causes include parvovirus and HIV infection.

Points to Remember About Immunodeficient States

- Severe congenital T-cell deficiency is most likely to occur during early infancy. AIDS and B-cell deficiency may occur at any age. Deficiency of the WBC phagocyte or complement system is usually evident in childhood.
- Chronic sinusitis, multiple pneumonias, sepsis, meningitis and repetitive skin abscesses are types of infections most likely to be associated with immune deficiency.
- Failure to thrive in an infant or "wasting" in an older child/adult, with increased susceptibility to infections (of any kind) should be an indication for screening for HIV.
- Recent onset of persistent sinopulmonary disease and/or diarrhea in an older child/adult may be a sign of common variable immuno-deficiency.
- Multiple URIs (with or without ear infections) in an otherwise healthy younger child are more likely secondary to early exposure to other children (e.g., day-care) than due to inmmunodeficiency.

Congenital neutropenia, Kostmann's syndrome, is due to maturation arrest of myelopoiesis in the bone marrow. Patients early in life have recurrent pneumonia, gingivitis, otitis, or urinary tract infections and severe neutropenia. Patients respond to recombinant human granulocyte colony-stimulating factor (G-CSF) with increased neutrophil counts.

Cyclic neutropenia is a disorder in which individuals have regular fluctuations in the number of peripheral blood neutrophils, with neutropenia occurring approximately every 3 wk. Typically, symptoms occur cyclically during times of neutropenia and include fever, malaise, periodontitis, mucosal ulcers, impetigo, sore throat or lymph node enlargement. Clinical improvement has been seen with use of G-CSF.

Chronic granulomatous disease (CGD) occurs as the result of a decrease in the granulocyte's ability to kill specific types of microorganisms because of dysfunction of the cytochrome enzyme, nicotinamide adenine dinucleotide phosphate (NADPH) oxidase. Recurrent, severe, life-threatening infections are often due to organisms such as *Staphylococcus aureus*, Gram-negative enteric bacteria like *Serratia marcescens*, *Proteus*, *Klebsiella*, *Escherichia coli* and others, including *Pseudomonas cepacia*, *Nocardia* species and *Aspergillus* species. Common types of infections include adenitis, abscesses including perianal abscesses, pneumonia and osteomyelitis. Lymphadenopathy, hepatosplenomegaly and ulcerative stomatitis are not uncommon findings. Granuloma formation may lead to obstruction in the gastrointestinal tract. Both systemic and discoid lupus erythematosus have been described in CGD. Inheritance pattern is both X linked and autosomal recessive.

Other disorders of intracellular killing include myeloperoxidase (MPO) deficiency and glucose-6 phosphate dehydrogenase deficiency. MPO deficiency is the most common neutrophil granule defect, and the immune problem associated with this enzyme deficiency, resulting from low levels of MPO activity, is usually mild. The clinical manifestations of the disease are usually seen in association with diabetes mellitus. Defective killing of *Candida albicans* results in increased susceptibility to infection with *Candida*.

Leukocyte adhesion deficiency (LAD) is due to impaired ability of cells to adhere to the vascular endothelium and migrate out of the intravascular space. The deficiency in LAD-1 results from lack of leukocyte adherence glycoproteins, CD11/CD18. The β-chain (CD18) of the adhesion heterodimer is not expressed, resulting in failure of expression of α-chains of the heterodimer also. Affected individuals have severe bacterial infections such as pneumonia, otitis, omphalitis, gingivitis, septicemia and recurrent skin infections. Umbilical cord separation may be delayed, and wound healing is impaired. Peripheral blood neutrophil counts are usually elevated, and the diagnosis is confirmed by abnormal expression of adhesion markers on cell surfaces. LAD-2 results from the absence of sialyl-Lewis[x] on the neutrophil, a ligand of E-selectin on the vascular endothelium. Sialyl-Lewis[x] mediates initial adhesion and rolling of the neutrophil on the vascular endothelium. Infections are similar to those found in LAD-1. Treatment includes very aggressive evaluation and treatment of infections.

Complement Defects

Complement deficiencies are rare and represent only 2% of the primary immunodeficiency disorders. Deficiency of one of the early components of the classic pathway (C1q, C1r, C1s; C4; C2; or C3) is associated with systemic lupus erythematosus–like symptoms, glomerulonephritis and pyogenic infections. Deficiency of an alternative pathway component, factor D, properdin, factor I or factor H is also associated with recurrent pyogenic infections. Recurrent serious infection with neisserial organisms is the classic presentation for a complement deficiency and is seen with deficiency of one of the terminal components common to both the classic and alternative complement pathways and with properdin deficiency. Hereditary complement component deficiency is autosomal recessive in inheritance and results in absence of the component. The CH_{50} assay is a good screen for the presence of all of the classic pathway components and for the terminal components of the alternative pathway of complement. The CH_{50} titer ranges from very low to 0 when one of these components is missing. The CH_{50} assay should be performed when the active infection is resolved, because neisserial as well as other infection causes consumption of complement and can result in low values. If a complement component deficiency is suspected, testing for specific component levels is available.

DIAGNOSTIC TESTS

The evaluation for immunodeficiency revolves around a complete and reliable history and family history. The evaluation should be tailored to reflect likely disorders, given the historical background. Secondary causes for recurrent infection should be sought. For individuals with recurrent pneumonia, a sweat chloride test or test for mutation in the cystic fibrosis gene should be carried out to look for cystic fibrosis. The differential diagnosis should also include gastroesophageal reflux (GER), and consideration should be given to evaluation for GER and possibly for ciliary dysfunction. If allergy is thought to be the predisposing factor for the individual's recurrent sinopulmonary infection, an allergy evaluation should be undertaken, possibly including immediate hypersensitivity skin testing to evaluate for specific hypersensitivity to common allergens. IgE measure has poor negative predictive value for allergy.

Hallmark findings of wasting or failure to thrive and opportunistic infection without evidence of a systemic disorder such as malignant disease should trigger extensive evaluation for a T-cell disorder. For the infant and young child, SCID should be suspected. For all ages, the evaluation should include a test for HIV infection. An evaluation of the adhesion markers on peripheral blood granulocytes is needed for the patient with poor wound healing or gingivostomatitis along with a high white blood cell (WBC) count without a malignant or metabolic disorder. Recurrent, serious neisserial infection should trigger an evaluation for a late component complement defect. The typical presentations for immunodeficiency disorders and tests used in evaluation are listed in Table 3. If suspicion for an immune problem is high because of, for example, opportunistic infection or severe, recurrent bacterial infection, early involvement of an immunologist is advisable for an expedient detailed evaluation.

The complete blood count (CBC) gives extensive information regarding the immune system and should be a part of every evaluation of the immune system. Lymphopenia occurs in many types of SCID. Leukocytosis occurs in CGD and in LAD. Depending on the clinical context, neutropenia sometimes reflects autoimmune disease or bone marrow suppression that can accompany immunodeficiency such as HIV infection. Alternatively, neutropenia may be a reflection of cyclic neutropenia. Rarely, an infant might have a congenital form of neutropenia. Other findings include anemia, often accompanying chronic illness or due to autoimmune disease, and thrombocytopenia, also due to autoimmune disease. Thrombocytopenia with small platelets is a hallmark of Wiskott-Aldrich syndrome. Abnormal forms from the blood smear can indicate absence of the spleen (Howell-Jolly bodies), malignant disease or HIV infection (atypical lymphocytes), Chédiak-Higashi syndrome (large granules in granulocytes) and MPO deficiency (unusual staining of granulocytes). Eosinophils are increased in allergy, in some infections that accompany immunodeficiency such as PCP or parasitic infection, and in some forms of SCID.

Antibody production should be studied as part of the immune workup of the individual with recurrent sinopulmonary tract infection. Quantitative immunoglobulin levels are helpful in this evaluation. However, immunoglobulin levels do not evaluate directly for antibody production, and antibody deficiencies do exist in individuals with normal immunoglobulin levels. Also, a percentage of the normal population has low antibody levels, produces specific antibody normally when challenged and does not benefit from intravenous antibody replacement therapy. To evaluate antibody production, the level of antibody produced to known antigenic exposures should be measured. Isohemagglutinins are antibodies produced to blood group antigens that are not present on the individual's RBCs. When a person is exposed to these antigens that are present in the environment, the normal response involves production of antibody against the antigens that are not recognized as self. Isohemagglutinin titers are detected in most individuals over 1 yr of age. In the individual with both A and B blood group antigens, both A and B antigens will be recognized as self and isohemagglutinins will not be produced.

Immunization elicits an antibody response, and measuring this response is another routine test of antibody production. Previous response to the tetanus vaccine is

Table 3: Evaluation and Referral

Disorder group	Example presentation	Screening tests	Detailed evaluation tests	Specialist referral
Antibody deficiency	Recurrent or severe infection with encapsulated bacteria	CBC with differential and platelets IgG, IgA, IgM Antibody titers to tetanus toxoid, diphtheria, pneumococcus	Response to immunization (required to exclude an antibody deficiency) Isohemagglutinins IgG subclasses in select cases B-cell and T-cell number in peripheral blood Bacteriophage ϕX174 Stool for α-1 antitrypsin; urinalysis if protein loss is suspected	Helpful in performance and interpretation of tests, especially when suspicion for deficiency is strong or detailed evaluation is required For family testing and genetic testing and counseling Prior to use of IVIG for confirmation and counseling As consultant for management
T-cell deficiency or combined deficiency	Recurrent or severe infection with bacteria or with opportunistic organism Wasting, failure to gain weight or diarrhea Dermatitis	CBC with differential and platelets HIV, ELISA IgG, IgA, IgM, IgE Delayed hypersensitivity skin test (>6 to 12 mo)	T-cell numbers and percentages in the peripheral blood B- and NK-cell numbers and percentages in the peripheral blood Lymphocyte proliferation to mitogen and antigen stimulation	Diagnosis of a T-cell or combined immunodeficiency, except HIV infection, should be done with the help of specialist trained in the diagnosis and management of the suspected disorder. If the patient is an infant, urgent referral is required.
Phagocytic cell deficiency	Organ abscesses, recurrent skin infection or abscesses, lymphadenitis, periodontitis Poor wound healing	CBC with differential (sometimes serial monitoring is required) Nitroblue tetrazolium (NBT) test	Adhesion marker presence and up-regulation Chemiluminescence Chemotaxis Bactericidal activity Granulocyte production and margination	Helpful in performance and interpretation of tests, especially when suspicion for deficiency is strong or detailed evaluation is required For family testing and genetic testing and counseling As consultant for management
Complement deficiency	Systemic lupus (C1, C4, C2) Recurrent pyogenic infections (early classic and alternative pathway components) Recurrent neisserial infections (C5–C9)	Serum total hemolytic complement (CH50)	Specific complement component levels Alternative pathway total hemolytic complement (AH50)	Helpful in performance and interpretation of tests, especially when suspicion for deficiency is strong or detailed evaluation is required For family testing and genetic testing and counseling As consultant for management

evidenced by expected titers of antibody to diphtheria and to tetanus toxoid. A challenge normally elicits at least a twofold increase in individuals with low baseline titers. A fourfold response or greater is typical. Response to tetanus toxoid challenge is usually measured 2 wk post immunization.

Response to polysaccharide antigens can be measured by challenge with the unconjugated pneumococcal vaccine. Expected results using a reliable laboratory would include a twofold to fourfold increase in antibody to at least one of the serotypes of pneumococcus contained in the vaccine. The test for response to pneumococcus is best done with a preimmunization specimen sent along with a specimen drawn 3–4 wk post immunization for processing on the same day to control for day-to-day variability in results. In normal children less than 2 yr of age, the response is not reliably present using the unconjugated vaccine. The pneumococcal vaccines containing a protein antigen conjugated to the polysaccharide antigen, which are not currently routinely available, will be useful to elicit a protective antibody response to pneumococcus in the less than 2-yr-old much like the conjugated hemophilus vaccine has done. However, these conjugated vaccines result in antibody production to the protein antigen conjugate rather than the pure polysaccharide antigen. Pneumococcus type 3 is one of the more antigenic serotypes present in the unconjugated vaccine.

The delayed-type hypersensitivity skin test (DTH) measures T-cell recall response and is a cost-effective measure of T-cell function. This intradermal skin test is commonly performed using 0.1 mL of an antigen such as Candida albicans (1:200 dilution), tetanus toxoid (1:10 dilution) or mumps. A positive test requires induration. The reported criteria for interpreting a DTH response as reactive vary. The usual indication of a positive DTH reaction is 10 mm of induration recorded at 48–72 hr; however, a recent study suggests that using a 2 mm cutpoint of DTH induration is useful for determination of immunocompetence in adult women with HIV infection.

For individuals suspected of having a disorder involving T- and/or B-lymphocyte dysfunction, in vitro study of lymphocyte function is in order. This testing is often done in specialized centers. Enumeration of peripheral blood lymphocyte surface markers is utilized to look for deficiencies or patterns suggestive of described disorders. For example, the presence of B-cells with the near-absence of helper and cytotoxic T-cells in an infant is suggestive for X-linked SCID. Likewise, the absence of B-cells with normal numbers and percentages of T-cells is found in X-linked agammaglobulinemia. CD40 ligand is not up-regulated on T-lymphocytes in hyper-IgM syndrome. Routine in the evaluation for degree of immunodeficiency and as a predictor of prognosis in HIV infection is the measure of the percentage and number of CD4 lymphocytes in the peripheral blood.

An example of in vitro functional studies of lymphocytes is the measure of the proliferation of the lymphocytes following stimulation. This test is performed by quantification of the incorporation of radiolabeled thymidine into the nucleus of cultured lymphocytes. Proliferation following mitogen stimulation occurs independent of the T-cell receptor. Antigen stimulation tests recall response and require recognition of the processed antigen on the antigen-presenting cell by the T-cell receptor complex. Experimental tests of lymphocyte responses to cytokine stimulation are also available in specialized centers.

The nitroblue tetrazolium (NBT) test is routinely used to test for CGD. When superoxide generation is normal, the NBT dye is reduced and the granulocytes on the test slide change from a having a yellow-appearing cytoplasm to blue. The blue is not present in the cytoplasm of CGD patients. Other tests of granulocytes, available at specialized centers, include chemilumenescence, a direct measure of superoxide production and energy release, and chemotaxis, an in vitro measure of granulocyte movement in the direction of chemoattractants. Testing for LAD involves the measure of the presence and up-regulation of adhesion markers on the surface of the granulocytes. MPO deficiency is diagnosed by measure of the MPO content of the granulocyte and is easily diagnosed with a routine CBC since the automated differential WBC counters identify granulocytes by MPO content. Glucose-6-phosphate dehydrogenase (G6PD) deficiency is diagnosed by a measure of the G6PD enzyme level.

The CH_{50} is an excellent screening test for complement component deficiencies of the classic pathway components and of the terminal components of both complement pathways. Consumption of components can result in a low value during active infection that normalizes in convalescence. This test requires proper handling of the specimen to avoid spuriously low results. Each of the specific components can be tested if the CH_{50} is confirmed to be low. A similar test, the AH_{50}, is available at specialized centers for use in individuals for whom an alternative pathway early component deficiency is suspected. Individual component testing for alternative pathway components, such as properdin, is available as well.

Genetic studies are available for some of the inherited immunodeficiency disorders. Fluorescence in situ hybridization (FISH) analysis of genetic material is widely available to probe for the genetic deletion found in DiGeorge anomaly. Select research centers offer genetic evaluation for immune disorders for which the genetic defect is known or can be mapped in a family, such as Wiskott-Aldrich syndrome, X-linked agammaglobulinemia, ADA-deficient SCID, other forms of SCID, X-linked lymphoproliferative syndrome and ataxia-telangiectasia. Genetic counseling for families with a member who has an inherited disorder is imperative.

TREATMENT

Treatment options for the primary immune deficiency disorders and HIV infection are complex and require the expertise of a specialist trained in the management of the suspected or proven disorder. Precautions regarding exposures to infection, an aggressive search for the source of infections and judicious use of antibiotics for infection are required in the management of these individuals. For children with a severe form of immunodeficiency, caretakers are cautioned to limit exposures and eliminate ill contacts. Practical advice includes frequent hand washing and bathing. Prophylactic antibiotics may be indicated for patients with recurrent otitis or chronic sinusitis. Routine sputum cultures and rotating antibiotics are useful in preventing further infection and damage in patients who have bronchiectasis. PCP prophylaxis is indicated for individuals with severe T-cell deficiencies. In HIV infection, guidelines exist for other types of prophylaxis, such as antibiotics to prevent infection with *Toxoplasma* and *Mycobacterium* in the severely immune compromised.

Live viral vaccines are to be avoided for individuals with severe immunodeficiency. However, in HIV infection, the measles, mumps and rubella vaccine is recommended for routine use, but should be avoided in severely immunocompromised patients. In contrast, routine immunizations and other vaccines, namely, the influenza vaccine and the pneumococcal vaccine, which are not live viral vaccines, should be used in individuals with immunodeficiency who have the capacity to mount a protective response.

The small number of T-cells that are given with packed RBC transfusions can cause graft vs host disease in individuals with T-cell immunodeficiency. Therefore, blood products should be irradiated. Also, individuals with very low IgA levels may make IgG antibody against IgA. Packed RBCs should be washed to remove the IgA for these individuals. Other products containing IgA such as intramuscular immune globulin, plasma and some of the IVIG products, can cause severe reactions in individuals who have made anti-IgA antibody.

Replacement of the missing component of immunity or correction of the immune defect is used whenever possible for the management of the immunodeficiency disorders. For HIV infection, combination antiretroviral therapy has been shown to restore CD4+ T-cell numbers and to prevent deterioration of the immune system in individuals with susceptible virus. Intravenous infusion of immunoglobulin has been lifesaving for individuals with immunodeficiency involving poor IgG antibody production. This therapy is reserved for individuals who have a proven deficiency of antibody production. The usual replacement dose is 400–600 mg/kg given every 4 wk. A higher dose or a shorter dosing interval is sometimes necessary for prevention of infection or during infection. CGD patients have fewer infections when injections of the cytokine γ-interferon are used in the treatment regimen in addition to prophylaxis against staphylococcal infection. Stem cell transplantation has been used successfully to correct the underlying immune defect for particular primary immunodeficiency disorders, including SCID and Wiskott-Aldrich syndrome. If gene therapy can be perfected, this therapy may be possible for use in those disorders for which the gene defects have been described.

SUGGESTED READING

Noroski LM, Shearer WT. Short analytical review: screening for primary immunodeficiences in the clinical immunology laboratory. *Clin Immunol Immunopath* 1998;86:237–245.

Paul ME, Shearer WT. The child with recurrent infection. In: Kelly KK, ed. *Immunol Allergy Clin North Am*, 1999.

Puck JM. Primary immunodeficiency diseases. *JAMA* 1997;278:1835–1841.

Shearer WT, Fleisher TA. The immune system. In: Middleton E, Reed CE, Ellis EF, Adkinson NF, Yunginger JW, Busse WW, eds. *Allergy: Principles and Practice*, 5th ed., St. Louis: Mosby, pp. 1–13, 1998.

Index

From: *Current Clinical Practice: Allergic Disease: Diagnosis and Treatment, 2nd Edition*
Edited by: P. Lieberman and J. Anderson © Humana Press Inc., Totowa, NJ

ABOUT THE EDITORS

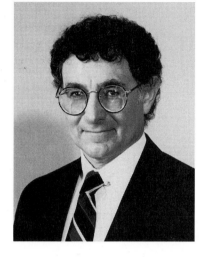

Dr. Phil Lieberman is currently Clinical Professor of Medicine and Pediatrics, Divisions of Allergy and Clinical Immunology, Departments of Medicine and Pediatrics at the University of Tennessee College of Medicine. He is also a member of the American Board of Allergy and Immunology and is past president of the American Academy of Allergy, Asthma, and Immunology and the Association of Certified Allergists.

His research interests are anaphylaxis, rhinitis, and asthma. He is currently involved with a long-term followup of patients with recurrent episodes of anaphylaxis and a longitudinal study of the irreversible decline in lung function of asthmatics.

Dr. Lieberman is the author of more than 66 peer-reviewed publications and 66 abstracts. In addition, he has authored 98 book chapters and edited 5 textbooks of allergy and clinical immunology. He is also a past member of the Board of Directors of the Asthma and Allergy Foundation of America and previous chairman of its Medical Advisory panel. He is presently chairman elect of the education and research trust of the American Academy of Asthma, Allergy, and Immunology, and he was recently named outstanding alumnus of the University of Tennessee College of Medicine for the year 2000.

He has been named in every edition of Woodward and White's *Best Doctors in America* since its inception. Dr. Lieberman lectures around the world on numerous topics in allergy and immunology.

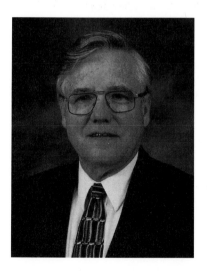

Dr. John A. Anderson is in the private practice of allergy with VIVRA, Asthma and Allergy of Arizona, in Tucson, AZ. He is the former Head of the Division of Allergy and Clinical Immunology, Department of Pediatrics and Internal Medicine, at Henry Ford Health System, having held that position for twenty-two years.

Dr. Anderson was a professor of pediatrics at Case Western Reserve University School of Medicine from 1994 to 1999. He is a past president of the American Academy of Allergy and Immunology and a past chairman of the Section on Allergy and Immunology of the American Academy of Pediatrics. He has held many other national professional positions, including that of secretary of the American Board of Allergy and Immunology, vice-president of research of the Asthma/Allergy Foundation of America, and member of its residency Review Committee for Allergy and Immunology.

Dr. Anderson is well recognized for his interest in adverse reactions to both foods and drugs. He is an accomplished speaker on many allergy subjects, including that of management of childhood asthma, allergies, and rhinitis. He is the author of over 60 scientific publications and 30 published abstracts. His recent research activities include principal investigator for NIH National Cooperative Inner City Asthma Study and a coinvestigator on an NHLBI-funded study concerning the control of asthma in a school population in Detroit.

Dr. Anderson is a busy practitioner of the specialty of allergy and immunology. He has been recognized in *Best Doctors in America* in 1993 and 1996, *Best Doctors in the Midwest* in 1996–1997, and *Who's Who in Medicine and Health Care,* 2000–2001.